Analysis of Sterols and Other Biologically Significant Steroids

Analysis of Sterols and Other Biologically Significant Steroids

Edited by

W. David Nes
Russell Research Center
U.S. Department of Agriculture
Athens, Georgia

Edward J. Parish
Department of Chemistry
Auburn University
Auburn, Alabama

Academic Press, Inc.
Harcourt Brace Jovanovich, Publishers
San Diego New York Berkeley Boston
London Sydney Tokyo Toronto

ACADEMIC PRESS, INC.
San Diego, California 92101

United Kingdom Edition published by
ACADEMIC PRESS LIMITED
24-28 Oval Road, London NW1 7DX

Library of Congress Cataloging-in-Publication Data

Analysis of sterols and other biologically significant steroids / edited by W. David Nes and Edward J. Parish.
p. cm.
Includes index.
ISBN 0-12-515445-3 (alk. paper)
1. Sterols—Analysis. 2. Steroids—Analysis. I. Nes, W. David. II. Parish, Edward J.
[DNLM: 1. Steroids—analysis. 2. Sterols—analysis. QU95 A532]
QP752.S75A53 1989
574.19'2431—dc19
DNLM/DLC
for Library of Congress 88-10516
CIP

PRINTED IN THE UNITED STATES OF AMERICA
89 90 91 92 9 8 7 6 5 4 3 2 1

To William R. Nes—
scientist, teacher, parent, and friend
May 16, 1926 – March 24, 1988

Contents

Contributors

Patricia Acuña-Johnson Escuela de Química y Farmacía, Universidad de Valparaiso, Valparaiso, Chile

Toshihiro Akihisa (née Itoh) College of Science and Technology, Nihon University, Kanda Surugadai, Chiyoda-ku, Tokyo 101, Japan

Pierre Benveniste Laboratoire de Biochimie Végétale, CNRS UA 1182, 67083 Strasbourg Cédex, France

Ian S. Butler Department of Chemistry, McGill University, Montreal, Quebec, Canada H3A 2K6

Clair Cheer Department of Chemistry, University of Rhode Island, Kingston, Rhode Island 02881

Monique Doyon Department of Chemistry, McGill University, Montreal, Quebec, Canada H3A 2K6

William L. Duax Medical Foundation of Buffalo, Inc., Buffalo, New York 14203

Erick J. Dufourc Centre de Recherche Paul Pascal, CNRS, Domaine Universitaire, Talence Cédex, France

Mark F. Feldlaufer Insect and Nematode Hormone Laboratory, United States Department of Agriculture, Agricultural Research Service, Beltsville, Maryland 20705

Gregeory Fenner Department of Microbiology, North Carolina State University, Raleigh, North Carolina 27695

Jane F. Griffin Medical Foundation of Buffalo, Inc., Buffalo, New York 14203

Claus Grunwald Department of Plant Biology and Illinois Natural History Survey, University of Illinois, Champaign, Illinois 61820

Kristen Haeckler Department of Biochemistry, North Carolina State University, Raleigh, North Carolina 27695

Rick C. Heupel Plant Development and Productivity Research Unit, Western Regional Research Center, Agricultural Research Service, United States Department of Agriculture, Albany, California 94710

Li-Shar Huang Department of Plant Biology and Illinois Natural History Survey, University of Illinois, Champaign, Illinois 61820

Arnis Kuksis Banting and Best Department of Medical Research, University of Toronto, Toronto, Ontario M5G 1L6, Canada

R. Todd Lorenz Department of Microbiology, North Carolina State University, Raleigh, North Carolina 27695

Trevor C. McMorris Department of Chemistry, University of California, San Diego, La Jolla, California 92093

Toshihiro Nohara Faculty of Pharmaceutical Sciences, Kumamoto University, Kumamoto 862, Japan

A. C. Oehlschlager Department of Chemistry, Simon Fraser University, Burnaby, British Columbia, Canada V5A 1S6

Stanley F. Osman United States Department of Agriculture, Eastern Regional Research Center, Wyndmoor, Pennsylvania 19118

Edward J. Parish Department of Chemistry, Auburn University, Auburn, Alabama 36849

Leo W. Parks Department of Microbiology, North Carolina State University, Raleigh, North Carolina 27695

Alain Rahier Laboratoire de Biochimie Végétale, CNRS UA 1182, 67083 Strasbourg Cédex, France

Ian C. P. Smith Division of Biological Sciences, National Research Council of Canada, Ottawa, Canada K1A OR6

James A. Svoboda Insect and Nematode Hormone Laboratory, United States Department of Agriculture, Agricultural Research Service, Beltsville, Maryland 20705

Malcolm J. Thompson Insect and Nematode Hormone Laboratory, United States Department of Agriculture, Agricultural Research Service, Beltsville, Maryland 20705

Philip L. Yeagle Department of Biochemistry, State University of New York at Buffalo, Buffalo, New York 14214

Preface

One of the miracles generated on planet Earth was the creation of life from nonlife. In order for life to have evolved into its present state of complexity, a variety of biomolecules, including steroids, were required for cell vitality. That we have learned so much about the chemistry, biosynthesis, phylogenetic distribution, and function of cholesterol and biogenetically related compounds is fascinating in light of the lack of a standardized course or textbook on the topic. Consequently, most students are not seriously introduced to the field of steroids until well into their graduate studies or, for some, much later in their career development. For many scientists, the field is self-taught, their formal training derived from a range of traditional disciplines—microbiology or botany to chemistry or medical physiology. At first glance, the steroid field is incredibly diverse and seemingly unfathomable to the untrained. But as is true of any scientific discipline, once one learns the rules, the subject is intellectually manageable. Between 1910 and 1985, fifteen Nobel Prizes have been awarded to scientists who have successfully exercised the mental gymnastics involved in becoming a ''steroidologist.''

The first step in steroid training is to master analysis. This book is devoted to the analysis of sterols and other biologically significant steroids. Because of space limitations and production deadlines the analysis of certain molecules is not covered. The excellent Academic Press book *Methods in Enzymology* (1985), edited by Law and Rilling, covers the analysis of many steroids not discussed here.

This book contains 13 chapters that review the spectroscopic and chromatographic properties of sterols and select steroids. After studying the latter material, the investigator not familiar with how to isolate and characterize sterols and steroid metabolites of plant, fungal, and insect origin will be able to do so. Additional chapters on lipoprotein analysis and the use of physical-analytical techniques are provided; these should be useful for the inquisitive student and the senior investigator who wish to be well informed on modern techniques used in medicine and the membrane field.

We would especially like to thank the authors who contributed to this book and Academic Press for their assistance in bringing the project to completion.

W. David Nes
Edward J. Parish

1

Isolation and Primary Characterization of Sterols

Rick C. Heupel
Plant Development and Productivity Research Unit
Western Regional Research Center
Agricultural Research Service
U.S. Department of Agriculture
Albany, California

I. INTRODUCTION

Steroids constitute a large group of compounds with a broad range of biological activities and physical properties. This group contains the naturally occurring polycyclic isopentenoids (Fig. 1) that possess the 1,2-cyclopentanophenthrene skeleton and which, either in their own biosynthesis or in the biosynthesis of one of their precursors, have passed through a state with a stereochemistry similar to the trans-syn-trans-anti-trans-anti configuration at their ring junctions (i.e., through the protosteroid cation by electron addition) (Nes and McKean, 1977). Sterols have been defined as "any hydroxylated steroid that retains some or all of the carbon atoms of squalene in its side chain and partitions almost completely into the ether layer when it is shaken with equal volumes of water and ether" (Nes and McKean, 1977).

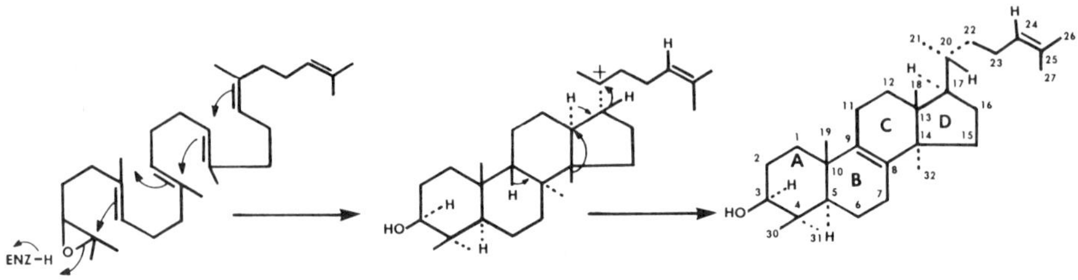

SQUALENE OXIDE — PROTOSTEROID CATION — LANOSTEROL (A STEROID)

Figure 1 Conversion of squalene oxide through the protosteroid cation to a steroid (lanosterol). The protosteroid cation structure shows the trans-syn-trans-anti-trans-anti stereochemistry at its ring junctions. The designations of the four rings characteristic of the sterol nucleus and the conventional carbon numbering system (Fieser and Fieser, 1959; W. R. Nes and McKean, 1977) are shown in the steroid/sterol lanosterol. Additional carbons at C-24 would be designated C-28 and C-29 in the numbering system.

Naturally occurring sterols usually have 27 to 30 carbon atoms, an oxygen atom at C-3, and a side chain of at least seven carbons at C-17 (Fig. 1). Sterols can differ from each other by both nuclear vartiations (differences within the ring system) and side-chain variations (W. R. Nes, 1984). Nuclear variations include the stereochemistry (5α or 5β) at C-5, the number and location of double bonds; the presence of methyl groups at C-4, C-14, and C-19; the contraction of ring A to a pentacycle (A-nor); and the presence of a cyclopropyl group at the C-9β,19 position (Fig. 1). Side-chain variations can include the number and position of double bonds; a shortened side chain (C-26 and/or C-27-nor); a lengthened side chain (C-26 and/or C-27-methyl); a broadened side chain with one to three carbon units (C_1–C_3) at C-22, C-23, C-24, and/or C-25; and the stereochemistry within the side chain, particularly at C-22 and C-24. It is also worth pointing out that β is dropped in common usage when referring to β-sitosterol, since α- and γ-sitosterol are not true entities (Nes and McKean, 1977).

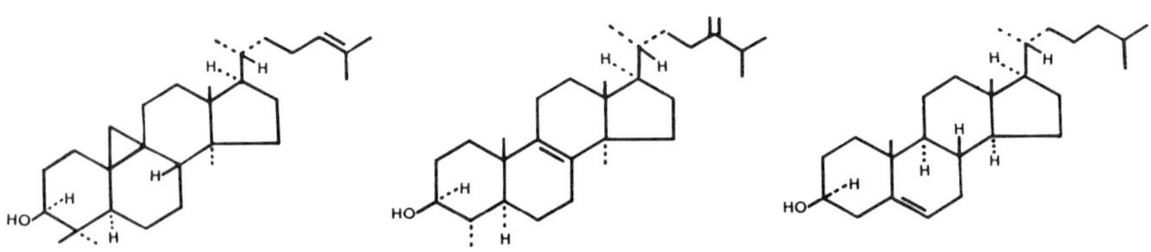

CYCLOARTENOL (4,4 - DIMETHYLSTEROL) — OBTUSIFOLIOL (4α - METHYLSTEROL) — CHOLESTEROL (4,4 DESMETHYLSTEROL)

Figure 2 Examples of the three subclases of sterols: 4,4-dimethylsterols (cycloartenol), 4α-methylsterols (obtusifoliol), and 4,4-desmethylsterols (cholesterol).

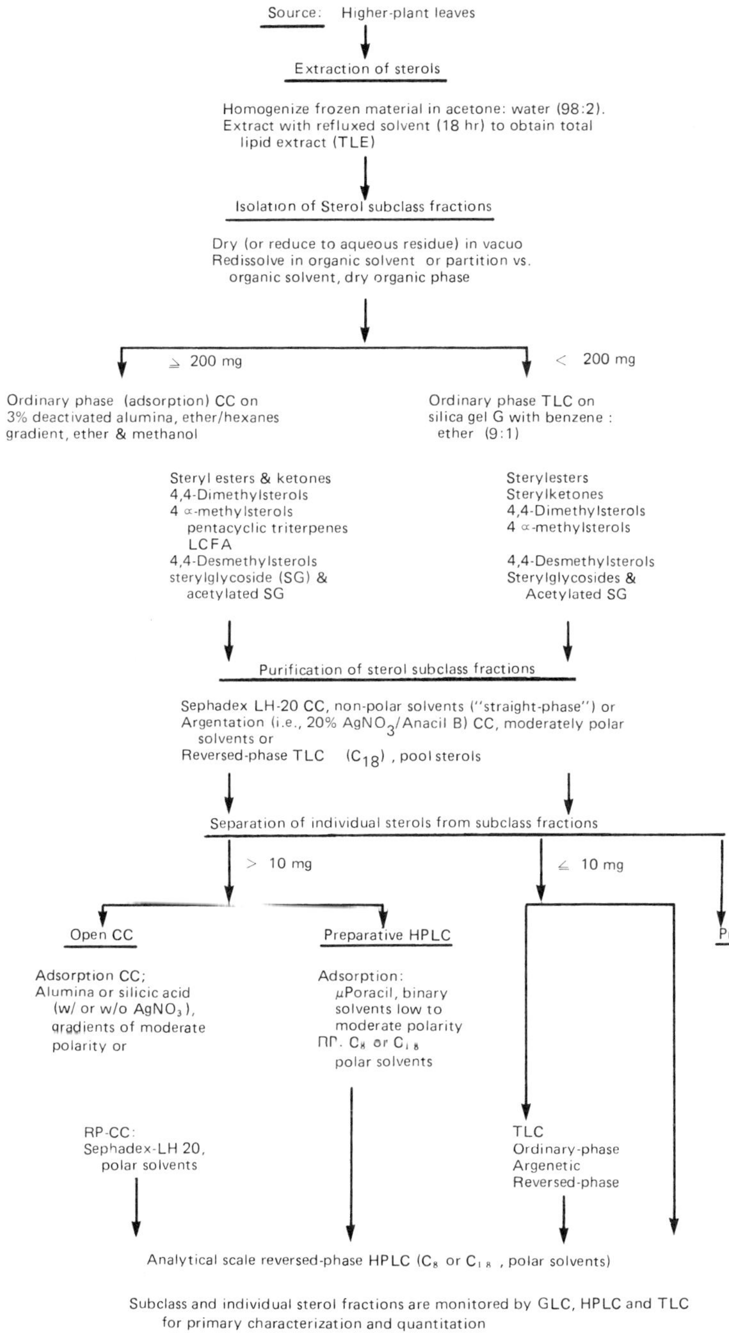

Figure 3 Flow chart describing the extraction, isolation, and separation of sterols from a higher-plant source. This generalized scheme depicts the procedures detailed in the text. A complex source (i.e., higher-plant leaf) is extracted to obtain a total liquid extract (TLE). The sterol subclasses are isolated from the TLE, purified (i.e., removal of LCFA and lipid pigments) by one of three described options, and individual sterols separated for identification. Although multiple options are listed for sterol separation, reversed-phase HPLC (preparative and analytical) is rapidly replacing the other procedures in popularity.

We divide the sterols into three subclasses: the 4,4-dimethylsterols, which retain both methyl groups at C-4; the 4α-methylsterols, which retain a methyl group at the C-4α position; and the 4,4-desmethylsterols, from which both methyl groups at C-4 have been removed (Fig. 2). In this chapter we consider the extraction, isolation, separation, primary characterization, and quantitation of these three sterol subclasses from a variety of sources. Figure 3 is a flow chart outlining these procedures. The analysis of sterol derivatives, metabolites, and related compounds will be discussed elsewhere in this book and will only be alluded to here in the cases of sterylesters and sterylglycosides.

II. EXTRACTION OF STEROLS

In spite of their importance in sterol analytical procedures and quantitative determinations, remarkably few studies have been made of sterol extraction methods. Most studies were designed for a comparison of the extraction of lipids in general from cells or tissues of a single source (e.g., Folch *et al.*, 1957; Bligh and Dyer, 1959) and have been applied subsequently to various plant and animal materials, without obtaining data on the absolute recovery of sterols (Crist *et al.*, 1983; Raederstorff and Rohmer, 1984; Kesselmeier *et al.*, 1985; Weete *et al.*, 1985; Devgun and Paterson, 1986). A few studies have attempted to compare the efficiency of various sterol extraction methods using the same source (Knights, 1971; Sobus and Holmlund, 1976; Gonzales and Parks, 1977; W. D. Nes *et al.*, 1981; Osagie and Kates, 1984); however, these studies do not encompass the entire range of extraction methods that have been employed or are in use today. Unfortunately, these evaluations of extraction efficiency are often based on quantitation of *fractions* obtained from isolation and separation procedures. However, the largest source of error in the quantitative analysis of sterols, which probably occurs at the extraction step, can be alleviated by using *in situ* labeling of key sterols and sterol intermediates, which can, in some cases, enable absolute efficiencies to be evaluated.

The choice of extraction technique is often determined by the nature of the source, the amount of information the investigator chooses to obtain concerning the forms of sterols present (i.e., free, glycosylated, and/or esterified), and tradition. The usual goal of the extraction is to obtain a total lipid extract (TLE) which, *inter alia*, includes sterols, sterol derivatives (conjugates through the 3β-hydroxyl), sterol metabolites, and other steroids. Irrespective of the nature of the source, one of four methods of sample preparation is usually employed: Samples can be extracted (1) directly, with little or no preparation; (2) after drying and powdering; (3) after homogenization of the fresh materials; or (4) after freeze-drying or fresh-freezing, followed by powdering, sonication, or homogenization. Sonication and homogenization are usually performed in the presence of the extraction solvent. Examples of these preparation methods are given in Table 1.

The solvents most frequently used for extracting sterols from nonphotosynthetic materials include chloroform-methanol mixtures (Folch *et al.*, 1957, Bligh and Dyer, 1959); chloroform, acetone, methylene chloride, petroleum ether, and ethanol. In

Table 1 Examples of material preparation and extraction procedures

Source[a]	Material Preparation[b]	Extraction Solvent[c]	Extraction Conditions[d]
Fungi			
Sc	Lyo, pwdr	$MeOH\text{-}H_2O$ (9:1)	Repeated extraction
An	Lyo, pwdr	$CHCl_3\text{-}MeOH\text{-}H_2O$	See Folch *et al.* (1957)
Gf	Dried, pwdr	$(CH_3)_2CO$	Soxhlet, 18 h
Td	Lyo, pwdr	$CHCl_3\text{-}MeOH\text{-}H_2O$	See Bligh and Dyer (1959)
Algae			
Ac	Homogenized	$CHCl_3\text{-}MeOH$ (1:1)	Repeated extraction
Ev	Homogenized	$CHCl_3\text{-}MeOH$ (1:1)	Repeated extraction
St	Dried, pwdr	$CHCl_3\text{-}MeOH\text{-}H_2O$	See Folch *et al.* (1957)
Bryophytes			
Cc	Dried, pwdr	CHCl-MeOH (2:1)	Soxhlet, 24 h
Higher plants			
Ha	Crushed	PE (40–60°)	Soxhlet, > 18 h
Sb	Dried, homogenized	$(CH_3)_2CO$	Soxhlet, > 18 h
Zm	Homogenized	$(CH_3)_2CO$	Repeated extraction (4 ×)
Ama	Homogenized	$CHCl_3\text{-}MeOH$ (1:1)	Repeated extraction (3 ×)
At	Dried, pwdr	$CHCl_3\text{-}MeOH$ (2:1)	Soxhlet, > 24 h
To	Freeze-Dried, Crumbled	EtOH	Soxhlet, 16 h
Pv	Vacuum dried	PE (40–60°); $(CH_3)_2CO$	Seq. extract (hot solvents), 5 min centrifugation
Invertebrates			
Ame	Frozen, homogenized	$CHCl_3\text{-}MeOH\text{-}H_2O$	See Bligh and Dyer (1959)
Sg	Homogenized	$(CH_3)_2CO$	Soxhlet, 18 h
Ap	Dried, crumbled	$CHCl_3\text{-}MeOH\text{-}H_2O$	See Bligh and Dyer (1959)
Hp	Frozen, homogenized	$(CH_3)_2CO$	Repeated extraction
Vertebrates			
Hs	No preparation	$CHCl_3\text{-}MeOH\text{-}H_2O$	See Bligh and Dyer (1959)

[a] Abbreviations: Sc = *Saccharomyces cervevisiae* (Parks *et al.*, 1986); An = *Aspergillus nidulans* (Ziogas *et al.*, 1983); Gf = *Gibberella fujikuroi* (W. D. Nes and Heupel, 1986); Td = *Taphrina deformans* (Weete *et al.*,1985); Ac = *Amphidinum carterae* (Kokke *et al.*, 1981); Ev = *Eutreptia viridis* (Zielinski *et al.*, 1982b); St = *Sargassum thumbegil* (Kobayashi *et al.*, 1985); Cc = *Conocephalum conicum* (Chiu *et al.*, 1985); Ha = *Helianthus annus* (Bianchini *et al.*, 1985); Sb = *Sorghum bicolor* (Heupel, 1985); Zm = *Zea mays* (Rendell *et al.*, 1986); Ama = *Avicennia marina* (Hogg and Gillan, 1984); At = *Amaranthus tricolor* (Xu *et al.*, 1986); To = *Taraxacum officinale* (Westerman and Roddick, 1981); Pv = *Phaseolus vulgaris* (Knights, 1971); Ame = *Apis mellifera* (Svoboda *et al.*, 1986); Sg = *Schizaphis graminum* (Campbell and Nes, 1983); Ap = *Aciculites pulchra* (Crist *et al.*, 1983); Hp = *Halocynthia papillosa* (Zollo *et al.*, 1986); Hs = *Homo sapiens* (Devgun and Paterson, 1986).

[b] Homogenized refers to homogenization in the presence of the extracting solvent in mortar and pestle, Waring blender, or polytron depending on the source. Abbreviations: lyo, lyophilized; pwdr, powdered.

[c] Abbreviations: $(CH_3)_2CO$, acetone; EtOH, ethanol; $CHCl_3$, chloroform; MeOH, methanol; PE, petroleum ether.

[d] Repeated extraction refers to mixing the material with solvent under various time and temperature conditions, filtering or centrifuging the particulate matter, resuspending the residue, and repeating. The organic phases are then combined. Soxhlet extraction refers to continuous extraction of the material with refluxed solvent in a soxhlet apparatus for the specified length of time. Bligh and Dyer (1959) and Folch *et al.* (1957) are references to solvent extraction/partitioning procedures that have been modified and used in the designated studies.

contrast, the solvents most frequently used for photosynthetic materials are only chloroform-methanol (2:1, v:v) and acetone. In both cases, a small percentage (2–7 %) of water added to the solvent when extracting from dried material, improves the sterol yield (cf. W. D. Nes, 1987). Because the HPLC-grade or glass-distilled solvents used in most extraction procedures lack water, it is advisable to add some to these solvents as opposed to using reagent-grade solvents, which contain varying amounts of water.

Extraction conditions range from simply mixing the prepared material with the extraction solvent for a short time (30 min to 1 h) and separating the organic solvent phases from the aqueous phases and debris by centrifugation (Devgun and Paterson, 1986), to extracting from homogenized material with refluxed solvent in a Soxhlet apparatus for 18 h (Heupel, 1985) or with boiling solvent for 1 h (Osagie and Kates, 1984). In most materials, sterols are believed to be associated mainly with membrane systems, including those containing light-harvesting pigments (W. R. Nes, 1974; Grunwald, 1975: Block, 1979, 1981; W. D. Nes and Heftmann, 1981). It has become accepted procedure, especially for materials that contain lipophyllic pigments, to continue the extraction until the material is bleached (W. R. Nes *et al.*, 1976; Heupel, 1985; Kesselmeier *et al.*, 1985).

In specific instances, the extraction procedures have been modified to enhance the extraction of sterols from the materials. For example, W. R. Nes and co-workers (1986) have reported an increase in the amount of sterols extracted from yeast cells by saponifying directly in 10 % KOH in 95 % ethanol. In this instance, the investigators were comparing free sterol and sterol released from esters by the saponification procedure with totals obtained by extracting the cells to obtain a total lipid extract, then saponifying, and subsequently recovering the neutral lipids. Gonzales and Parks (1977) have reported an increase in extractable sterols of yeast by first treating the cells with acid. Nakanishi *et al.* (1984) have used pyrogallol saponification, under basic conditions, as the primary step in the extraction of sterols from yeast. These modifications all involve conditions under which the entire contribution of sterylglycosides may not be included in the quantitations; sterylglycosides would not be hydrolyzed under basic conditions and would partition mainly into the aqueous phase during subsequent solvent extraction of the free sterols and the sterols released from esters. These studies were concerned with single-celled organisms. A protocol for the isolation of sterols from mycelial fungi has been developed by W. D. Nes *et al.* (1981), which can be used to determine total sterol content, including the contribution of sterylglycosides.

When sterols endogenous to the sample are unknown, and little material is available or small aliquots are analyzed, it is recommended that heat and strongly basic or acidic conditions be avoided at every stage of the extraction procedure. Although many sterols are very stable, trace levels of polyunsaturated sterols and sterols that contain additional functional groups can be altered or lost during prolonged exposure to heat and high or low pH. The material, fresh or fresh frozen, should be homogenized and extracted with solvent. Solvent choice is somewhat arbitrary. Chloroform-methanol mixtures and acetone are routinely used for most materials, but more studies comparing solvents on the basis of their ability to extract sterols specifically would be useful.

III. CHROMATOGRAPHIC ISOLATION AND PURIFICATION OF STEROL SUBCLASSES

The isolation of the sterol subclasses is dependent on the complexity of the total lipid extract, which of course reflects the nature of the source. The primary isolation techniques described in this section isolate and purify the three sterol subclasses and 3β-hydroxy derivatives (e.g., esters and glycosides). Furthermore, many of these techniques have been modified to achieve the subsequent separation of individual sterols from each subclass (see Section IV). The design of an isolation protocol can also yield important structural information. Several recent reviews of the chromatography of sterols aid in the design of an appropriate protocol (e.g., Heftmann, 1975, 1976; W. R. Nes, 1985, and this book).

Solvent partitioning plays a minor role in many isolation protocols. The extract is often reduced to an aqueous residue and partitioned against the extraction solvent (e.g., Zielinski *et al.*, 1982a) or some other organic solvent such as ether (e.g., Zollo *et al.*, 1986). In some instances, the aqueous residue is first saponified with methanolic or ethanolic potassium hydroxide (5–10% w/v) and then partitioned against ether to obtain a nonsaponified lipid fraction (NLF) that would contain, *inter alia*, free sterols and sterols released from esters, as noted earlier. Sterylglycosides and some polar sterol metabolites would not be retained in the organic phase.

Early investigators employed digitonin precipitation as a primary isolation technique. Digitonin, a sapogenin, forms an insoluble 1:1 complex with cholesterol, with only 14 mg in 100 ml of 95% ethanol being soluble. Digitonin seems to be specific for 3β-hydroxysteroids in the 5α series. Dissociation of the complex is accomplished with pyridine. The major drawback to the use of digitonin precipitation is that a thorough systemic study of structural effects has not been made to determine if the three subclasses of sterols are equally precipitable. Despite this drawback, digitonin precipitation still can be employed when only 4-desmethylsterols in the 5α series are being analyzed (Davis and Poneleit, 1974; Kadkade *et al.*, 1983; Huang and Grunwald, 1986). It is important to keep in mind, however, that this particular technique can fail to indicate the presence of trace (i.e., microgram or less) components.

A. Open Column Chromatography

Open column chromatography (CC), whether ordinary-phase (adsorption), reversed-phase, or argentation, is still important in most isolation protocols, especially when the TLE or the NLF (e.g., from higher-plant materials) is complex or high in weight (i.e., 200 mg or more).

Ordinary-phase (adsorption) chromatography is used here to isolate the sterol subclasses. Reversed-phase and argentation column chromatography techniques are discussed with respect to their usefulness in the purification of these isolated subclasses.

1. Ordinary-Phase (Adsorption) Chromatography

This chromatographic method involves the binding of a substrate to the surface of a stationary polar phase (i.e., silica gel or alumina) through hydrogen-bonding and other electronic attractions (e.g., dipole-dipole interactions), followed by elutions with mobile phases of moderate polarity (Wren, 1961; Heftmann, 1967; W. R. Nes, 1985). Alumina and silica-gel systems provide "straight phase" separations, with the more nonpolar compounds eluting first; the influence of groupings on the rate of movement will be alkyl < ketone < hindered hydroxyl < unhindered hydroxyl. To produce this kind of separation by alumina column chromatography, a gradient of diethyl ether into mixed hexanes such as skelly solv B (10% increments up to 70%) is used, followed by elution with 100% ether and 100% methanol. The alumina is usually dried and deactivated with 3% water (w/w). The amount of TLF or NLF applied is usually 1 g/100 g of alumina. The usual order of elution is 100% hexane: hydrocarbons and squalene; 10–30% ether (E): steryl esters, steryl ketones, squalene oxide, and waxes; 40–50% E: 4,4-dimethylsterols, 4α-methylsterols, pentacyclic triterpenoids, and long-chain fatty alcohols (C_{22}–C_{32}); 60–70% E: 4,4-desmethylsterols; and 100% E to 100% MeOH: sterylglycosides, acetylated sterylglycosides, polar steroids, organic acids, and phospholipids. The elution profile is routinely monitored by gas-liquid or thin-layer chromatography. Permutations of this procedure have been used by others to obtain sterols from TLFs or NLFs (Westerman and Roddick, 1981; Campbell and Nes, 1983; Chiu *et al.*, 1985; Heupel, 1985; McNamara *et al.*, 1985; Rendell *et al.*, 1986).

Silica-gel column chromatography can be used as a preliminary clean-up step prior to alumina chromatography (Popov *et al.*, 1983) or as the primary isolation procedure (Davis and Poneleit, 1974; Zielinski *et al.*, 1982a; Itoh *et al.*, 1983; Volkman *et al.*, 1984; Akihisa *et al.*, 1986). A routine procedure is to apply 1 g TLF to a column (39 cm × 25 mm i.d. containing 60 g silicic acid, 100–200 mesh) and elute as follows: 100% hexane: hydrocarbons, squalene, waxes, and so on; hexane/benzene (50/50): pentacyclic triterpenes (PT), long-chain fatty alcohols (C_{22}–C_{32}), steryl esters, PT esters; benzene, as hexane/benzene (50/50); 100% ether: long-chain fatty alcohols, 4,4-dimethylsterols, 4α-methylsterols, 4,4-desmethylsterols; and 100% methanol: acetylated sterylglycosides, sterylglycosides, polar compounds such as phospholipids, polar steroids, and so on (W. D. Nes, personal communication). The hexane/benzene, benzene, and ether fractions can then be combined and chromatographed on alumina for further purification and separation of the sterol subclasses. If the weight has been reduced sufficiently, preparative thin-layer chromatography (Section III.B.) can be used on these combined fractions to isolate the sterol subclasses.

2. Reversed-Phase Column Chromatography

These systems employ lipophyllic hydrophobic sephadex derivatives [i.e., alkyloxy covalently bonded to lipophyllic dextran (Ellingboe *et al.*, 1970)] as the stationary phase and have been developed for both the purification and separation of bulk sterol fractions. Materials, such as Sephadex LH-20 or Lipidex 5000, eluted with nonpolar solvents (e.g., 5 % methanol in hexane) will separate compounds in order of increasing polarity (Ellingboe *et al.*, 1970). This "straight-phase" system was perfected by W. D. Nes and Bach (1985) and used to isolate 4,4-dimethylsterols from long-chain fatty alcohols in fractions obtained from alumina column chromatography (Heupel and Nes, 1985). Columns of this material (e.g., Lipidex 5000 eluted with 5 % hexane in methanol) have also been used to separate preparative quantities of individual sterols that differ, for instance, in the extent of C-24 alkylation in the sterol side-chain (W. R. Nes, 1985, and references cited therein).

3. Argentation Column Chromatography

Argentation column chromatography, in which silica (e.g., Anacil B) is impregnated with a solution of $AgNO_3$ and dried, is most often used in the separation of sterols as their acetates (see Section IV); however, the technique can be modified to separate acetylated sterols, particularly 4,4-desmethylsterols, from contaminants such as long-chain fatty alcohols (C_{22}–C_{32}) and lipid pigments prior to further analysis. For example, a 20% $AgNO_3$-Anacil B (w/w) column eluted sequentially with one column volume each of (1) hexane, (2) hexane/benzene (9:1), (3) hexane/benzene (50/50), and (4) benzene has been used to separate long-chain fatty alcohol (LCFA) acetate (fractions 1 and 2) and 4,4-desmethylsteryl acetates (fraction 3) (R. C. Heupel and W. D. Nes, unpublished results).

B. Thin-Layer Chromatography

Thin-layer chromatography (TLC) systems can be used as the primary technique for isolating and separating the sterol subclasses from complex TLEs or NLFs that weigh less than 200 mg. Additionally, these systems can be used to separate or further characterize the sterol subclasses from the open column systems described in the preceding section.

1. Ordinary-Phase (Adsorption) Thin-Layer Chromatography

These systems most often use silica gel as the adsorbent though systems employing other adsorbents (e.g., alumina) have been developed (Heftmann, 1976). A variety of analytical plates ($\leq$0.25 mm in thickness) or preparative plates ($\geq$0.50 mm) are commercially available and are usually more convenient and uniform than those prepared in the laboratory. Most investigators use partially deactivated plates (i.e., plates equilibrated with the laboratory atmosphere). Thin-layer chromatograms are most frequently developed by a single solvent ascent, but separations can be improved by multiple developments. For instance, Δ^5-sterols can be separated from Δ^7-sterols by changing the ratio of benzene to ether or by multiple developments (Heupel *et al.*, 1986). It is also important not to overload the plates; a general rule of thumb is 1 mg or less per centimeter for analytical plates or 2 mg per 0.50 mm

Table 2 Retention values of selected sterols and derivatives in selected TLC, GLC, and RP–HPLC systems

Sterol Subclasses	TLC[a] R_f	SE-30	GLC[b] (RRT$_c$) OV-17	SP-1000	HPLC 4 % AqMeOH	(α_c)[c] 100 % MeOH
4,4-Desmethylsterols	0.3–0.4					
Cholest-4-en-3β-ol	0.38	0.97	—	—	0.94	—
Cholest-5-en-3β-ol	0.33	1.0 (1.43)	1.0 (1.39)	1.0 (1.15)	1.0 (2.44)	1.0 (1.0)
Cholest-8-en-3β-ol	0.33					
24α-Methylcholest-5-en-3β-ol (campesterol)	0.33	1.29 (1.82)	1.33 (1.78)	1.29 (—)	1.14 (2.79)	1.20 (1.15)
24β-Methylcholest-5-en-3β-ol (dihydrobrassicasterol)	0.33	1.29 (1.82)	1.33 (1.78)	1.29 (—)	1.14 (2.79)	1.20 (1.15)
24α-Ethylcholest-5-en-3β-ol (sitosterol)	0.33	1.61 (2.26)	1.68 (2.26)	1.54 (—)	1.32 (—)	1.42 (1.29)
24α-Ethylidienecholesterol (stigmasterol)	0.33	1.40 (1.98)	1.47 (1.98)	1.37 (0.99)	1.14 (2.68)	1.20 (1.10)
4α-Methylsterols	0.4–0.50					
24α-Methylenelophenol	0.45	1.63 (2.27)	1.83 (2.54)	—	— (1.0)	—
Obtusifoliol	0.43	1.49	1.54	—	— (0.82)	—

4,4-Desmethylsterols	0.50–0.60					
Lanosterol	0.55	1.65 (2.20)	1.79 (2.22)	1.41 (1.19)	1.0	—
Lanosta-8-en-3β-ol	0.55	1.52	—	—	1.26	—
Cycloartenol	0.55	1.92 (2.35)	2.06 (2.61)	1.63 (1.46)	1.15 (2.44)	1.18
24-Methylenecycloartenol	0.55	2.13 (2.87)	2.32 (2.93)	1.85 (1.59)	—	—
3β-Ketones	0.60–0.85					
Cholest-5-en-3one	0.63	1.30	—	—	1.02	—
Ergosta-4,6,22-triene-3one	0.64	1.57	—	—	0.79	—
Sterylesters	0.85–1.0					
Cholesterol oleate	0.98	—	—	—	—	—
Cholesterol cinnamate	0.98	—	—	—	—	—
Cholesterol acetate	0.98	1.43	1.39	1.15	—	—
Sterylglycosides	0.0–0.1					
Cholesterylglycosides	0.00	—	—	—	—	—
Acetylatedsterylglycoside	0.0–0.1					
Acetylated cholesylglucoside	0.00	—	—	—	—	—

Note: The physical constants (chromatographic) listed were obtained in the following studies: W. D. Nes *et al.* (1982); Heupel *et al.* (1986); Le and Nes (1986); R. C. Heupel and W. D. Nes, unpublished data.

[a] Thin-layer chromatography (TLC); silica gel G (250 μm × 20 cm × 20 cm) developed once with benzene-diethylether (9:1, v/v).

[b] Gas-liquid chromatography (GLC); flame-ionization detector (300°C); 3% SE-30 (on gas chrome Q 100/120 mesh, 1.8 m × 2 mm i.d.), 3% OV-17 (on gas chrome Q 100/120 mesh, 1.8 m × 2 mm i.d.), and 1% SP-1000 (on supelcoport, 100/120 mesh, 1.8 m × 2 mm i.d.); oven temp 240°C (except SP-1000), 255°C); flow rate of He 30 ml min^{-1}; RRT_c = relative retention time to cholesterol. Parenthetical values are of the 3β-acetates.

[c] Reversed-phase high-performance liquid chromatography (RP-HPLC): Altex column packed with Ultrasphere ODS (5 μm particle size), 4.6 mm i.d. × 250 mm; 100% methanol (flow rate 1.0 ml min^{-1}) or 4% aqueous methanol (flow rate 1.6 ml min^{-1}); detector 205 nm. Parenthetical values are of the 3β-acetates.

thickness per centimeter for preparative plates. A variety of detection systems is available (Heftmann, 1976), ranging from the inclusion of inorganic fluorescent indicators in the prepared plates and detecting the sterols under UV light to spraying of the plates with an ethanolic solution of Rhodamine-6G and visualizing directly. A common method is to spray the plates with 50 % sulfuric acid in ethanol followed by heating; although this method is destructive, detection is rapid and is done without inclusion of inorganic indicators that might interfere with further analysis. For analytical or preparative TLC, a stationary phase of silica gel G and a mobile phase of benzene/ether (9:1, v:v) can be used to separate the three sterol subclasses and their C-3 ketones, C-3 glycosides, C-3 esters, and polar metabolites (Table 2) (Campbell and Nes, 1983; Heupel, 1985; Heupel *et al.*, 1986; Le and Nes, 1986; W. D. Nes and Heupel, 1986; W. R. Nes *et al.*, 1986). After separation, the silica from the appropriate bands is scraped from the plate and eluted sequentially with solvents of varying polarity (i.e., acetone, benzene, and ether). It should be noted that although long-chain fatty alcohols (C_{22}–C_{32}) usually elute at R_f 0.53 (the approximate R_f of 4,4-dimethylsterols, see Table 2), considerable tailing of each occurs when loaded at levels greater than 10 μg/cm (Stafford and Nes, 1983). Consequently, each of the sterol subclasses may contain LCFA contaminants in addition to sterol intermediates, the related pentacyclic triterpenoids, and other lipid compounds. These can be removed by $AgNO_3$–silica-gel column chromatography, previously described, by reversed-phase thin-layer chromatography, or by argentation thin-layer chromatography. Another approach, especially with 4,4-desmethylsterol fractions, is to use digitonin precipitation. Other adsorption TLC systems for the isolation of sterols have been and are continuously being used (Westerman and Roddick, 1981; Zielinski *et al.*, 1982a; Osagie and Kates, 1984; Akihisa *et al.*, 1986; Garg and Paleg, 1986; Rendell *et al.*, 1986).

2. Reversed-Phase Thin-Layer Chromatography

This is a method of chromatography in which the stationary phase is nonpolar. It usually employs C_{18} or C_8 plates [i.e., plates on which octadecyldimethylsiloxy (C_{18} or ODS) or octasylidimethyl (C_8) is attached to one of the Si atoms of the silica gel]. When eluted with polar solvents, the more polar compounds move faster than the less polar compounds. By manipulating the solvent systems, it is possible to separate the sterol subclasses, and individual sterols, from each other (De Souza and Nes, 1969; Domnas *et al.*, 1983). The major drawback of this technique is that the amount of material that can be loaded on the plates (0.25 mm thickness) is much less than that of ordinary silica gel. Additionally, rigorous extraction of the scraped silica, even with moderately polar solvents, can cause considerable support bleed, thereby contaminating the sample. This technique can be useful in separating long-chain fatty alcohols from sterol fractions obtained by adsorption open-column chromatography or adsorption TLC (Campbell and Nes, 1983; W. D. Nes and Bach, 1985).

C. High-Performance Liquid Chromatography

High performance liquid chromatography (HPLC) (normal-phase, reversed-phase, or adsorption) has been used as a primary technique for the isolation of the sterol subclasses from TLEs or NLFs that are simple and low in mass, for example, extracts from enzyme assays employing subcellular components (Noshino *et al.*, 1985) or from blood serum (Matsuoka *et al.*, 1985; Devgun and Paterson, 1986). The technique is rarely used as the primary isolation method for complex extracts such as those from higher plants. Hogg and Gillan (1984) have reported the isolation of 4,4-desmethylsterols directly from the NLF of several mangrove species using normal-phase HPLC and their quantitation by capillary gas-liquid chromatography (GLC). In such complex samples, nonsteroidal contaminants (e.g., long-chain fatty alcohols) that may co-chromatograph with sterols could affect the results. HPLC is most frequently used to separate individual sterols and as an aid in their primary characterization prior to subsequent identification.

IV. CHROMATOGRAPHIC SEPARATION OF INDIVIDUAL STEROLS FROM STEROL SUBCLASSES

The ultimate goal, of course, of the aforementioned extraction and isolation procedures is the separation of sterols into the three subclasses prior to quantification and identification of specific sterols. An inherent characteristic in the procedures for obtaining the sterol subclasses is that various individual sterols can (and do) co-chromatograph with each other and with nonsteroidal contaminants, which makes it difficult to identify and quantify specific sterols. Consequently, the separation of individual sterols may be necessary for their quantification and preparation for identification. Chromatographic techniques can separate sterols; and the degree of separation is strongly influenced by structure, presence of polar groups, and stereochemistry. Thus, the mobility of a sterol in a given system, coupled to an analysis of the degree of separation from standards in different systems, can be correlated with structural characteristics.

A. Open Column Chromatography

Open column chromatography is usually used to separate individual sterols from subclass fractions that are high in mass (>10 mg). Adsorption systems, both with and without silver ions (argentation chromatography), and reversed-phase systems have been developed and used (for guides to this literature, see Wren, 1961; Heftmann, 1967, 1975, 1976; W. R. Nes, 1985).

As discussed earlier (Section III.A.1), adsorption systems (alumina or silica gel) eluted with gradients of moderate polarity (straight phase) separate sterols in order of increasing polarity. Hydrogen bonding and other electronic interactions of functional groups with the support reduce the rates of movement of the sterol; the influence of the groups on the rates of movement will follow the order of alkyl $<$ ketone $<$ hindered hydroxyl $<$ unhindered hydroxyl groups. Adsorption systems are good methods for separating sterols according to the kind and number of their oxygen functions (W. R. Nes, 1985). Size can also be a contributing factor in the separation of sterols with adsorption systems (Hunter *et al.*, 1979). Double bonds have a small but definite effect on the mobility of sterols in adsorption systems (W. R. Nes *et al.*, 1978; Hunter *et al.*, 1979; Thowsen and Schroefer, 1979); for example, W. R. Nes and co-workers (1978) have used a 10% deactivated alumina column eluted with a gradient of ether into mixed hexanes to separate Δ^5 from $\Delta^{5,7}$-4,4-desmethylsterols. Argentation systems have been developed that enhance the influence of the double bond by the inclusion of 5–30% $AgNO_3$ into the silica gel or alumina (Vromen and Cohen, 1967) and have been used in the separation of sterols differing in the number and position of double bonds from a variety of sources (e.g., Lutsky *et al.*, 1971, 1975; Popov *et al.*, 1983; and references cited in W. R. Nes 1985). In general, the more a double bond can interact with the silver ions, usually associated with decreased substitution or steric hinderance about the double bond, the greater the adsorption and the slower the rate of movement; multiple double bonds also retard mobility. The influence of the double bond is enhanced by acetylation with pyrimidine/acetic anhydride (1:1 or 2:1), before chromatography in argentation systems. Polar solvents (e.g., gradients of benzene in hexane or chloroform in hexane with small amounts of acetone or acetic acid) are usually used. Reversed-phase systems that employ materials such as Sephadex LH-20 or Lipidex 5000 eluted with polar solvents separate sterols in order of decreasing polarity and increasing size (Ellingboe *et al.*, 1970). These systems are more sensitive to structural changes than are normal systems (W. R. Nes, 1985). Such systems have been employed by W. R. Nes *et al.* (1976) and Chiu *et al.* (1985) in the isolation of sterols with C-24 methyl and ethyl groups from a variety of plant sources. The advent of preparative high-performance liquid chromatography employing bonded silica phases [i.e., phases in which octadecyldimethylsiloxy (ODS or C_{18}) or octasylidimethylsiloxy (C_8) is attached to one of the Si atoms in the silica] is rapidly replacing reversed-phase column chromatography as a separatory technique (see Section IV.C). In addition to its greater number of theoretical plates, preparative reversed-phase high-performance liquid chromatography is faster than the Sephadex LH-20 system; the former requires a few hours of elution time compared with a few days for the latter.

B. Thin-Layer Chromatography

Thin-layer chromatographic (TLC) systems (adsorption, argenetic, and reversed-phase) have been developed that can be used in the separation of sterols from subclass fractions that are less than 10 mg in mass. The same characteristics of the sterols and supports that result in their separation in open-column chromatography apply to TLC separation. The drawbacks in using TLC separation include: (1) losses during recovery from the layers; (2) generation of artifacts from bulk sterols or loss of trace sterols by interaction of the compounds with the support; and (3) the reduced number of theoretical plates relative to open column chromatography or high-performance liquid chromatography, which results in less than total separation. The major advantages in the use of TLC systems are in (1) speed, relative to open column chromatography; (2) ability to chromatograph several samples simultaneously (which can be important in metabolic and/or developmental studies); and (3) ease in system manipulation (i.e., altering solvents or supports). W. R. Nes and co-workers (1977) have reported the separation of Δ^5- and Δ^7-4,4-desmethylsterols using thin or thick layers of silica gel G developed 3–6 times using 15 % ether in benzene as solvents; they have also obtained the separation of Δ^5-, $\Delta^{5,22}$-, $\Delta^{5,7}$-, and $\Delta^{5,7,22}$-4,4-desmethylsterol acetates (in order of decreasing R_f values) using silica gel impregnated with 10 % $AgNO_3$ and developed with chloroform/hexane/acetone (100:40:0.75, ratio by volume) (W. R. Nes *et al.*, 1978, 1981). Raederstorff and Rohmer (1984) have reported the separation of dienic 4,4-desmethylsterol acetates that differ only in the alkylation at C-22. A reversed-phase TLC (RP-TLC) system (C_{18} plates developed with acetone/H_2O; 94:6 v/v) that separates ergosta-8(9),14(15),22(23)-triene-3β-ol and ergosta-5(6),8(9),22(23)-triene-3β-ol from ergosta-5(6),7(8),22(23)-triene-3β-ol and ergosta-6(7),8(14), 22(23)-triene-3β-ol has been used in sterol isolations from *Gibberella fujikuroi* (W. D. Nes *et al.*, 1985).

C. High-Performance Liquid Chromatography

High-performance liquid chromatography (HPLC), adsorption or reversed-phase, is becoming the most commonly used technique for the separation of individual sterols from subclass fractions. Although HPLC is discussed in this section as a preparative technique, the comments herein apply equally to its use, in conjunction with suitable detectors, as a purely analytical tool in the primary characterization of sterols (Section V).

In adsorption HPLC, microspheres of silica (silicic acid such as μ-Poracil) are employed. As in adsorption, open column, and thin-layer chromatography, this method is characterized by hydrogen bonding and other electronic attractions between the sterol and the stationary phase. The small diameter (3–5 μm) and high porosity of these microspheres create a very large effective surface area and a great increase in the number of theoretical plates. TLC solvent systems can be used directly for adsorption HPLC. In general, the solvents that give best separations are binary (or trinary) systems of mostly low-to-moderate polarity solvents with a small amount of a strongly polar solvent such as hexane/benzene (9:1), dichloromethane/n-hexane/ethyl acetate (94:5:1) (Hunter *et al.*, 1979; Thowsen and Schroepfer, 1979; Tsai and Hudson, 1981). The influence of the alkyl groupings, double bonds, stereochemistry, and size on the mobility of sterols in these systems are the same as in other adsorption systems. For example, Thowsen and Schroepfer (1979) have reported the baseline separation of C_{27} cholesterol precursor acetates differing in the number and position of double bonds using four μ-Porasil columns in series eluted with hexane/benzene (9:1). The order of mobility observed was $\Delta^0 > \Delta^5 > \Delta^{8(14)} > \Delta^{8(9)} > \Delta^7 > \Delta^{5,7} > \Delta^{8(14)} > \Delta^{7,14}$. A UV monitor is used as the detector in most systems; however, refractive index detectors are preferred when monitoring for sterols lacking a chromophore (e.g., cholestanol) or when the solvents have high absorbance in the UV region (e.g., benzene).

In reversed-phase HPLC systems, alkyl groups (C_8 or C_{18}) have been chemically bonded to microspheres of silica. These small diameter (2–5 μm), highly porous particles give the stationary phases very large effective surface areas for the interaction of the sterols with the bonded alkyl groups. This large area in turn, makes possible rapid equilibration of the sterol between the stationary phase and an appropriate mobile phase, yielding columns with as much as 10^4 theoretical plates (W. R. Nes, 1985). A variety of polar mobile phases have been employed in RP-HPLC [e.g., 100% acetonitrile, acetonitrile-water mixtures (0–20%), and methanol-water mixtures (2–20% water]. Samples are usually injected onto the analytical column at levels of 1–100 μg per component (up to 1.0 mg total) for routine separations. Retention volumes of eluted sterols are usually expressed relative to cholesterol; the α_c (DiBussolo and Nes, 1982) for representative sterols are shown in Table 2. For improved column life, it is recommended that HPLC-grade or glass-distilled solvents be degassed prior to use and that samples be prefiltered through a commercial C_{18} Sep-Pack (Parks *et al.*, 1986) or that guard columns be employed.

Complex systems are now available that employ computer-controlled solvent metering systems for gradient elutions with multicomponent mobile phases and diode-array multiple wavelength detectors for obtaining UV spectra of the components as they elute from the column.

Simple and complex reversed-phase HPLC systems have been used to isolate individual sterols from a variety of sources (Kokke *et al.*, 1981, 1982; Zielinski *et al.*, 1982b; Crist *et al.*, 1983; Itoh *et al.*, 1983; Garg and Nes, 1984; Bianchini *et al.*, 1985; Heupel, 1985; Kesselmeier *et al.*, 1985; Matsuoka *et al.*, 1985; W. D. Nes *et al.*, 1985; Poll *et al.*, 1985; Akihisa *et al.*, 1986; Devgun and Paterson, 1986; Heupel *et al.*, 1986; W. D. Nes, and Heupel, 1986).

D. Gas–Liquid Chromatography

Gas–liquid chromatography (GLC) is most frequently used as an analytical technique to monitor fractions during the isolation and separation of sterols; however, this technique can also be used in preparative separations. The use of GLC as an analytical and preparative technique for sterols and related steroids has been discussed in numerous reviews (e.g., Fumagalli, 1969; Heftmann, 1975, 1976; Knights, 1982; Paterson, 1984; W. R. Nes, 1985).

The separation of sterols in gas–liquid systems depends on the polarity and molecular weight (frequently correlating with size and volume) of the molecule. The contributions that molecular weight makes to the mobility of the sterols depend mainly on how vaporization is altered, whereas the way changes in the compound's polarity influence mobility also depends on the liquid phase (W. R. Nes, 1985). The effects of molecular weight can be influenced through derivatization of the molecule and by altering the operating temperatures, and the effects of changes in polarity are influenced through the use of liquid phases differing in polarity. With the advent of high-temperature liquid phases of varying polarities, derivatization to increase volatility of the sterols prior to GLC is becoming unnecessary (Patterson, 1984). However, an examination of the effect of derivatization on retention times can give useful information for the primary characterization of a sterol.

The liquid phases in common use are of two types: (1) the nonpolar silicones (e.g., SE-30, methylsilicone), in which silicon atoms of the polymer bear alkyl groups and (2) polar phases of the silicone and other types. In polar silicones, one or more of the alkyl groups are replaced by a polar group (e.g., OV-17, phenyl-methyl silicone). The overall polarity of the phases is measured by McReynolds constants (McReynolds, 1970), which increase as the polarity increases. The influence of the polarity of the liquid phase and the molecular features of sterols on their mobility has been investigated by a number of workers (Patterson, 1971; W. R. Nes *et al.*, 1976; Homberg and Bielefeld, 1979; see also W. R. Nes, 1985, for a key to the literature). As with HPLC, mathematical formulas have been developed, employing retention times (relative to standards; i.e., cholesterol), that can be used with other information to help characterize an unknown sterol mixture during the separation of the individual components (see Section V).

In the preliminary analysis of sterol fractions, it is advisable to dissolve samples in ethanol and then inject 1–2 μg onto packed columns (columns in which the liquid phase has been coated onto an inert support) that are operated isothermally at 235°C. Helium is used as the carrier gas (30 ml/min). Samples should routinely be chromatographed on three packed columns covering the range of McReynolds constants. Although several types of detectors are available, such as thermal conductivity (TC), electron capture (EC), and flame ionization (FI) detectors, flame ionization detection is preferred in many laboratories because of its sensitivity (potentially, nanogram quantities can be detected), its linearity in response over a wide mass range, and its universality (its response to most sterols is nearly equivalent on a per-mass basis). The theory and usage of each type of detector has been described by Fumagalli (1969) and others (e.g., Heftmann, 1976). Because of possible fluctuations of the chromatographic and detector variables (e.g., column age and gas flow rates), retention times of the peaks in the chromatogram of a sterol fraction are expressed relative to that of cholesterol, either as an internal standard or injected immediately prior to the sample (Patterson, 1971). These relative retention times to cholesterol (RRT_c) of some selected sterols under these conditions are shown in Table 2. Similar systems have been employed by a number of workers for monitoring fractions during sterol purification and for primary characterization of the sterols (e.g., Kokke *et al.*, 1981; W. R. Nes *et al.*, 1981, 1986; Campbell and Nes, 1983; W. D. Nes, *et al.*, 1985; Berquist *et al.*, 1986; Garg and Paleg, 1986; Rendell *et al.*, 1986).

Capillary columns are particularly useful in the analytical separation of structurally similar sterols (Patterson, 1984). Two types of capillary columns are generally used: (a) those in which the liquid phase has been bound to the inside surface (about 0.3-μm thick film) of a capillary column (e.g., columns with i.d. about 0.3 mm and lengths about 30 m), called a wall-coated open tubular column (WCOT); or (b) those in which the inert support (coated with liquid phase) has been bound to the inner surface, called a support-coated open tubular columns (SCOT). The WCOT and SCOT methods allow a much more efficient mass transfer of sterol to the liquid phase, resulting in truer equilibria between the gas and liquid phases and thereby sharpening the bands. Longer (100 m) and more polar columns can be employed, making available more theoretical plates for the separation. Analyses employing these columns have been run under isothermal or programmed temperature conditions and at various flow rates (e.g., Hogg and Gillan, 1984; Raederstorff and Rohmer, 1984; Bianchini *et al.*, 1985; Akihisa *et al.*, 1986).

Conditions employed in the analysis of a fraction can be modified and used in the separation of sterols (Van Lier and Smith, 1968; Kokke *et al.*, 1982; Ha *et al.*, 1982). In general, packed columns with greater internal diameters (e.g., 6 mm) are used to allow for greater sample loading (0.1–1.0 mg); splitters are usually placed between the column and flame-ionization detectors so that the column effluent can be monitored while fractions are collected. Electron-capture detectors, which are non destructive, can be used and fractions collected after detection.

V. PRIMARY CHARACTERIZATION OF STEROLS

It would not be possible in this section to discuss in detail the influence of sterol structure on chromatography or the application of spectroscopic techniques (NMR, MS, UV, IR, and X-ray) to the final identification of sterols. The purpose here is simply to demonstrate that the chromatographic and spectral information accumulated during the extraction, isolation, and separation of sterols can be used in the primary characterization of these sterols. Primary characterization can indicate the presence of known sterols (i.e., sterols whose structures are known), indicate the presence of novel sterols, and provide clues for the elucidation of the full structure of new sterols.

A. Chromatographic Characterization

Modern chromatographic systems, including those employed in the isolation and separation of sterols, can provide reliable structural clues, based on chromatographic mobilities, for the identification of compounds. At present, however, no single chromatographic system can separate each of the known sterols. Consequently, multiple chromatographic systems are used to provide corroborative information to characterize a suspected sterol. There are many reported instances of the identification of known and novel sterols from materials, based on their chromatographic properties in multiple systems. At best, these should be considered tentative identifications or primary characterizations. As noted by W. R. Nes (1985), "Identification cannot be achieved by the use of a single method, although NMR, especially ^{13}C-NMR comes close to providing a pattern of information unique enough to represent a fingerprint."

Combined chromatographic characters can be used to monitor changes in sterols in developmental studies after their identity has been established; easily the most useful chromatographic characters are obtained from thin-layer, gas–liquid, and high-performance liquid chromatography.

1. Thin-Layer Chromatography

As noted earlier, TLC, adsorption or reversed-phase, can be used as a primary technique for the isolation of the three sterol subclasses from extracts or to separate the sterol subclasses obtained through open-column chromatography (e.g., silica-gel column fractions, Section III.B). Additionally, aliquots of sterol fractions obtained from alumina column chromatography of total lipid extracts or nonsaponifiable lipid fractions can be monitored by TLC and the presence of sterols of the suspected subclass corroborated. Thus, using TLC, samples can be characterized as containing mainly 4-desmethyl-, 4α-monomethyl-, or 4,4-dimethylsterol compounds (Tables 2 and 3).

It has also been noted that TLC can separate individual sterols from subclass fractions (see Section IV.B). For example, sterols differing in the number and positions of double bonds can be separated by argentation TLC; the systems mentioned (see also Heftmann, 1975, 1976, for keys to the literature) can be used to monitor the sterol subfractions for components that differ in their degrees of saturation.

A common method for detection of sterols and other steroids on thin layers is to spray the plate with 50% sulfuric acid; then, after heating, lipids char black. Under controlled temperature conditions (careful heating at 78°C), sulfuric acid has been shown to elicit characteristic color and fluorescence responses from sterols and steroids. The color and fluorescence responses for a wide range of sterols have been tabulated (see Heftmann, 1975, 1976, for data and as keys to the literature) and can be used in the primary characterization of sterol mixtures and isolated individual sterols. Fluorescent sprays are available to aspirate on plates for visualization under UV lamps, allowing nondestructive characterization of samples.

2. Gas–Liquid Chromatography

Information from the analysis of sterol fractions during their extraction, isolation, and separation by GLC on packed (or capillary) columns with a wide range of McReynolds' constants (Section IV.D) can be used to further characterize the compounds present. The necessity for the use of multiple columns is illustrated in Fig. 4. In this figure, the separation of an equal-mass mixture of five 4,4-desmethylsterols on four packed columns is shown. Conditions of the chromatography in each case (described in Section IV.D) were adjusted so that cholesterol eluted in ~10 min. Only SP-1000 was able to resolve the five sterols. With a mixture of unknowns, the peaks would be assigned a retention time relative to cholesterol (RRT_c) for each column; the retention time of cholesterol can be determined immediately before sample injection or from cholesterol added to the sample aliquot prior to injection. The resolution of the various mixture components would then be monitored through continued fraction analysis during the isolation and separation procedures. Tentative assignments of structure can be made by comparing the RRT_c of the components with those of standards analyzed under the same conditions (Tables 2 and 3) or with lists of reported RRT_c determined under similar conditions. Additionally, compilations of contributions of selected molecular features to retention times, σ^G, of sterols on various columns are available (see W. R. Nes, 1985, for more details and keys to the literature). Thus, the relative retention time of a suspected unknown (RRT_u) can be used to formulate the

Table 3 Retention values of selected sterol precursors, long-chain fatty alcohols, and pentacyclic triterpenenes in TLC, GLC, and RP-HPLC.

	TLC[a]	GLC[b] (RRT$_c$)			RP–HPLC[c] (α_c)	
Sterol intermediates	R_f	SE-30	OV-17	SP-1000	4 % AqMeOH	100 % MeOH
Mevalonate	0.00					
Geraniol	0.43					
Farnesol	0.47					
Squalene	0.97					
Squalene oxide	0.97					
Fatty alcohols	0.50–0.60					
Decosanol (C22)	0.53	0.22 (0.30)	0.14 (—)	0.15 (—)	—	—
Tetracosanol (C24)	0.53	0.38 (0.52)	0.32 (—)	0.22 (—)	—	—
Hexacosanol (C26)	0.53	0.66 (0.90)	0.42 (—)	0.34 (—)	—	—
Octacosanol (C28)	0.53	1.16 (—)	0.75 (—)	0.64 (—)	—	—
Tricontanol (C30)	0.53	1.98 (2.60)	1.34 (1.84)	1.05 (—)	—	—
Pentacyclic triterpenes	0.50–0.60					
α-Amyrin	0.53	1.79 (2.29)	2.10 (2.55)	1.77 (1.47)	1.28 (3.19)	1.12 (—)
β-Amyrin	0.53	1.64 (2.17)	1.83 (2.25)	1.55 (1.29)	1.15 (2.10)	— (—)
δ-Amyrin	0.53	1.89 (—)	2.06 (—)	1.72 (—)	1.15 (—)	1.09 (—)

Note: The physical constants (chromatographic) listed were obtained from the following studies: W. D. Nes and Bach (1985); Heupel (1985); R. C. Heupel and W. D. Nes, unpublished.

[a] Thin-layer chromatography (TLC); silica gel G (250 μm) × 20 cm × 20 cm) developed once with benzene-diethylether (9:1, v/v).

[b] Gas–liquid chromatography (GLC); flame-ionization detector (310°C); 3 % SE-30 (on gas chrome Q 100/120 mesh, 1.8 m × 2 mm. i.d.); 3 % OV-17 (on gas chrome Q 100/120 mesh, 1.8 m × 2 mm i.d.); 1 % SP-1000 (on supelcoport 100/120 mesh, 1.8 m × 2 mm i.d.; oven temp. 240°C (except 1 % SP-1000, 255°C); flow rate of He 30 ml min^{-1}. RRT$_c$ = retention time relative to cholesterol. Parenthetical values are of 3β-acetates.

[c] Reversed-phase high-performance liquid chromatography (RP-HPLC); Altex column packed with ultrasphere ODS (5 μm particle size), 4.6 mm i.d. × 250 mm; 100 % methanol or 4 % aqueous methanol (flow rate 1.0 ml min^{-1} and 1.6 ml min^{-1} respectively), detector 205 nm, parenthetical values are of 3β-acetates.

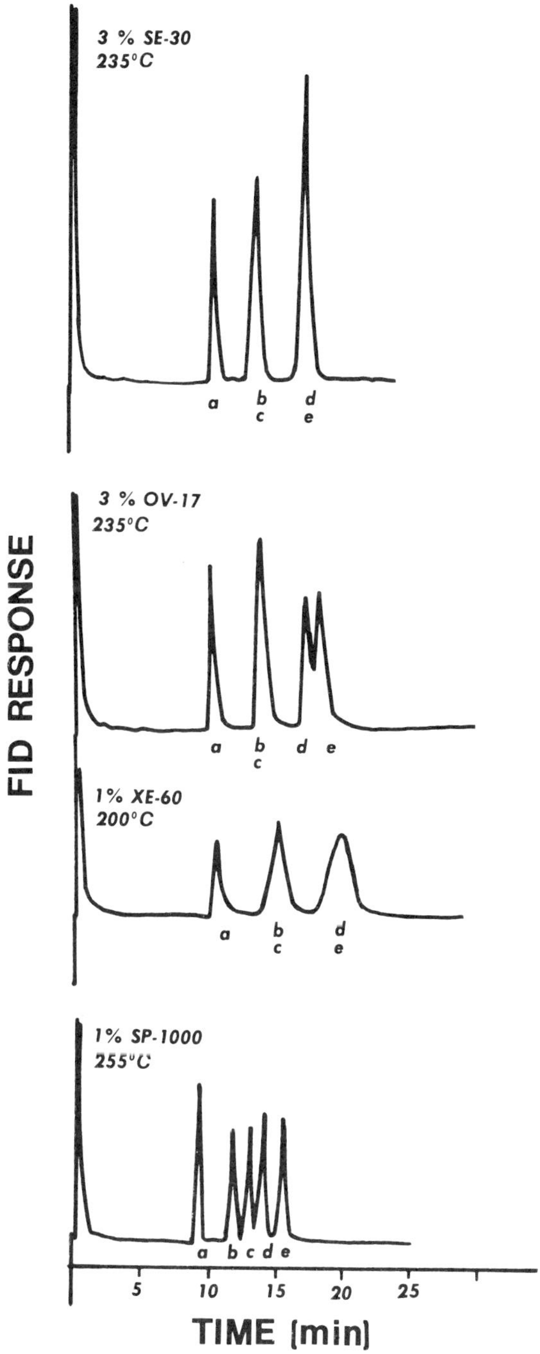

Figure 4 Gas-liquid chromatograms of an equal mass (1 μg/μl) injection of sterols on four columns. Each 1-μl sample contained 0.2 μg of (a) cholesterol, (b) 24-methylcholesterol, (c) 24-methylenecholesterol, (d) 24-ethylcholesterol, and (e) 24-ethylidienecholesterol. Carrier gas (He) flow rate for each column was 30 ml/min. Temperature was adjusted as indicated so that cholesterol eluted from each column in approximately 10 min. The chromatograms were prepared by W. D. Nes. The author appreciates the use of this information prior to publication.

nature of its molecular features. These relationships are shown by the following series of equations:

$$\sigma^G = \text{RRT with feature/RRT without feature} \tag{1}$$

$$\text{RRT}_u = \text{RRT}_p \times \text{product of } \sigma^G \text{ values} \tag{2}$$

$$\text{RRT}_u/\text{RRT}_p = \text{product of } \sigma^G \text{ values} \tag{3}$$

where RRT is the relative retention time, u the unknown, p the parent, and σ^G the contribution of molecular feature. As shown in Fig. 4, cholesterol, campesterol, sitosterol, 24(28)-methylenecholesterol, and 24-ethylidenecholesterol are completely separable only on a very polar GLC column.

3. *High-Performance Liquid Chromatography*

As mentioned earlier, reversed-phase (RP) chromatography is more sensitive to the presence of structural features and effective molecular size than is adsorption chromatography. The relationship between the rate of movement of a sterol and its structure in RP-HPLC systems has been explored by a number of workers (see Hansbury and Scallen, 1978; DiBussolo and Nes, 1982; Holen, 1985; W. R. Nes, 1985). The regularities observed have allowed the development of mathematical formulas that can be used to predict, *a priori*, whether a sterol mixture can be separated in a given system (Heftmann and Hunter, 1979; DiBussolo and Nes, 1982; Ritter *et al.*, 1982; W. R. Nes, 1985). Conversely, these same formulas can be used to indicate the presence of a known sterol or help characterize an unknown sterol during its separation from other components in a mixture. W. R. Nes (1985) has presented a detailed discussion of these formulas. As in gas-liquid chromatography, the rate of movement of a sterol in RP-HPLC is expressed relative to cholesterol, α_c (DiBussolo and Nes, 1982). This chromatographic constant can be defined by the following equations,

$$\alpha_c = \frac{K' \text{ of test sterol}}{K' \text{ of cholesterol}} \tag{4}$$

$$K' = \frac{V_s - V_0}{V_0} = \frac{t_s - t_0}{t_0} \tag{5}$$

where K' is the capacity factor of the column for a sterol, V_0 is the void volume (expressed in time as t_0), V_s (t_s) is the total elution volume (time) of the compound in question. The contribution that a molecular feature σ makes to the rate of mobility of a sterol in a RP-HPLC system can be treated in terms of α_c:

$$\sigma = \frac{\alpha_c \text{ of sterol with feature}}{\alpha_c \text{ of sterol without feature}} \tag{6}$$

The α_c of an unknown can then be used to characterize its molecular features through the following formulas.

$$\alpha_c^u = \alpha_c^p \times \text{product of the } \sigma \text{ values} \tag{7}$$

$$\frac{\alpha_c^u}{\alpha_c^p} = \text{product of the } \sigma \text{ values} \tag{8}$$

where α_c^u is the α_c of the unknown, α_c^p the α_c of the parental sterol (usually cholesterol or cholestanol), and σ the contribution of the molecular feature. A long list of σ values has been compiled (DiBussolo and Nes, 1982), and others can be obtained from current literature. It is apparent, then, that monitoring the α_c of the components of a suspected sterol mixture during their separation is a tool in their characterization; the α_c can be and are used to corroborate information obtained from GLC.

B. Spectral Characterization

For a full discussion of the identification of sterols with nuclear magnetic resonance, mass, ultraviolet, infrared, and X-ray spectrographic techniques, the reader is referred to other chapters in this book. The purpose of this section is to discuss the expansion of the chromatographic structural clues by coupling the systems of choice to appropriate detectors.

1. GLC/Mass Spectroscopy

Mass spectrometers can be coupled to gas-liquid chromatographs (employing packed or capillary columns) for use as reliable and sensitive monitors that can provide information concerning the molecular weight of the components of a sterol mixture or of isolated sterols. An important feature of most present-day GLC/mass spectroscopy (GLC/MS) systems is computerized data acquisition and processing, essential additions to GLC/MS for analyzing complex sterol mixtures. This combination enables the use of specialized techniques such as single-ion current monitoring (SICM or SIM) and multiple ion monitoring (MIM) to increase the sensitivity of the mass spectrometer as a detector for minor sterol components in mixtures. The GLC/mass spectrometer is also invaluable for determining the purity of isolated samples prior to other spectral analyses requiring 0.1 mg or more quantities (i.e., NMR, UV, IR, and X-ray). At high ionization voltages (70 eV), sterols fragment, giving reliable structural information (e.g., characteristic ring fragments and side-chain fragments). Full mass spectra can be obtained from sterols in mixtures by GLC/MS or from isolated sterols by direct probe techniques. However, for the increasing number of sterol stereoisomers that are being found and that (as yet) are not easily resolved by chromatography and have similar mass spectra [i.e., 24α- and 24β-methylcholesterol in sorghum (Heupel *et al.*, 1986)], mass spectroscopy alone is not sufficient for definitive identification of full structures.

2. HPLC/UV Spectroscopy

The simplest HPLC systems, employed most often, use variable UV wavelength detectors. In monitoring sterol fractions, advantage is taken of the fact that all but a few sterols contain at least one carbon-carbon double bond, and that this chromophore exhibits the phenomenon of end absorption, to use UV monitors set from 205–210 nm as relatively nonspecific sterol detectors. After determination from α_c and σ factors that a fraction contains a sterol with a possible conjugated double-bond system (i.e., a $\Delta^{5,7}$-homoannular system), the fraction can then be rerun at a wavelength determined by Woodward's rules (i.e., 283 nm) to be characteristic of the system. Modern diode array multiple-wavelength detectors, with computer controlled data acquisition and processing equipment coupled to HPLC columns, are capable of rapidly monitoring the full UV spectra of samples as they elute from the column (W. D. Nes *et al.*, 1985). Thus, the purity of a peak in a mixture can be monitored and/or the entire spectrum of an isolated sterol can be obtained simultaneously with its chromatographic data.

C. Characterization of Cholesterol in Samples

Cholesterol is widespread in the animal and plant kingdoms; but in many instances, especially in plants, its level of occurrence is quite low. As noted above, cholesterol is frequently used as a standard, either external or internal, for the chromatographic characterization of sterols (Section V.A) and in many cases is added to extracts as an aid in sterol quantification (Knights, 1982).

It is necessary to determine if cholesterol is present in a source early in the extraction-isolation-separation protocols. If the total lipid extract of the sample contains little contaminating substance, aliquots should be analyzed by GLC on packed columns of varying McReynolds constants (i.e., SE-30, OV-17, SP-100) coupled to an FI detector. An aliquot of the sample should then be analyzed by RP-HPLC on a C_{18} column, eluted with a polar solvent (e.g., methanol/water, 96:4) coupled to a UV monitor set at 205 nm. The retention times of the sample components (peaks in the chromatogram) should be compared with those of cholesterol (the external standard) analyzed immediately before sample injection. Should a peak elute at the retention time (volume) of the external standard, a known amount of pure standard can then be added to another aliquot of the sample and the mass response of the detector to this peak compared with that of the peak prior to standard addition (see Section VI of this chapter). If the peak in question is indeed cholesterol, then the mass response of the FI detector or UV monitor should be enhanced by an amount proportional to the pure standard added.

If available, an aliquot of the extract without added standard can be examined by GLC-single-ion monitoring or GLC–multiple-ion monitoring for the presence of ions characteristic of cholesterol [e.g., m/z 386 (M^+), 371 (M^+-CH_3), 273 (M^+-side chain), 275 (M^+-111, characteristic of Δ^5 sterols)] at the appropriate retention time with the same relative intensities as those of the standard under the same conditions.

This analysis by GLC-SIM or GLC-MIM is particularly useful for detecting trace cholesterol in complex mixtures. These same procedures can be performed on the isolated 4,4-desmethylsterol subclass fraction should the total lipid extract prove too complex (e.g., higher-plant extracts) for direct analysis.

If the presence of cholesterol in the fraction is indicated, then an alternative internal standard should be added to the extract for the estimation of recoveries during the isolation and separation procedures (Knights, 1982). Alternatively, cholesterol labeled at 100% isotopic dilution with, for example, several deuterium atoms, can be added to the extract and used in conjunction with GC/MS both to monitor the quantity of cholesterol in the extract and to estimate recoveries during subsequent procedures (Knights, 1982, and references cited therein; Section VI of this chapter).

VI. QUANTITATIVE ANALYSIS OF STEROLS

Quantification of naturally-occurring compounds, especially sterols, depends on two factors: the sensitivity and selectivity of the detection method and the estimation of recoveries during extraction, isolation, and separation. The physicochemical nature of sterols requires high-resolution chromatographic procedures for selectivity. Detectors, though sensitive, vary in their selectivity.

A. Gas–Liquid Chromatography

Gas–liquid chromatography is most frequently used to quantitate sterols in extracts, subfraction mixtures, and isolated sterol fractions. Selectivity is provided by the gas–liquid partitioning (See section IV). In general, three different detectors have been employed for quantitation: flame-ionization detectors (FID), electron-capture detectors (ECD), and mass detectors (MD) (e.g., Bernini *et al.*, 1986; Knights, 1982). However, FID is by far the most commonly employed because (a) it is relatively insensitive to temperature changes during analysis and to minor structural differences in sterols and related steroids and (b) it has a large linear mass range of response. For quantitative analysis it is necessary to determine the linear range of response for each FID, and accompanying chromatographic system, to a sterol standard such as cholesterol or β-cholestanol. For sample analysis, dried fractions are routinely weighed, dissolved in a known amount of solvent to give a mass-to-volume ratio within the linear range of the detector, and the samples injected onto the column. Modern computer-controlled integrators can then relate detector response to mass for each peak, based on a value determined for the standard. The amount of suspected sterol per fraction can then be computed. As noted previously (Section V.A.2), samples should be monitored on multiple columns and the masses and RRT_c of the suspected sterols correlated, thereby aiding in their primary characterization and quantification.

B. High-Performance Liquid Chromatography

Quantification of sterols in extracts, subclass fractions, or isolated sterol fractions by high-performance liquid chromatography is somewhat limited. The selectivity provided by either adsorption or reversed-phase chromatography is in many cases greater than that provided by GLC. Most frequently, UV detectors are employed and are set at end absorption wavelengths (e.g., Heupel, 1985; Poll *et al.*, 1985). These detectors have limited sensitivity, with monochromatic detectors being most sensitive. Additionally, UV detectors cannot be considered universal sterol detectors. Most sterols differ significantly in their UV absorption properties, even in end-absorption regions. Thus, it would not be possible to select a single wavelength for the quantitation of complex sterol mixtures (Bianchini *et al.*, 1985). Conversely, HPLC coupled to variable wavelength detectors or multidiode detectors can be used to quantitate specific sterols in a mixture if the compound in question has a unique absorption spectrum relative to other members of the mixture. By setting the detector at a unique maximum within the compound's spectrum and by the use of an appropriate standard, a dose-response curve for the sterol in the HPLC system can be obtained and used to quantitate the compound (e.g., W. D. Nes *et al.*, 1985; Devgun and Paterson, 1986; W. D. Nes and Heupel, 1986).

C. Methods for Estimating Recoveries

Quantification of the sterols originally present in an extract requires the correction of the final analytical result to account for losses during isolation and separation. For trace components, of course, these losses may be significant; thus these factors must be considered when estimating total sterol content of an extract. Some investigators have accomplished this by using internal standards (e.g., Knights, 1982), which are commonly added to the initial extract prior to isolation. These standards usually are sterol-like compounds not found in the particular organism's sterol complement and/or are radioisotope or heavy isotope labeled to permit the estimation of losses during isolation and separation of the sterols. It is important to remember that this permits only an estimation of recoveries.

The greatest potential source of error in estimating the sterol content of extracts is the extraction efficiency. This problem can be approached by evaluating extraction procedures to determine best efficiency, by then repeating the extraction procedure of choice to analyze the repeatibility of its efficiency, or by using an internal standard as discussed above.

An alternate approach represents a variation of traditional pulse-chase experiments. Radiolabeled sterol precursor or sterol is introduced into the organism itself and the label followed through extraction and isolation (e.g., W. D. Nes *et al.*, 1981).

VII. CONCLUSIONS

The isolation and primary characterization of the large group of compounds known as sterols involves a series of complex experimental problems. Solutions to some of these problems (i.e., isolation, separation, and primary characterization) have been accomplished and are described in this chapter. However, despite its importance to subsequent analytical procedures and quantitative determinations, the evaluation of the efficiency of extraction in quantitative studies is relatively uncommon. Nevertheless, if careful attention is paid to extraction efficiency, total sterol content can be determined. It is this knowledge that will ultimately lead to a better understanding of the physiological role(s) of sterols.

REFERENCES

Akihisa, T., Thakur, S., Rosenstein, F. U., and Matsumoto, T. (1986). Sterols of Cucurbitaceae: The configurations at 24-alkyl Δ^5-Δ^7- and Δ^8-sterols. *Lipids* **21**, 39–47.

Bergquist, P. R., Lavis, A., and Cambie, R. C. (1986). Sterol composition and classification of the porifera. *Biochem. Syst. Ecol.* **14**, 105–112.

Bernini, F., Sangiovanni, G., Pezzotta, S., Galli, G., Fumagalli, R., and Paoletti, P. (1986). Selected ion monitoring technique for the evaluation of sterols in cerebrospinal fluid: A new approach to desmosterol test for central nervous system tumors. *J. Neuro-Oncol.* **4**, 31–35.

Bianchini, J.-P., Gaydou, E. M., Sigóillot, J.-C., and Terrom, G. (1985). Determination of sterol and triterpene alcohol acetates in natural products by reversed-phase liquid chromatography and gas chromatography-mass spectrometry. *J. Chromatogr.* **329**, 231–246.

Bligh, E. G., and Dyer, W. J. (1959). A rapid method of total lipid extraction and purification. *Can. J. Biochem. Physiol.* **37**, 911–917.

Block, K. E. (1979). Speculations on the evolution of sterol structure and function. *CRC Crit. Rev. Biochem.* **7**, 1–5.

Block, K. E. (1981). Sterol structure and membrane function. *CRC Crit. Biochem.* **14**, 47–92.

Campbell, B. C., and Nes, W. D. (1983). A reappraisal of sterol biosynthesis and metabolism in aphids. *J. Insect Physiol.* **29**, 149–156.

Chiu, P. L., Patterson, G. W., and Fenner, G. P. (1985). Sterols of Bryophytes. *Phytochemistry* **24**, 263–266.

Crist, B. V., Li, X., Bergquist, P. R., and Djerassi, C. (1983). Sterols of marine invertebrates. 44. Isolation, structure elucidation, partial synthesis, and determination of absolute configuration of pulchrasterol. The first example of double bialkylation of the sterol side chain at position 26. *J. Org. Chem.* **48**, 4472–4479.

Davis, D. L., and Poneleit, C. G. (1974). Sterol accumulation and composition in developing *Zea mays* L. Kernels. *Plant Physiol.* **54**, 794–796.

De Souza, N. J., and Nes, W. R. (1969). Improved separation of sterols by reversed phase thin-layer chromatography. *J. Lipid Res.* **10**, 240–243.

Devgun, M. S., and Paterson, C. R. (1986). Measurement of blood levels of 7 dehydrocholesterol in man by high performance liquid chromatography. *J. Chromatogr.* **353**, 169–173.

DiBussolo, J. M., and Nes, W. R. (1982). Structural elucidation of sterols by reverse phase liquid chromatography. 1. Assignments of retention coefficients to various groups. *J. Chromatogr. Sci.* **20**, 193–202.

Domnas, A. J., Warner, S. A., and Johnson, S. L. (1983). Reversed-phase thin layer chromatography of some common sterols. *Lipids* **18**, 87–89.

Ellingboe, J., Nyström, E., and Sjövall, J. (1970). Liquid–gel chromatography on lipophillic-hydrophobic sephadex derivatives. *J. Lipid Res.* **11**, 266–273.

Fieser, L. F., and Fieser, M. (1959). "Steroids." Reinhold, New York.

Folch, J., Lees, M., and Stanley, G. H. (1957). A simple method for the isolation and purification of total lipids from animal tissues. *J. Biol. Chem.* **226**, 497–509.

Fumagalli, R. (1969). Gas chromatography of cholesterol and sterol precursors. *In* "Lipid Chromatographic Analysis" (G. V. Marinetti, ed.), Vol. 2, pp. 187–213.

Garg, V. K., and Nes, W. R. (1984). Codisterol and other Δ^5-sterols in the seeds of *Cucurbita maxima*. *Phytochemistry* **23**, 2925–2929.

Garg, V. K., and Paleg, L. G. (1986). Changes in the levels and composition of sterols in different tissues of *Lolium tumulentum* plants during floral development. *Physiol. Plant.* **68**, 335–341.

Gonzales, R. A., and Parks, L. W. (1977). Acid-labilization of sterols for extraction from yeast. *Biochim. Biophys. Acta* **489**, 507–509.

Grunwald, C. (1975). Plant sterols. *Annu. Rev. Plant Physiol.* **26**, 209–236.

Ha, T. B., Kokke, W. C. M., and Djerassi, C. (1982). Minor sterols of marine invertebrates 37. Isolation of novel coprostanols and 4α-methyl sterols from the tunicate *Asidia nigra*. *Steroids* **40**, 433–453.

Hansbury, E., and Scallen, T. J. (1978). Resolution of desmosterol, cholesterol and other sterol intermediates by reversed-phase high pressure liquid chromatography. *J. Lipid Res.* **19**, 742–746.

Heftmann, E. (1967). Chromatography of steroids. *In* "Chromatography" (E. Heftmann, ed.), 2nd ed., pp. 539–572. Reinhold, New York.

Heftmann, E. (1975). Chromatography of steroids, *In* "Chromatography" (E. Heftmann, ed.), 3rd ed., pp. 611–636. Van Nostrand-Reinhold, New York.

Heftmann, E. (1976). Chromatography of steroids. *J. Chromatogr. Libr.* **8**, 1–203.

Heftmann, E., and Hunter, I. R. (1979). High pressure liquid chromatography of sterols. *J. Chromatogr.* **165**, 283–299.

Heupel, R. C. (1985). Varietal similarities and differences in the polycyclic isopentenoid composition of sorghum. *Phytochemistry* **24**, 2929–2937.

Heupel, R. C., and Nes, W. D. (1985). The biosynthesis, metabolism and translocation of β-Amyrin in *Sorghum bicolor*. *Phytochemistry* **24**, 2905–2909.

Heupel, R. C., Sauvaire, Y., Le, P. H., Parish, E. J., and Nes, W. D. (1986). Sterol composition and biosynthesis in Sorghum: Importance to developmental regulation. *Lipids* **21**, 69–75.

Hogg, R. W., and Gillan, F. T. (1984). Fatty acids, sterols and hydrocarbons in the leaves from eleven species of mangrove. *Phytochemistry* **23**, 93–97.

Holen, B. (1985). Rapid separation of free sterols by reversed-phase high performance liquid chromatography. *J. Am. Oil Chem. Soc.* **62**, 1344–1346.

Homberg, E., and Bielefeld, B. (1979). Gas chromatographische trennung unpolarer und oxidier ter sterine. *J. Chromatogr.* **180**, 83–91.

Huang, L.-S., and Grunwald, G. (1986). Comparative study of *In vivo* stigmasterol biosynthesis in *Nicotiana tabacum* and *Hordeum vulgare*. *Phytochemistry* **12**, 2779–2781.

Hunter, I. R., Walden, M. K., Bailey, G. F., and Heftmann, E. (1979). High pressure liquid chromatography and ultraviolet spectrometry of ketonic C_{27} sterols. *Lipids* **14**, 687–690.

Itoh, T., Sica, D., and Djerassi, C. (1983). Minor and trace sterols in marine invertebrates. Part 35. Isolation and structure elucidation of seventy-four sterols from the sponge *Axinella cannabina*. *J. Chem. Soc., Perkin Trans.* **1** pp. 147–153.

Kadkade, P. G., Lujan, C., and Rolz, C. (1983). Studies on the distribution of phytosterols in Dioscorea species tubers. *J. Naturforsch., C: Biosci.* **38**, 488–499.

Kesselmeier, J., Eichenberger, W., and Urban, B. (1985). High performance liquid chromatography of molecular species from free sterols and sterylglycosides isolated from oat leaves and seeds. *Plant Cell Physiol.* **26**, 463–471.

Knights, B. A. (1971). Sterols in chloroplasts: A description of two qualitatively different forms. *Lipids* **6**, 215–218.

Knights, B. A. (1982). Quantitative analysis of plant sterols. *Lipids* **17**, 204–208.

Kobayashi, M., Hasegawa, A., and Mitsuhashi, H. (1985). Marine sterols. XV. Isolation of 24-vinyl-oxycholesta-5,23-dien-3β-ol from the brown alga *Sargassum theimbergii*. *Chem. Pharm. Bull.* **33**, 4012–4013.

Kokke, W. C. M. C., Fenical, W., and Djerassi, C. (1981). Sterols with unusual nuclear unsaturation from three cultured marine dinoflagellates. *Phytochemistry* **20**, 127–134.

Kokke, W. C. M. C., Fenical, W., and Djerassi, C. (1982). Sterols of the cultured dinoflagellate *Pyrocystii lunula*. *Steroids* **40**, 307–317.

Le, P. H., and Nes, W. D. (1986). Sterols: Tritium-labeling and selective oxidations. *Chem. Phys. Lipids* **40**, 57–69.

Lutsky, B. N., Martin, J. A., and Schroepfer, G. J. (1971). Studies of the metabolism of 5α-cholesta-8,14-dien-3β-ol and 5α-cholesta-7,14-dien-3β-ol in rat liver homogenate preparation. *J. Biol. Chem.* **246**, 6737–6744.

Lutsky, B. N., Hsiung, H. M., and Schroepfer, G. J., Jr. (1975). Inhibition of enzymatic reduction of Δ^{14}-double bond of 5α-cholesta-8,14,-dien-3β-ol and 5α-cholesta-7,14-dien-3β-ol. *Lipids* **10**, 9–11.

McNamara, D. J., Bloch, C. A., Botha, A., and Mendelsohn, D. (1985). Sterol synthesis *in vitro* in freshly isolated blood mononuclear leukocyles from familial hypercholesterolemic patients treated with probucol. *Biochim. Biophys. Acta* **833**, 412–416.

McReynolds, W. O. (1970). Characterization of some lipid phases. *J. Chromatogr. Sci.* **8**, 685–691.

Matsuoka, C., Nohta, J., Kuroda, W., and Ohkura, Y. (1985). Simultaneous determination of cholestanol and cholesterol in human serum by high performance liquid chromatography with fluorescence detection. *J. Chromatogr.* **341**, 1432–1436.

Nakanishi, S., Nishino, T., Yabusaki, Y., Fujisaki, S., and Katsuki, H. (1984). Preparation of ^{14}C-labeled and unlabeled sterol intermedites from yeast using metabolic inhibitions. *J. Biochem. (Tokyo)* **96**, 1665–1672.

Nes, W. D. (1987). Biosynthesis and requirement for sterols in growth and reproduction of oomycetes. *ACS Symp. Ser.* **325**, 303–328.

Nes, W. D., and Bach, T. J. (1985). Evidence for a mevalonate shunt in a tracheophyte. *Proc. R. Soc. London, Ser. B* **225**, 425–444.

Nes, W. D., and Heftmann, E. (1981). A comparison of triterpenoids with steroids as membrane components. *J. Nat. Prod.* **44**, 377–400.

Nes, W. D., and Heupel, R. C. (1986). Physiological requirement for biosynthesis of multiple 24β-methylsterols in *Gibberella fujikuroi*. *Arch. Biochem. Biophys.* **244**, 211–217.

Nes, W. D., Saunders, G. A., and Heftmann, E. (1981). Metabolic discriminations between cholesterol and β-amyrin by *Phytophthora cactorum*. *Lipids* **16**, 744–748.

Nes, W. D., Yavin, Z., and Heftmann, E. (1982). Translocation of cholesterol from leaves to ripening fruits of *Solanum khasianum*, *Phytochemistry* **21**, 581–583.

Nes, W. D., Heupel, R. C., and Le, P. H. (1985). Biosynthesis of Ergosta-6(7),8(14),22(23)-triene-3β-ol by *Gibberella fujikuroi*: Its importance to ergosterol's metabolic pathway. *J. Chem. Soc., Chem. Commun.* pp. 1431–1433.

Nes, W. R. (1974). Roles of sterols in membranes. *Lipids* **9**, 596–612.

Nes, W. R. (1984). University vs. diversity in the structure, biosynthesis and functions of sterols. *In* "Isopentenoids in Plants: Biochemistry and Function" (W. D. Nes, G. Fuller, and L.-S. Tsai, eds.), pp. 325–347. Dekker, New York.

Nes, W. R. (1985). A comparison of methods for the identification of sterols. *In* "Methods in Enzymology" (J. H. Laio and H. C. Rilling, eds.), Vol. 111, pp. 3–37. Academic Press, New York.

Nes, W. R., and McKean, L. (1977). "Biochemistry of Steroids and Other Isopentenoids." University Park Press, Baltimore, Maryland.

Nes, W. R., Krevitz, K., and Behzadan, S. (1976). Configuration of C-24 of 24-methyl and 24-ethylcholesterol in tracheophytes. *Lipids* **11**, 118–126.

Nes, W. R., Krevitz, K., Joseph, J., Nes, W. D., Harris, B., Gibbons, G. F., and Patterson, G. W. (1977). Phytogenetic distribution of sterols in tracheophytes. *Lipids* **12**, 511–527.

Nes, W. R., Joseph, J. M., Landrey, J. R., and Connors, R. L. (1978). The steric requirements for the metabolism of sterols by *Tetrahymena pyriformis*. *J. Biol. Chem.* **253**, 2361–2367.

Nes, W. R., Joseph, J. M., Landrey, J. R., Behzada, S., and Conner, R. C. (1981). Steric effects of C-20 and C-24 on the metabolism of sterols by *Tetrahymena pyriformis*. *J. Lipid Res.* **22**, 770–777.

Nes, W. R., Dhanuka, I. C., and Pinto, W. J. (1986). Evidence for facilitated transport in the absorptions of sterols by *Saccharomyces cerevisiae*. *Lipids* **21**, 102–106.

Noshiro, M., Ishida, H., Hayashi, S.-I., and Okuda, K. (1985). Assays for cholesterol 7α-hydroxylase and 12α-hydroxylase using high performance liquid chromatography. *Steroids* **45**, 539–551.

Osagie, A. U., and Kates, M. (1984). Lipid composition of millet (*Pennisetum americanum*) seeds. *Lipids* **19**, 958–965.

Parks, L. W., Rodriguez, R. J., and Low, C. (1986). An essential fungal growth factor derived from ergosterol. A new product of sterol biosynthesis in fungi. *Lipids* **21**, 89–91.

Paterson, G. W. (1971). Relations between structure and retention time of sterols in gas chromatography. *Anal. Chem.* **43**, 1165–1170.

Paterson, G. W. (1984). Chemical and physical methods in the analysis of plant sterols. *In* "Isopentenoids in Plants: Biochemistry and Function" (W. D. Nes, G. Fuller, and L.-S. Tsai, eds.), pp. 293–323. Dekker, New York.

Poll, D., Harding, D. R. K., and Hancock, W. S. (1985). The use of reversed-phase high performance liquid chromatography to analyze the cholesterol ester profiles in lipoproteins of patients exhibiting hyperalphalipoproteinaemia or hypoalphalipoproteinaemia (Tangier disease). *J. Chromatogr.* **343**, 149–154.

Popov, S., Carlson, R. M. K., and Djerassi, C. (1983). Occurrence and seasonal variation of 19-noncholest-4-en-3-one and 3β-monohydroxysterols in the California Gorgonian, *Muricea california*. *Steroids* **41**, 537–549.

Raederstorff, D., and Rohmer, M. (1984). Sterols of the unicellular algae *Nematochrysopsis roscoffensis* and *Chrysotila lamellosa*: Isolation of (24)-24-n-propylidene cholesterol and 24-n-propylcholesterol. *Phytochemistry* **23**, 2835–2838.

Rendell, N., Misso, N. L. A., and Goad, L. J. (1986). Biosynthesis of 24-methyl-cholest-5-en-3β-ol and 24-ethylcholest-5-en-3β-ol in *Zea mays*. *Lipids* **21**, 63–68.

Ritter, K. S., Weiss, B. A., Norrbom, A. C., and Nes, W. R. (1982). Identification of $\Delta^{5,7}$-24-methylene and methylsterols in the brain and whole body of *Atta cephaloles isthmicola*. *Comp. Biochem. Physiol. B* **71B**, 345.

Sobus, M. T., and Holmlund, C. E. (1976). Extraction of Lipids from Yeast. *Lipids* **11**, 341–348.

Stafford, A. E., and Nes, W. D. (1983). Biosynthesis of long-chain fatty alcohols in *Phytophthora cactorum*. *Exp. Mycol.* **7**, 374–379.

Svoboda, J. A., Herbert, E. W., Jr., Thompson, M. J., and Feldlaufer, M. F. (1986). Selective sterol transfer in the honey bee: Its significance and relationship to other *Hymenoptera*. *Lipids* **21**, 97–101.

Thowsen, J. R., and Schroepfer, G. J., Jr. (1979). Sterol synthesis. High-pressure liquid chromatography of C27 sterol precursors of cholesterol. *J. Lipid Res.* **20**, 681–685.

Tsai, L. S., and Hudson, C. A. (1981). High performance liquid chromatography of oxygenated cholesterols and related compounds. *J. Am. Oil Chem. Soc.* 931–934.

Van Lier, J. E., and Smith, L. L. (1968). Crystalline sterols obtained by gas chromatography. *J. Chromatogr.* **36**, 7–17.

Volkman, J. K., Gagosian, R. B., and Wakeman, S. G. (1984). Free and esterified sterols of marine dinoflagellate *Gonyaulax polygramme*. *Lipids* **19**, 457–464.

Vroman, H. E., and Cohen, C. F. (1967). Separation of sterol acetates by column and thin layer argentation chromatography. *J. Lipid Res.* **8**, 150–153.

Weete, J. D., Kulifaj, M., Montant, C., Nes, W. R., and Sancholle, M. (1985). Distribution of sterols in fungi. II. Brassicasterol in Tuber and Terfesiza species. *Can J. Microbiol.* **31**, 1127–1130.

Westerman, L., and Roddick, J. G. (1981). Annual variation in sterol levels in leaves of *Taraxaccum officinale* Weber. *Plant Physiol* **68**, 872–875.

Wren, J. J. (1961). Chromatography of lipids on silicic acid. *Chromatogr. Rev.* **3**, 111–133.

Xu, S., Patterson, G. W., and Schmid, K. (1986). Sterols of amaranthaceae. *Phytochemistry* **25**, 1883–1886.

Zielinski, J., Mikova, T., Popov, S., Marekoo, N., and Djerassi, C. (1982a). Minor and trace sterols in marine invertebrates. 34. Isolation and structure elucidation of 24-methyl-5α-cholesta-7,9(11),24(28)triene-3β-ol, the first naturally occurring sterol. *Steroids* **39**, 675–678.

Zielinski, J., Kokke, W. C. M. C., Fenical W., and Djerassi, C. (1982)b). Sterols of the cultured euglenoid *Eutreptia viridis:* A novel Δ^{23}-unsaturated sterol. *Steroids* **40**, 403–411.

Ziogas, B. N., Sisler, H. D., and Lusby, W. R. (1983). Sterol content and other characteristics of pimaricin-resistant mutants of *Aspergillus nidulans*. *Pestic. Biochem. Physiol.* **20**, 320–329.

Zollo, F., Finamore, E., Gargiulo, D., Riccio, R., and Minale, L. (1986). Marine sterols. Coprostanols and 4α-methylsterols from Mediterranean tunicates. *Comp. Biochem. Physiol.* **85B**, 559–560.

2

Analysis of Steryl Esters

R. Todd Lorenz, Gregeory Fenner, and Leo W. Parks
Department of Microbiology
North Carolina State University
Raleigh, North Carolina

Kristen Haeckler
Department of Biochemistry
North Carolina State University
Raleigh, North Carolina

I. INTRODUCTION

Steryl esters frequently account for a large portion of cellular lipids. Their synthesis by acyl-coenzyme A: sterol *o*-acyltransferase or a phospholipid sterol acyltransferase represents a substantial expenditure of energy by an organism. Yet, steryl esters are generally dismissed as "storage products," and minimal attention is paid to their physiological roles. As better understanding of the functions of sterols develops, there is an increasing awareness that steryl esters represent a dynamic pool of material that is responsive to the physiological state of the cell (Taylor and Parks, 1978). In this chapter we review the extraction, isolation, separation, and analysis of steryl esters. It

Analysis of Sterols and Other Biologically Significant Steroids

is not our intent to review comprehensively the literature in this field; rather, we want to present procedures that are relevant to steryl ester analysis, which we hope will facilitate additional research in the area of steryl ester metabolism and physiology. Figure 1 outlines the procedures used by this laboratory for steryl ester analysis of *Saccharomyces cerevisae*.

Steryl esters have been reported in a variety of organisms such as plants (Bush *et al.* 1971), mammals (Glomset, 1968), and microorganisms (Elliot *et al.*, 1974) and have received a variety of different terminologies: spherosomes from peanuts (Jacks *et al.*,

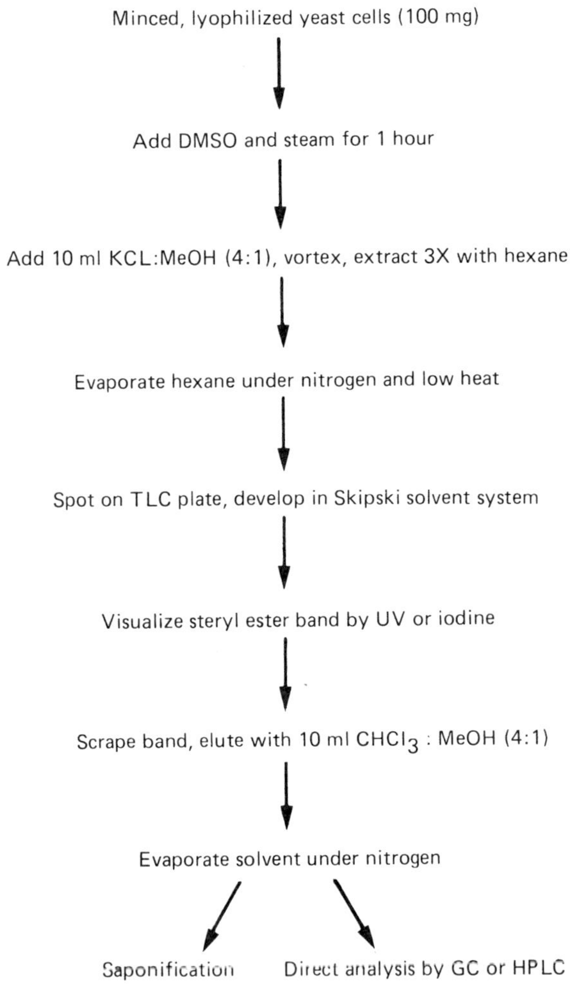

Figure 1 Schematic of the procedures used in this laboratory to extract, purify, and analyze steryl esters (see text for detail).

1967), simple lipid vesicles from bush beans (Mollenhauer and Totten, 1971; Allen *et al.*, 1971), mature oil droplets from castor beans (Harnwood *et al.*, 1971), and lipid droplets from liver (DiAugustine *et al.*, 1973) and from kidney medulla (Anggard *et al.*, 1972).

In *Saccharomyces cerevisiae,* sterols are esterified predominately to unsaturated C_{16} and C_{18} fatty acids (Madyastha and Parks, 1969), and the cellular ester content rapidly increases upon entry of the yeast culture into stationary phase. Additionally, significant changes occur in the composition of steryl esters during the growth cycle. The percentage of ergosterol precursors increases as the culture cycle progresses into stationary phase whereas the ergosterol concentration decreases relative to the total sterol pool. It has also been demonstrated that esterified sterol intermediates cannot be further converted to ergosterol until they are hydrolyzed (Bailey and Parks, 1975).

Sterol-ester synthetase (acyl-CoA: sterol *o*-acyltransferase EC 2.3.1.26) is located in the microsomal fraction of *Saccharomyces cerevisiae* (Taketani *et al.*, 1979) and has a broad range of substrate specificity for sterols and acyl-CoAs. The same type of enzyme is known to be present in liver and adrenal glands of animals as cholesterol esterase (Goodman *et al.*, 1964; Shyamala *et al.*, 1966). In yeast, steryl esters are deposited exclusively in cytosolic lipid droplets along with triacylglycerols in a nearly equivalent concentration (Clausen *et al.*, 1974).

II. EXTRACTION OF LIPID FROM SAMPLE MATERIAL

A. Homogenization

There are no published procedures for extracting steryl esters specifically, but they can be efficiently removed from a sample as part of the total lipid extract and separated by various methods. Most procedures include initial homogenization of the sample to facilitate cell breakage and increase the surface area available for solvent extraction. The extraction and recovery of the steryl esters from samples is critical because incomplete recovery leads to inaccurate quantitation, even if perfect technique is applied at later stages of the analysis.

The two basic requirements in extracting steryl esters from intact cells are (1) as efficient and complete recovery of the lipid as possible and (2) minimal degradation of the steryl ester. Thus, a balance must be achieved so that cell walls are disrupted and complexes of the steryl esters with other components are broken, without altering the association and composition of the sterol or fatty acid.

B. Folch Procedure

A simplified method of lipid extraction was proposed by Folch *et al.* (1957) that consisted of homogenizing tissue in a 2:1 chloroform methanol (v/v) mixture and washing the extract by adding 20% of the total volume of either water or salt solution. The resultant mixture separates into two distinct phases with the lower phase containing the total crude lipid extract. The washing procedure removes nearly all nonlipid contaminants with a very small loss of lipids (minimized with the use of an aqueous salt solution). The Folch procedure has been used successfully in *Candida albicans* (Ghannoum *et al.*, 1986), the flowering parts of *Narthecium ossifragum* (Holen and Stabursvik, 1986), rat liver cells (Stokke and Norum, 1970), and human tissues (Gregg *et al.*, 1986). Modifications to the Folch procedure have included lyophilization of the tissue prior to extraction to obtain dry weights in tissues of *Lolium temulentum* (Garg and Paleg, 1986), or by extraction in three successive intervals with chloroform-methanol mixtures of increasing polarity (2:1, 1:1, and 1:2, v/v) in mouse organs (Schoephoerscher *et al.*, 1985) and chicken epidermis (Wertz *et al.*, 1986). It is recommended that the ratio of solvent to tissue be at least 20:1 (v/v) for the best results. A reextraction step of the original sample is required for quantitative lipid recovery. The loss of lipid is reported to be less than 5 % if the residue is washed with extra solvent in the filtration step.

C. Bligh and Dyer Procedure

A variation of the Folch procedure published by Bligh and Dyer (1959) is another standard in lipid extraction protocol currently used. Their report emphasized the critical importance of the ratios of solvents to water and took into account the variation of water content in different tissues; they also used less solvent volume per extraction. For example, a 100-g sample (80 % water) is homogenized for 2 min with a mixture of 300 ml chloroform/methanol (1:2, v/v); then 100 ml of chloroform is added and the mixture homogenized an additional 30 sec. Distilled water (100 ml) is added, and the sample is blended for 30 sec. The resulting mixture is filtered and allowed to separate and clarify in a graduated cylinder. The volume of the chloroform layer is recorded, and the aqueous methanol layer is removed by aspiration. A second extraction can be performed by reblending the residue and the filter paper with 100 ml chloroform, refiltering, and rinsing with a total of 50 ml of chloroform. The second filtrate is mixed with the original filtrate prior to removal of the alcoholic layer. Variations of this procedure can be used, but it is critical that the volumes of chloroform, methanol, and water, before and after dilution, be kept at 1:2:0.8 and 2:2:1.8, respectively. This includes the water present in the sample, which can be compensated either by sample size or by solvent volumes to give the proper proportions. A solvent-to-sample ratio of 25:1 should facilitate nearly complete extraction of lipids in one step. The Bligh and Dyer technique has been widely successful in such systems as mangrove leaves (Ghosh *et al.*, 1985), *Dictyostelium discoideum* (MacDonald and Weeks, 1985), and hepatoma cells (Van Heusden *et al.*, 1985).

D. Yeast: A Model System

A third procedure for extracting steryl esters from *Saccharomyces cerevisiae* calls for pelleted cells to be frozen and lyophilized. This dried pellet is ground to a powder with a glass rod, and just enough dimethyl sulfoxide (DMSO) is added to the powder to saturate it. The DMSO acts as a permeabilizing agent. The sample is then steamed for 1 h and cooled before adding 10 ml *n*-hexane and vortexing the suspension for 30 sec. A 10-ml volume of 2-M KCl/methanol (4 : 1) is added and the sample vortexed for an additional 30 sec. After the suspension is centrifuged at 500 g for 3 min, the upper hexane layer is removed by pipette to a clean test tube. The mixture is reextracted two more times with 10-ml volumes of hexane in the same manner. This procedure has been compared with the previously described methods, and it was found that the DMSO-hexane extraction efficiency for sterol and steryl esters is over 95 % (unpublished data). The extraction system involving hexane and an aqueous salt phase is quicker and much easier to separate than the systems previously described.

The extraction solvent containing the lipids is typically dried by rotary evaporation under vacuum at 15°C or less or by a stream of nitrogen gas under low heat. Solvents are usually redistilled prior to use to remove impurities and peroxides that may cause auto-oxidation of double bonds in the sterol or fatty acid. The pH of the steryl ester environment should be less than 7 to avoid hydrolysis of the ester bond. The lipids are stored in the dark under freezing conditions.

III. SEPARATION OF STERYL ESTERS FROM TOTAL LIPID

A. Supports

The lipids in the extract must be separated to obtain purified steryl esters. The lipid separatory capacity of silica, either in column form or bonded to glass plates, has been used. Organic solvents, in mixtures or singly, separate the lipid classes according to the polar interactions of the lipids, solvent(s), and silica. Detection of the lipid classes and quantitation follows the separation process.

Silica has been used extensively to form the matrix for lipid separation (Hirsch and Ahrens, 1958). The use of silica appears to have become standardized over that of Factice chromatography for the separation of major lipid classes (Hirsch, 1963). Silica open-flow columns (Nicolaides and Santos, 1985) have become almost obsolete for routine determination of lipid due to the recent advances that have been made in the production of silica thin-layer chromatographic (TLC) plates. Large-scale industrial preparation of steryl esters include a silica-column chromatographic separatory step to process large volumes of lipid extract. The lipid extract is applied to the top of the silica column, and organic solvent mixtures are used to elute specific lipid classes from the column (Popov *et al.*, 1985). High- and low-pressure liquid chromatography have also been used with silica columns for resolution of lipid classes (Holen and Stabursvik, 1986). For the smaller-scale routine lipid preparations, thin-layer and preparative thin-layer plates suffice.

B. Thin-Layer Chromatography

Silica gel G or H analytical plates (20 × 20 cm, 0.25 mm thickness) are currently used for most lipid separations. Preparative plates (2 mm thickness) of the same type can be used when recovery of more than 250 μg of sample is needed. Typically, the lipid extract is dissolved in a volatile solvent such as diethyl ether or chloroform and applied in a thin line to lanes scored on the plate. It is essential that the sample be fully dissolved in the solvent when applying the sample, and repeated washings of the sample vial may be necessary.

After the sample is applied to the plate, all solvent traces are allowed to evaporate, and the plate is placed in a closed chamber that contains a saturating environment of the appropriate developing solvent(s). For a comprehensive review of lipid thin-layer separatory systems, the *Handbook of Chromatography* published by CRC Press Inc. is most helpful (Mangold, 1984). This laboratory has found the method of Skipski and Barclay to be the most practical for separating steryl esters from a crude yeast lipid extract (Skipski *et al.*, 1958). The developing uses two solvent systems: the first, consisting of isopropyl ether/acetic acid acid (96:4, v/v), is run 10 cm up the plate, followed by a drying period of 10 min. The plate is then developed to the top in the same dimension using the second solvent system of diethyl ether/hexane/acetic acid (90:10:1, v/v/v). We have found this system to be very efficient, with less than 1.5 h being required. Free sterols and steryl esters are well separated on the basis of polarity, with a 50% increase in the movement of steryl esters over free sterols. Optimal sample quantities for these plates range from 5–250 μg/lipid class, but overloading of the plates with up to 3 mg/lipid class has not affected the resolution of the steryl esters from free sterol. Preparative TLC plates can be developed in the same manner as the analytical plates, but the solvent volume and developing time must be increased. After development of the plate in the second solvent system, it is allowed to air dry, and the steryl ester band is marked by pencil.

IV. DETECTION OF STERYL ESTERS

A. Nondestructive Detection

Visual detection of bands on a thin layer plate can be done in a variety of ways. Appropriate standards are usually developed in lanes adjacent to the lipid samples and can be used to locate the band of interest. Detection can be achieved in a destructive or nondestruve manner, and this choice is dependent upon the information needed from the sample after the TLC phase. Iodine vapor and ultraviolet light are the two most common nondestructive methods.

Iodine reversibly stains organic compounds by association with π electrons and is useful because the stained bands can be marked with pencil and the plates placed in a fume hood to sublimate the iodine. Iodine may create artifacts in further analysis of unsaturated fatty acids. When more information is needed, iodine staining should be avoided (Radwan, 1984). A sealed developing chamber with a teaspoon of iodine crystals in the bottom can be used repeatedly for several months, and staining is usually complete after 1–3 min of exposure. Palumbo and Zullo (1987) have recently devised a method that uses spray reagents and iodine vapor to quantitate lipids directly. Under certain conditions, ultraviolet (UV) light can also be used to locate steryl ester bands. Conjugated double bonds absorb UV light, and steryl esters that contain this feature are made visible by this method. This method should not be used when the steryl ester components are not known.

Other nondestructive means of identification of steryl ester bands on a thin-layer plate can be achieved with the use of spray reagents. Examples are berberine, fluoresceine, and G-6 rhodamine (Vioque, 1984). Typically, these are made as an alcohol solution and sprayed on the plate. The standard lane can be used alone to identify the sample bands.

B. Destructive Detection

For qualitative research, destructive means of identification of the ester band can be done. Charring the thin-layer plate (250°C) after spraying with 50% (v/v) sulfuric acid or dichromate solution enables visualization of all organic material (Freeman and West, 1966). In some instances, steryl esters can be quantitated using a densitometric scan to relate char intensity to concentration, but the interpretation of data is sometimes limited.

C. Elution from Thin-Layer Plates

The separated steryl ester band must be eluted from the silica to characterize a composition. Two techniques have been used successfully by this laboratory. The first involves scraping the band off the glass backing onto weigh paper and transferring it to a glass tube. Five milliliters of $CHCl_3$/MeOH (4:1, v/v) is added to the tube and vortexed. The tube is centrifuged, and the solvent transferred to another tube. This is repeated three times. Since some unwanted particulate silica will be present in the solution, another step is required. A Pasteur pipette is stuffed with a small piece of cotton (hexane and acetone washed), and 3–4 cm of finely ground sodium sulfate is placed on top. The solvent fraction is eluted through the column and collected in a clean test tube. In the second technique, the steryl ester band is scraped from the TLC plate, minced with a glass rod, and transferred directly to the prepared sodium sulfate column. Ten milliliters of $CHCl_3$MeOH (4:1, v/v) is passed through the column and collected in another test tube. The purified steryl ester solution is then evaporated with nitrogen gas and low heat. The dried samples can be stored under freezing conditions in a stoppered test tube.

The most straightforward analysis of steryl esters is a direct determination of the sterol and fatty acid component of the steryl ester. Methods for this type of analysis are described later.

Indirect analysis of the steryl ester component is achieved by determining the sterol and/or fatty acid moiety of the steryl ester. The ester bond can be hydrolyzed by saponification or thin-layer enzymatic lipase digestion (Mistra *et al.*, 1984).

D. Saponification

The well-described base-catalyzed ester cleavage (saponification) is by far the most commonly used method of steryl ester cleavage (Morrison and Boyd, 1973). Various methods have been described that differ only in the concentration of reagents. For the yeast system, steryl ester saponification of TLC-purified steryl esters is performed after extraction of the esters from the silica. We have found that an efficiency of only 10–20 % is achieved if saponification is attempted directly from silica (R. Griffiths, unpublished communication). Thus, the purified steryl ester extract is suspended in a mixture of 3 ml of methanol, 2 ml of 6 % methanolic KOH, and 2 ml of 2 % methanolic pyrogallol, an antioxidant necessary for ergosterol stability. This mixture is heated under reflux at 75–80°C for 2–3 h. The nonsaponifiable lipids are then extracted from this solution with hexane or diethyl ether (Taylor and Parks, 1978).

V. ANALYSIS OF STERYL ESTERS BY GAS CHROMATOGRAPHY, HIGH-PERFORMANCE LIQUID CHROMATOGRAPHY, AND MASS SPECTROMETRY

A. Indirect Approach

1. Fatty Acids

A variety of techniques use flame-ionization detection (FID) gas chromatography (GC) for analyzing sterols and fatty acids obtained from the saponification of steryl esters. The aqueous phase, containing the fatty acid salts produced during saponification, is allowed to react with dilute HCl to render free fatty acids (Chiu *et al.*, 1985). Following their extraction from the aqueous phase, the free fatty acids are treated with a methylating agent such as boron trichloride-methanol (Chiu *et al.*, 1985; Lepage and Roy, 1984; MacCarthy and Stumpf; 1980; Tremolieres and Mazliak, 1974) to yield the fatty acid methyl esters. Experiments conducted by Lepage and Roy (1984) suggest that more accurate analyses of fatty acids are achieved by direct transesterification from the crude sample prior to extraction or purification. The methyl esters are resuspended in an appropriate solvent and are ready for GC analysis. Choices of the appropriate GC column depend upon the application, but more-polar columns such as the cyanopropyl-phenyl methyl silicones are generally thought to provide the best results (Myher *et al.*, 1974). By comparing data from unknowns with standards of known composition and quantity, very reproducible results can be obtained. In this manner the contribution of fatty acid esters to the total fatty acid composition can be determined.

2. Sterols

Free Sterols from saponification of steryl esters can be extracted by washing the saponification mixture with an organic solvent, preferably ether or hexane (Chiu *et al.*, 1985; Taylor and Parks, 1978). The successful application of gas chromatography to sterol analysis was pioneered by Beerthuis and Recourt (1960) and Clayton (1962). One of the GC methods uses glass columns packed with small, inert spherical particles coated with the stationary phase. Many phases have been developed, and depending on the application, one or more may be necessary for an analysis. Patterson (1971) performed extensive studies with various stationary phases and published data suggesting the use of cholesterol as a reference compound for the analysis of C-24 alkylated sterols. Cholesterol, unlike other previously used reference sterols such as cholestane, migrates close enough to unknowns to provide reproducible relative retention times (RRT), that is, the retention time of a sterol by a stationary phase relative to the retention time of cholesterol. This ratio is determined by dividing the retention time of the unknown by the retention time of cholesterol. Since cholesterol is seldom a major component of the sterol profile in nonmammalian systems, it can be incorporated into samples as an internal standard for accurate analyses.

Currently, most GC applications employ high-resolution capillary columns, which are usually composed of glass or fused silica, with the stationary phase coated or chemically bonded to the surface. These columns have led to increased sensitivity and greater resolution because of increased sterol-column interaction, which results in greater efficiency. With relatively simple mixtures, sterols can be chromatographed as the free alcohol. However, with complex mixtures or in the interest of improving the resolution for simple mixtures, sterols are converted to trimethylsilyl ether (TMSE) derivatives (Patterson, 1984; Thompson *et al.*, 1981). Figure 2 shows a completely resolved mixture of TMSE derivatives of C-24 alkylated sterols analyzed by capillary GC with cholesterol as an internal standard. The same mixture, chromatographed as free sterols or on a packed GC column of the same phase, resulted in partial overlap of peaks (data not shown). Recently, high-performance liquid chromatography (HPLC) has proven to be a powerful tool in sterol and fatty acid research (DiBussolo and Nes, 1982; Lin *et al.*, 1981; Rodriguez and Parks, 1982; Taylor and Parks, 1981). This

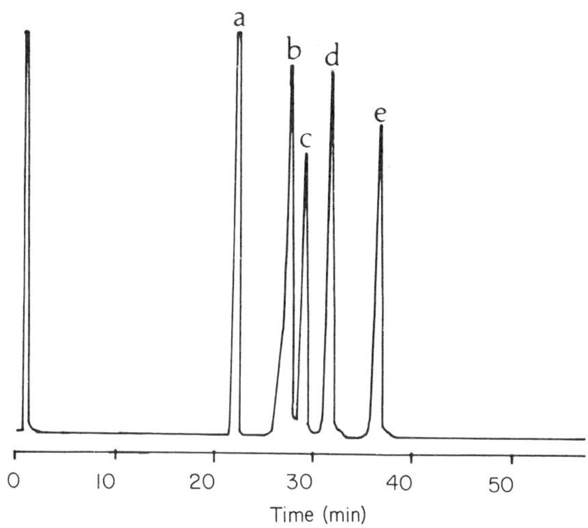

Figure 2 Separation of a mixture of C-24 alkylated sterol derivatives (TMSE) by capillary gas chromatography on a nonpolar column (SPB-1), Supelco Inc., Belfonte, Pa.) Peaks are a, cholesterol (internal standard); b, ergosterol; c, campesterol; d, stigmasterol; and e, sitosterol.

nondestructive method is advantageous because resolved mixtures can be collected after separation. Reversed-phase liquid chromatography (RPLC) employs metal columns of various dimensions that contain small spheres coated with a C_{18} hydrocarbon (commonly octadecylsilane) or hydrocarbons of other chain lengths. *Reverse phase* refers to the finding that, contrary to conventional chromatographic methods, the more-polar sterols have retention coefficients lower than nonpolar sterols and thus elute earlier (DiBussolo and Nes, 1982). Figure 3 illustrates how a mixture of sterols is resolved by RPLC. Various modifications to the ring or the side chain causes some sterols to elute "early" when cholesterol is designated as the reference compound. Detection of sterols by HPLC is usually based on UV absorption at 200–210 nm for most sterols or 282 nm for conjugated dienes such as ergosterol (DiBussolo and Nes, 1982; Patterson, 1984). The choice of solvent systems is important and can vary, but most are mixtures of methanol, acetonitrile, ethanol, and water (DiBussolo and Nes, 1982; Lin *et al.*, 1981; Rodriguez and Parks, 1982; Taylor and Parks, 1981). When RPLC analyses are performed, fatty acids are analyzed as the methyl esters whereas the sterols remain as the free alcohol form.

Various contributions to the sterol molecule, such as methyl groups, C-24 alkyl substituents, or various sites of unsaturation, can influence retention behavior. Even with some of the best systems, GC and HPLC have to be aided by other means for unequivocal identification. Electron-impact mass spectroscopy (MS) coupled to GC or HPLC is preferred by most sterol biochemists. Sterols or fatty acids subjected to ionizing voltages at 70 eV (Myher *et al.*, 1974; Knights, 1967; Wyllie and Djerassi, 1968) after separation by chromatography have led to the identification of many new compounds. Most applications employ extensive computer searches for compound identification because under similar conditions, sterols and fatty acids fragment in characteristic patterns. Fragmentation data from previously identified sterols can be used to construct an MS library for reference. When computerized searches are not possible, published data can be consulted.

B. Direct Analysis of Steryl Esters

In certain instances it can be important to determine specific kinds of steryl esters. The previous section showed how different lipid classes can be resolved by TLC. Other investigators (Hirsch, 1963; Tsai *et al.*, 1974) have used hydrophobic polymers to separate nonpolar lipids. In an attempt to circumvent many of the separation and purification steps, researchers have conducted studies that bypass traditional TLC, HPLC, or column (alumina or silica) chromatographic methods (Kaluzny *et al.*, 1985). These experiments involved an aminopropyl bonded-phase column and very strict but efficient solvent systems to elute different lipid classes. Such methods yield little information in terms of the quality of steryl esters. Likewise, saponification provides insight only on the total composition and quantity of sterols and fatty acids in the esters but not on specific pairings of sterols and fatty acids. When this information is needed, direct steryl ester analysis is preferred. The forerunners in this technology may be Kuksis and associates, who in the 1960s began experimenting with GC

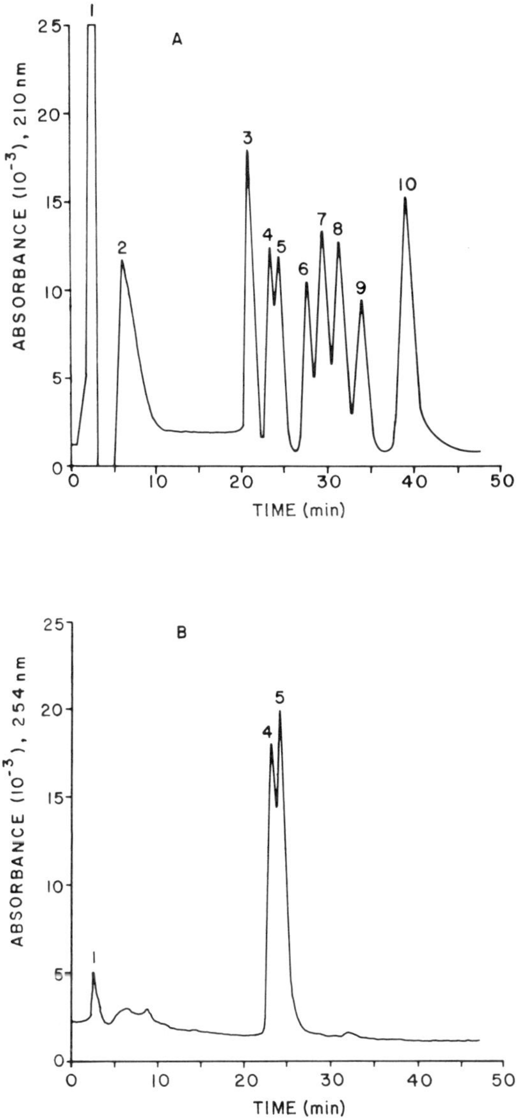

Figure 3 (a) HPLC separation of sterol standards monitered at 210 nm. Peaks 1 and 2 are solvent; 3, zymosterol; 4, ergosterol; 5, 7-dehydrocholesterol; 6, brassicasterol; 7, cholesterol; 8, lanosterol; 9, stigmasterol; and 10, sitosterol. (b) HPLC separation of the same standards monitored at 254 nm. Peak 1, solvent; 4, ergosterol; and 5, 7-dehydrocholesterol.

applications aimed at simultaneously separating different classes of nonpolar lipids and identifying members of each class (Kuksis, 1964a,b; Kuksis *et al.*, 1969). Their efforts have shown that GC methods provide data quite comparable to the Autoanalyzer methods frequently employed for lipid determination (Kuksis *et al.*, 1975, 1978). Following the advent of capillary GC systems, various kinds of steryl esters have been resolved from nonpolar lipids and from each other with some degree of success by GC (Kuksis *et al.*, 1986b; Myher and Kuksis, 1984).

An example of the application of direct steryl ester analysis is seen in the study of phytosterolemia, a rare disease in man that is characterized by an unusually high level of plant sterols. In experiments to determine steryl ester profiles associated with this disease (Kuksis *et al.*, 1986a), it was important to find out if plant sterols were esterified to a greater extent than cholesterol or if specificity existed between certain sterols and fatty acids. For a more in-depth analysis the esters were separated from the other lipids by TLC. However, in this case they were not saponified but analyzed directly on a 50% cyanopropyl-50% phenylmethyl silicone GC column, RPLC column, or by RPLC/MS. Their results showed that in addition to GC, RPLC also provided results regarding quantity and quality of intact steryl esters (Kuksis *et al.*, 1986a). Direct analyses using GC/MS have also been conducted, as shown in the study of esterified lipids from a marine organism (Cranwell *et al.*, 1985).

No reports to date were found in the literature concerning the application of the direct analytical method to steryl esters from yeast systems. However, this method could prove invaluable in gaining qualitative and quantitative data on this class of lipids. As Kuksis pointed out, the advantages are minimal if only one sterol moiety is present but are maximal in cases of mixed steryl esters (Kuksis *et al.*, 1986a). Some problems with overlap can arise when fatty acids of similar polarity exists (chain length versus unsaturation). These problems can be overcome by argentation TLC prior to GC or HPLC analysis (Kuksis *et al.*, 1986a). In the future, as column technologies are improved, argentation TLC may even become unnecessary.

ACKNOWLEDGMENTS

Research in the authors' laboratory was supported in part by grants PCM 854394 from the National Science Foundation and AM 37222 from the National Institute of Health of the U.S. Public Health Service. This is paper number 11756 of the Journal Series of the North Carolina Agricultural Research Service, Raleigh, N.C. 27695-7601.

REFERENCES

Allen, C. F., Good, P., Mollenhauer, H. H., and Totten, C. (1971). Lipid composition of bean cotyledon vesicles. *J. Cell Biol.* **48**, 542–546.

Anggard, E., Bohman, S. O., Griffin, J. E., Larsson, C., and Maunsbak, A. B. (1972). Subcellular localization of the prostaglandin system in the rabbit renal papilla. *Acta Physiol. Scand.* **84**, 231–246.

Bailey, R. B., and Parks, L. W. (1975). Yeast sterol esters and their relationship to the growth of yeast. *J. Bacteriol.* **124**, 606–612.

Beerthuis, R. K., and Recourt, J. H. (1960). Sterol analysis by gas chromatography. *Nature (London)* **186**, 372–374.

Bligh, E. G., and Dyer, W. J. (1959). A rapid method of total lipid extraction and purification. *Can. J. Biochem. Physiol.* **37**, 911–917.

Bush, P. B., Grunwald, C., and Davis, D. L. (1971). Sterol changes during germination of *Nicotiana tabacum* seeds. *Plant Physiol.* **50**, 69–72.

Chiu, P. L., Patterson, G. W., and Fenner, G. P. (1985). Sterols of bryophytes. *Phytochemistry* **24**, 263–266.

Clausen, K., Christiansen, K., Jensen, P. K., and Behnke, O. (1974). Isolation of lipid particles from bakers yeast. *FEBS Lett.* **43**, 176–179.

Clayton, R. B. (1962). Gas chromatography of sterol methyl ethers and some correlations between molecular structure and retention data. *Biochemistry* **1**, 357–366.

Cranwell, P. A., Robinson, N., and Eglinton, G. (1985). Esterfied lipids of the freshwater dinoflagellate *Peridinium lomnickii*. *Lipids* **20**, 645–651.

DiAugustine, R. P., Schaeffer, J. M., and Fouts, J. R. (1973). Hepatic lipid droplets, isolation, morphilogy and composition. *Biochem. J.* **132**, 323–327.

DiBussolo, J. M., and Nes, W. R. (1982). Structural elucidation of sterols by reversed-phase liquid chromatography. I. Assignment of retention coefficients to various groups. *J. Chromatogr. Sci.* **20**, 193–202.

Elliot, C. G., Knight, B. A., and Freeland, J. A. (1974). Sterols of *Neurospora crassa* and the pattern of their binding during the growth cycle. Biochim. Biophys. Acta **360**, 339–347.

Folch, J., Lees, M., and Sloane Stanley, G. H. (1957). A simple method for the isolation and purification of total lipides from animal tissues. *J. Biol. Chem.* **226**, 497–509.

Freeman, C. P., and West, D. (1966). Complete separation of lipid classes on a single thin-layer plate. *J. Lipid Res.* **7**, 324–329.

Garg, V. K., and Paleg, L. G. (1986). Changes in the levels and composition of sterols in different tissues of *Lolium temulentum* plants during floral development. *Physiol. Plant.* **68**, 335–341.

Ghannoum, M. A., Janini, G., Khamis, L., and Radwan, S. S. (1986). Dimorphism-associated variations in the lipid composition of *Candida albicans*. *J. Gen. Microbiol.* **132**, 2367–2375.

Ghosh, A., Mistra, S., Dutta, A. K., and Choudhury, A. (1985). Pentacyclic triterpenoids and sterols from seven species of mangrove. *Phytochemistry* **24**, 1725–1727.

Glomset, J. A. (1968). The plasma lecithin:cholesterol acyltransferase reaction. *J. Lipid Res.* **9**, 155–167.

Goodman, D. S., Dekkin, D., and Shiratori, T. (1964). The formation of cholesterol esters with rat liver enzymes. *J. Biol. Chem.* **239**, 1335–1345.

Gregg, R. E., Conner, W. E., Lin, D. S., and Brewer, H. B., Jr. (1986). Abnormal metabolism of shellfish sterols in a patient with sitosterolemia and xanthomatosis. *J. Clin. Invest.* **77**, 1864–1872.

Harnwood, J. L., Sodja, A., and Stumpf, P. K. (1971). On the origin of oil droplets in maturing castor bean seeds, *Ricinos communis*. *Lipids* **6**, 851–854.

Hirsch, J. (1963). Factice chromatography: An automatically monitored, liquid-gel system for the separation of nonpolar lipids. *J. Lipid Res.* **4**, 1–10.

Hirsch, J., and Ahrens, E., Jr. (1958). The separation of complex lipide mixtures by the use of silicic acid chromatography. *J. Biol. Chem.* **233**, 311–320.

Holen, B., and Stabursvik, A. (1986). (22*R*)-22-hydroxycholesteryl esters from *Narthecium ossifragum*. *Phytochemistry* **25**, 759-760.

Jacks, T. J., Yatsu, L. Y., and Altschul, A. M. (1967). Isolation and chracterization of peanut spherosomes. *Plant Physiol.* **42**, 585–597.

Kaluzny, M. A., Duncan, L. A., Merrit, M. V., and Epps, D. E. (1985). Rapid separation of lipid classes in high yield and purity using bonded phase columns. *J. Lipid Res.* **26**, 135–140.

Knights, B. A. (1967). Identification of plant sterols using combined GLC/Mass Spectrometry. *J. Gas Chromatogr.* **5**, 273–282.

Kuksis, A. (1964a). Gas chromatographic fractionation of natural steryl ester mixtures. *Can. J. Biochem.* **42**, 407–417.

Kuksis, A. (1964b). Direct gas chromatographic fractionation of mixed neutral lipids of natural origin. *Can. J. Biochem.* **42**, 419–430.

Kuksis, A., Stachnyk, O., and Holub, B. J. (1969). Improved quantitation of plasma lipids by direct gas-liquid chromatography. *J. Lipid Res.* **10**, 660–667.

Kuksis, A., Myher, J. J., Marai, L., and Geher, K. (1975). Determination of plasma lipid profiles by automated gas chromatography and computerized data analysis. *J. Chromatogr. Sci.* **13**, 423–430.

Kuksis, A., Myher, J. J., Geher, K., Hoffman, A. G. D., Brekenridge, W. C., Jones, G. J. L., and Little, J. A. (1978). Comparative determination of plasma cholesterol and triacylglycerol levels by automated gas-liquid chromatographic and autoanalyzer methods. *J. Chromatogr.* **146**, 393–412.

Kuksis, A., Myher, J. J., Marai, L., Little, J. A., McArthur, R. G., and Roncari, D. A. K. (1986a). Fatty acid composition of individual plasma esters in phytosterolemia and xanthomatosis. *Lipids* **21**, 371–377.

Kuksis, A., Myher, J. J., Marai, L., Little, J. A., McArthur, R. G., and Roncarni, D. A. K. (1986b). Usefulness of gas chromatographic profiles of plasma total lipid in diagnosis of phytosterolemia. *J. Chromatogr.* **381**, 1–12.

Legage, G., and Roy, C. C. (1984). Improved recovery of fatty acid through direct transesterification without prior extraction or purification. *J. Lipid Res.* **25**, 1391–1396.

Lin, J., Nes, W. D., and Heftmann, E. (1981). High performance liquid chromatography of triterpenoids. *J. Chromatogr.* **207**, 457–463.

MacCarthy, J. J., and Stumpf, P. K. (1980). Fatty-acid composition and biosynthesis in cell suspension cultures of *Glycine max* (L.) Merr., *Catharanthus roseus* G. Don and *Nicotiana tobacum* L. *Planta* **147**, 384–388.

MacDonald, J. I. S., and Weeks, G. (1985). The biosynthesis and turnover of lipid during differentiation of *Dictyostelium discodeum*. *Biochim. Biophys. Acta* **834**, 301–307.

Madyastha, P. B., and Parks, L. W. (1969). The effect of cultural conditions on the ergosterol ester components of yeast. *Biochim. Biophys. Acta* **176**, 858–862.

Mangold, H. K. (1984). Fractionation of complex lipid mixtures. *In* "CRC Handbook of Chromatography" (H. Mangold, ed.), pp. 47–55. CRC Press, Boca Raton, Florida.

Misra, S., Choudhury, A., Dutta, A. K., and Ghosh, A. (1984). Sterols and fatty acids from three species of mangrove. *Phytochemistry* **23**, 2823–2827.

Mollenhauer, H. H., and Totten, C. (1971). Isolation and structure of lipid containing vesicles. *J. Cell Biol.* **48**, 533–541.

Morrison, R. T., and Boyd, R. N. (1973). Reactions of esters. *In* "Organic Chemistry," pp. 675–680. Allyn & Bacon, Boston, Massachusetts.

Myher, J. J., and Kuksis, A. (1984). Determination of plasma total lipid profiles by capillary gas-liquid chromatography. *J. Biochem. Biophys. Methods* **10**, 13–23.

Myher, J. J., Marai, L., and Kuksis, A. (1974). Identification of fatty acids by GC-MS using polar siloxane liquid phases. *Anal. Biochem.* **62**, 188–203.

Nicolaides, N., and Santos, E. C. (1985). The di- and triesters of the lipids of steer and human meibomian glands. *Lipids* **20**, 454–467.

Palumbo, G., and Zullo, F. (1987). The use of iodine staining for the quantitative analysis of lipids separated by thin layer chromatography. *Lipids* **22**, 201–205.

Patterson, G. W. (1971). Relation between structure and retention time of sterols in gas chromatography. *Anal. Chem.* **43**, 1165–1170.

Patterson, G. W. (1984). Chemical and physical methods in the analysis of plant sterols. *In* "Isopentenoids in Plants: Biochemistry and Function" (W. D. Nes, G. Fuller, and L. Tsai, eds.), pp. 293–323. Dekker, New York.

Popov, S. S., Marekov, N. L., Konaklieva, M. I., Panayotova, M. I., and Dimitrova-Konaklieva, S. (1985). Sterols from some Black Sea ulvaceae. *Phytochemistry* **24**, 1987–1990.

Radwan, S. S. (1984). Glycerophospholipids. *In* "CRC Handbook of Chromatography" (H. Mangold, ed.), pp. 481–508. CRC Press, Boca Raton, Florida.

Rodriguez, R. J., and Parks, L. W. (1982). Application of high-performance liquid chromatographic separation of free sterols to the screening of yeast sterol mutants. *Anal. Biochem.* **119**, 200–204.

Schoephoersher, R. T., Wertz, P. W., Madison, K. C., and Downing, D. T. (1985). A survey of polar and non-polar lipids of mouse organs. *Comp. Biochem. Physiol. B* **82B**, 229–232.

Shyamala, G., Lossow, W. J., and Chaikoff, I. L. (1966). Esterification of cholesterol by rat adrenal gland homogenates and subcellular components. *Biochim. Biophys. Acta* **116**, 543–554.

Skipski, G. P., Smolowe, A. F., Sullivan, R. C., and Barclay, M. (1958). Separation of lipid classes by thin-layer chromatography. *Biochim. Biophys. Acta* **106**, 386–396.

Stokke, K. T., and Norum, K. R. (1970). Subcellular distribution of acyl-CoA:cholesterol acyltransferase in rat liver cells. *Biochim. Biophys. Acta* **210**, 202–204.

Taketani, S., Nishino, T., and Katsuki, H. (1979). Characterization of sterol-ester synthetase in *Saccharomyces cerevisiae. Biochim. Biophys. Acta* **575**, 148–155.

Taylor, F. R., and Parks, L. W. (1978). Metabolic interconversion of free sterols and steryl esters in *Saccharomyces cerevisiae. J. Bacteriol.* **136**, 531–537.

Taylor, F. R., and Parks, L. W. (1981). An assessment of the specificity of sterol uptake and esterification in *Saccharomyces cerevisiae. J. Biol. Chem.* **256**, 13048–13054.

Thompson, R. H., Jr., Patterson, G. W., Thompson, M. J., and Slover, H. T. (1981). Separation of pairs of C-24 epimeric sterols by glass capillary gas liquid chromatography. *Lipids* **16**, 694–699.

Tremolieres, A., and Mazliak,, P. (1974). Biosynthesis of α-linolenic acid in developing pea leaves. *In vivo* and *in vitro* study. *Plant Sci. Lett.* **2**, 193–201.

Tsai, L. B., Patterson, G. W., Cohen, C. F., and Klein, P. D. (1974). Metabolism of 2,4-^{3}H-14α-methyl-5α-ergost-8-enol and 2,4-^{3}H-5α-ergosta-8,14-dienol in *Chlorella ellipsoidea. Lipids* **9**, 1014–1017.

Van Heusden, G. P. H., Souren, J., Geelen, M. J. H., and Wirtz, K. A. (1985). The synthesis and esterification of cholesterol by hepatocytes and H35 hepatoma cells are independent of the level of nonspecific lipid transfer protein. *Biochim. Biophys. Acta* **846**, 21–25.

Vioque, E. (1984). Spray reagents for thin-layer chromatography (TLC) and paper chromatography (PC). *In* "CRC Handbook of Chromatography" (H. Mangold, ed.), pp. 309–317. CRC Press, Boca Raton, Florida.

Wertz, P. W., Stover, P. M., and Downing, D. T. (1986). A survey of polar and non-polar lipids from epidermis and epidermal appendages of the chicken (*Gallus domesticus*). *Comp. Biochem. Physiol. B* **84B**, 203–206.

Wyllie, S. G., and Djerassi, C. (1968). Mass spectrometry in structural and stereochemical problems. CXLVI. Mass spectrometric fragmentations typical of sterols with unsaturated side chains. *J. Org. Chem.* **33**, 305–313.

3

Analysis of Steryl Glycosides

Claus Grunwald and Li-Shar Huang*
Department of Plant Biology and
Illinois Natural History Survey
University of Illinois
Champaign, Illinois

I. INTRODUCTION

The first isolation and characterization of a steryl glycoside (SG) was by Power and Salway in 1913. Fifty years later Lepage (1964) was the first investigator to isolate the esterified (acetylated) steryl glycoside (ASG). Since these reports, SG and ASG have been isolated from many vascular plants (Aneja and Harries, 1974; Elbein and Forsee, 1975; Duperon *et al.*, 1984); indeed they probably occur in all plants. SG and ASG have also been isolated from mycoplasma (Rothblat and Smith, 1961; Smith and Mayberry, 1968), yeast (Esders and Light, 1972), fungi (McMorris and White, 1977), slime mold (Wojciechowski *et al.*, 1977), green, brown, and red algae (Duperon *et al.*, 1983), and starfish (Mackie and Turner, 1970).

Analysis of vascular plants has revealed that SG and ASG occur in all tissues, and probably all cells are able to synthesize these sterol forms (Grunwald, 1980; Mudd, 1980). At the cellular level, the largest amount of SG has been found in the microsomal fraction and the largest amount of ASG in the mitochondria.

To form the glycosides, the 3-position of the sterol moiety is linked through the C-1 hydroxyl of the carbohydrate (Fig. 1). In most cases it is a β-glycoside bond, but the α-glycoside bond has also been reported (Gupta *et al.*, 1971). So far, only the 4-demethyl sterols (sitosterol, stigmasterol, campesterol, α spinasterol, etc.) have been

* Present address: Donner Laboratory, University of California, Berkeley, CA 94720.

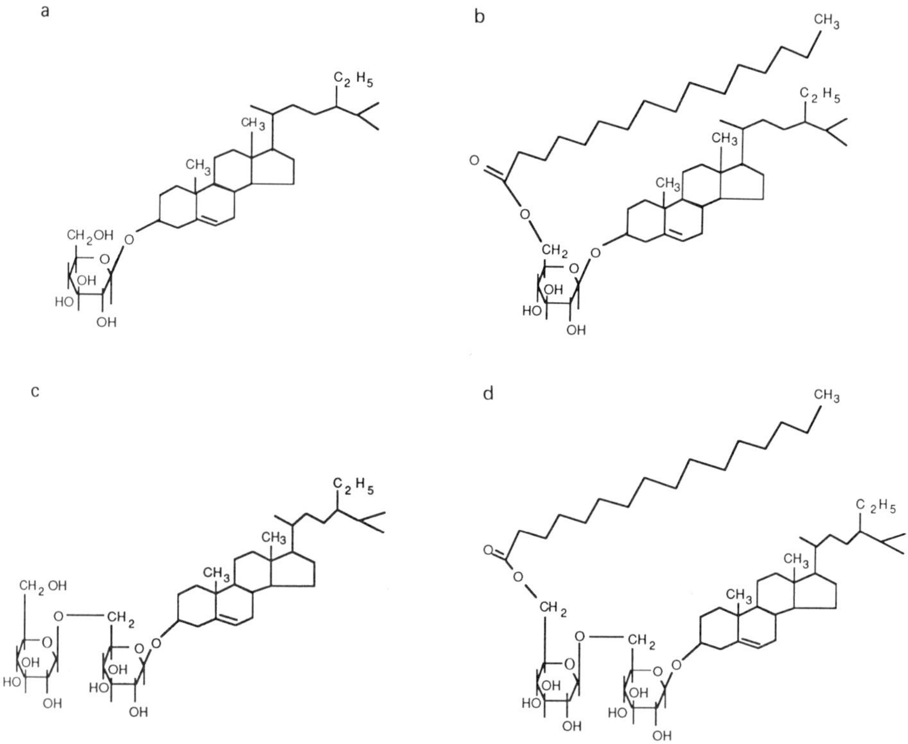

Figure 1 Plant steryl glycosides and acylsteryl glycosides:
(a) β-D-glucopyranosyl(1 → 3)sitosterol,
(b) palmitoyl-β-D-glucopyranosyl(1 → 3)sitosterol,
(c) β-D-glucopyranosyl(1 → 6)-β-D-glucopyranosyl(1 → 3)sitosterol, and
(d) 6-*O*-palmitoyl-β-D-glucopyranosyl(1 → 6)-β-D-glucopyranosyl(1 → 3)sitosterol.

found to form SG and ASG. The sugar isolated most often is glucose (Lepage, 1964; Ohnishi and Fujino, 1981); but, other monosaccharides such as galactose (Thompson *et al.*, 1970; Köstens and Willuhn, 1973), mannose (Eichenberger and Menke, 1966), and xylose have also been found (Tin-Wa *et al.*, 1971; Iribarren and Pomilio, 1984). The di- and trisaccharides are less common; however, Khanna *et al.* (1974) and Ghosal (1985) have identified β-D-glucopyranosyl(1 → 6)-β-D-glucopyranosyl sterols (gentiobiose sterols) as the SG carbohydrate in green tea (*Thea sinensis*) and banana (*Musa paradisiaca*), respectively. Fujino and Ohnishi (1979) found β-D-glucopyranosyl(1 → 4)-β-D-glucopyranosyl sterols (celloboise sterols) and β-D-glucopyranosyl(1 → 3)-β-D-glucopyranoside in rice straw (*Orya sativa*); cellobiosyl sitosterol was the major diglycosylsterol isolated from this source sterol. Other sterol disaccharides that have been characterized are α-L-rhamnopyranosyl(1 → 4) β-D-glucopyranoside, and α-L-rhamnopyranosyl(1 → 5)α-L-arabinofuranoside from the Indian annual herb *Lindenbergia indica* (Tiwari and Choudhary, 1979), and myo-inosityl(1 → 6)-β-D-glucopyranoside from banan (Ghosal, 1985). The triglycosylsterol, β-D-glucopyranosyl(1 → 4)-β-D-glucopyranosyl(1 → 4)-β-D-glucopyranosyl(1 → 3) sitosterol (cellotriosyl sitosterol) has been isolated from rice by Fugino and Ohnishi (1979) and Ohnishi and Fujino (1981), who suggested that tetra- and pentaglycosyl sterols may also exist.

In the ASG, fatty acid is attached to C-6 of the carbohydrate to form the 6-acyl-D-glycosides (Lepage, 1964; Kiribuchi *et al.*, 1966; Aneja and Harries, 1974). The fatty acids are those found as lipids in the same plant; the most common are palmitic, stearic, oleic, linoleic, and linolenic acid. Lauric, myristic, pentadecylic, palmitoleic, arachidic, gadoleic, and behenic acid are less common (Wojciechowski and Zimowski, 1975). The carbohydrates isolated most often from ASG are of the monosaccharide type, but acylated disaccharides such as 6-*O*-palmitoyl-β-D-glucopyranosyl(1 → 6)-β-D-glucopyranoside and 2-*O*-pamitoyl-myo-inosityl(1 → 6)-β-D-glucopyranoside have been reported (Ghosal, 1985).

II. EXTRACTION

For quantitative analysis, the steryl glycosides are most often extracted with (1) 2:1 (v/v) chloroform/methanol (Lepage, 1964; Duperon *et al.*, 1983); (2) hot (Soxhlet) acetone (Kiribuchi *et al.*, 1966; Grunwald, 1970); or (3) hot 80–95% aqueous ethanol (Sucrow, 1966; Tunmann and Frank, 1972). The chloroform/methanol extraction is particularly effective if small samples of tissue are to be quantitatively extracted. Hot acetone extraction has the advantage that the solvent can be easily removed under vacuum.

Basically, the weighed amount of tissue is homogenized with the desired solvent, usually 5–15 times the weight of the tissue, until a fine suspension is obtained. For hot extraction, the homogenate is transferred to a Soxhlet apparatus and continuously extracted for 15 to 20 h. The extract may need to be filtered to remove small particles before the sample is further processed. To deactivate the glycosidases, a hot solvent treatment of the tissue can precede the extraction (Lepage, 1964; Duperon *et al.*, 1984). If chloroform/methanol is the extraction solvent, hot alcohol is used for enzyme deactivation.

With choroform/methanol, if the solvent-to-tissue ratio is too small, especially with fresh tissue, two phases may be obtained; additional solvent will be required to form a single phase. A solvent-to-tissue ratio that is too high, particularly in the initial homogenizing step, can lower the water content to a point at which some of the more polar steryl glycosides (i.e., di- and triglycosylsterols) cannot be completely extracted. If dry tissue is used, tissue hydration may be required. After the suspension is filtered, the residue should be reground with the same solvent. A third extraction may be desirable, particularly if the more apolar sterols (free and esters) are also to be extracted. Tissues containing chlorophyll should be extracted until all of the pigments are removed. If the sample is to be analyzed for other lipid classes, chloroform/methanol is an excellent solvent for extracting total lipids (Folch *et al.*, 1957).

If only the glycosides are desired, the sample can be defatted before extraction. A common approach to defatting tissue is to dry the sample and extract it for 3 to 5 h in a Soxhlet apparatus with petroleum ether (Sucrow, 1966; Tunmann and Frank, 1972; Iribarren and Pomilio, 1984). If large quantities of biological materials must be extracted for qualitative work and the neutral lipids must be removed, the crude extract can be taken to dryness and defatted in a Soxhlet using petroleum ether (Ghosal, 1985).

If nonlipids (i.e., radioactive carbohydrates in biosynthetic SG studies) are to be removed, the filtered chloroform/methanol extract can be vigorously shaken with 0.2 volumes of water. Separation into two phases usually occurs within a reasonable amount of time; however, centrifugation will expedite the process and reduce the probability of contaminating the chloroform (lower) phase with aqueous microdroplets. Caution is in order because some of the highly polar steryl glycosides (e.g., triglycosylsterols) can be lost to the aqueous wash (upper) phase. Substitution of 3-mM $CaCl_2$ for water can reduce or eliminate this problem. When chloroform/methanol is used, the procedure can conveniently be carried out in solvent-resistant centrifuge tubes or bottles, thus minimizing contamination and loss of sample. If the hot acetone extraction procedure is used, the sample must be dried before the nonlipids can be removed, by partitioning the sample between chloroform and water.

To separate the SG and ASG from each other and from the free sterols (FS) and steryl esters (SE), the extract is subjected, without further purification, to thin-layer chromatography (TLC), high-performance liquid chromatography (HPLC), or column chromatography (CC). If the sample is small (25–30 mg of lipid), TLC is the preferred method; however, preparative CC has also resulted in excellent separation of the components (see below for a complete discussion). Biological tissue that is high in neutral lipid content may present a problem during sample purification by TLC or CC and may require defatting.

III. SEPARATION

Three chromatographic procedures (TLC, CC, and HPLC) have been used to separate the steryl glycosides, and each has its advantages and disadvantages. Selection of the proper procedure depends on a number of factors, but sample size and level of resolution are the most important.

A. Thin-Layer Chromatography

The method used most often to separate SG and ASG is TLC. The advantages are that it is rapid and inexpensive and gives excellent resolution of SG and ASG by number of carbohydrate units (Fujino and Ohnishi, 1979) and by degree of acylation (Eichenberger and Grob, 1969, 1970; Grunwald, 1978). The disadvantages are (1) that TLC does not enable the separation of an individual ASG or SG that differs in sterol moiety (e.g., stigmasteryl glucoside from sitosteryl glucoside) or type of saccharide (e.g., sitosteryl glucoside from sitosteryl mannoside) and (2) that recovery of the separated components is tedious and time consuming.

Table 1 R_f values of various sterol forms on silica-gel plates using various solvent systems

Sterol Form	Solvent 1[a]	2[b]	3[c]	4[d]	5[e]
Ester	—	—	0.96	0.91	—
Free	0.83	—	0.88	0.72	0.84
Glycoside					
Acylated	0.68	0.81	0.67	0.32	0.67
Nonacylated	0.43	0.55	0.47	0.14	0.46

[a] Chloroform/methanol (6:1, v/v) (Eichenberger and Grob, 1970).
[b] Chloroform/methanol/acetic acid (90:8:1, v/v) (Forsee *et al.*, 1976).
[c] Chloroform/methanol/acetic acid/water (80:15:3:2, v/v) (Hou *et al.*, 1967).
[d] Chloroform/methanol/acetic acid/water (90:8:1:1, v/v) (Grunwald, 1978).
[e] Diisobutyl ketone/acetic acid/water (80:50:10, v/v) (Lepage, 1964).

In most TLC applications, the absorbent of choice is heat-activated (80–110°C) silica gel (silicic acid), and the most often used solvent systems are various mixtures of chloroform and methanol. A 6:1 (v/v) mixture of chloroform/methanol gives good resolution of the FS, ASG, and SG; however, the SE usually move with the solvent front and are contaminated with pigments. A higher proportion of chloroform has been used, but the resolution of the various sterol components is not usually improved. Solvents of greater polarity, such as acetic acid and/or acetic acid/water mixtures (Table 1) have improved resolution. The solvent systems diisobutyl ketone/ acetic acid/water (Lepage, 1964; Grunwald, 1978) and methylene chloride/methanol/ water (85:15 80.5, v/v) have also been used successfully (Hartmann *et al.*, 1977).

Separation of ASG and SG by two-dimensional TLC has been reported. Ongun and Mudd (1970) developed activated silica-gel plates in the first direction with chloroform/methanol/7-N NH_4OH (65:30:4, v/v) and followed in the second direction with a chloroform/methanol/acetic acid/water (170:25:25:6, v/v) mixture. Eichenberger and Newman (1968) developed the plates in the first direction with chloroform/methanol/water (65:25:4, v/v) and in the second with diisobutyl ketone/ acetic acid/water (80:50:10, v/v). Both solvent systems gave excellent resolution for the SG and ASG, and the SG and ASG were free of other glycolipids.

Fujino and Ohnishi (1979) used silica-gel TLC to separate monoglycosyl-, diglycosyl-, and triglycosylsterols. The solvent was a chloroform/methanol/water (65:25:4, v/v) mixture. Eight sterol-positive components were detected; the R_f values were monoglycosylsterols 0.75, diglycosylsterols 0.57 and 0.53, and triglycosylsterols 0.29. They suggested that the four other sterol-positive spots were tetra- and pentaglycosylsterols.

Visualization of the glycosides can be either destructive or nondestructive. A destructive spray reagent, such as 20% aqueous perchloric acid or 5–50% sulfuric acid in ethanol, is acceptable if the separated glycoside components are not needed for further chemical characterization. After the chromatogram plate is sprayed with the destructive reagent, it is usually heated for 10 to 15 min at 100–150°C or until characteristic maximum color is reached. The glycosides fluoresce under long-wave UV light, and if the chromatogram is charred, black spots develop. A more specific reagent for glycosides is α-naphthol-sulfuric acid (Jacin and Mishkin, 1965). The reagent is made by dissolving 3 g of α-naphthol in 100 ml of 90% aqueous ethanol and adding 12 ml of sulfuric acid. The sprayed plate is heated at 100°C for 3 to 6 min or until reddish-brown spots appear on a white backgbround. Phospholipids, if present, are yellow. All lipids turn brown after about 2 to 3 h.

Nondestructive visualization is required if the separated components are needed for further chemical characterization. A number of sprays have been used for this purpose, and 0.01 to 0.1% of rhodamine 6G or berberine in 95% aqueous ethanol is excellent, though not specific for steryl glycosides. The chromatogram is sprayed until slightly wet and then is dried; the fluorescent spots are observed under long-wave UV radiation. Another reagent often used to visualize lipids nondestructively is iodine vapor. Crystals of iodine are placed in a closed vessel with the chromatogram, and the vapor forms brownish spots wherever lipids are present. However, iodine cannot be used with silver nitrate-impregnated plates.

If the SG and ASG are needed for further chemical characterization, the visualized zones are marked and scraped off the plate with a spatula or similar instrument and subsequently extracted with methanol. Iodine visualization has the advantage that the vapor-treated chromatogram loses its color, if not treated too long, and no interfering reagents are carried forward.

B. Column Chromatography

The preferred method for separating large amounts of lipid material is CC, particularly if sufficient quantities of ASG and/or SG are needed for further chemical analysis. The disadvantages of CC are that it is time consuming and requires relatively large volumes of solvent; however, separation of ASG and SG from each other, and from the SE and FS, is very good (Lepage, 1964; Kiribuchi *et al.*, 1966; Ongun and Mudd, 1970; Grunwald, 1971). Two types of adsorbents, silica gel and Florisil, have been used. Silica gel is a hydrated silica, $SiO_2 \cdot X\,H_2O$, with a large number of hydroxyl groups. It is a polar acidic adsorbent that preferentially adsorbs basic lipids. Florisil (magnesium silicate) is a coprecipitated mixture of silicic acid and magnesia. Because of the chemical nature of Florisil, highly polar solvents may result in column "bleeding."

1. Silica-Gel Column Chromatography

Ever since Lepage (1964) used silica-gel CC to isolate and purify ASG, a number of laboratories (Ongun and Mudd, 1970; Grunwald, 1971; Izzo and Navari-Izzo, 1981) have employed this procedure with excellent success. Several solvent systems have been used, generally in a stepwise gradient, to separate the glycosides from each other as well as from the FS and SE.

Lepage (1964) used a 5.5-cm i.d. column filled to a height of 14 cm with 100 mesh silica gel. The adsorbent is best packed as a slurry, which gives more even packing and results in a more consistent solvent flow. The following stepwise gradient was used: 500 ml *n*-hexane to recover the SE contaminated with pigments, followed by 1000 ml of 1:1 (v/v) *n*-hexane in diethyl ether to elute the FS. The hexane-ether fraction also contained the triglycerides and free fatty acids. The ASG were eluted next with 500 ml of 3:7 (v/v) *n*-hexane/ether, followed with 500 ml chloroform (discard) and 500 ml of chloroform/methanol. The chloroform/methanol fraction contained the SG as well as other glyco- and phospholipids. A 19:1 (v/v) chloroform/methanol eluent is of sufficient polarity to remove the SG (Ongun and Mudd, 1970; Grunwald, 1971) and leave most of the phospholipids behind (Newman *et al.*, 1961).

More recently, a second solvent system has been developed for stepwise elution of sterols from silica-gel columns (Grunwald, 1971). The column (1.5 cm i.d.) was packed with 30 g of heat-activated (20 h at 100°C) silica gel (70–325 mesh) in an *n*-hexane slurry. The lipid sample was applied as a suspension in *n*-hexane and washed into the column with 150 ml of 10% benzene in *n*-hexane (discarded). The SE were eluted with 700 ml of 40% benzene in *n*-hexane, the FS next with 150 ml benzene followed by 800 ml of chloroform, the ASG with 700 ml of 2% methanol in chloroform, and the SG with 600 ml of 5% methanol in chloroform.

With large lipid samples, especially those that are high in neutral lipids, poor solvent flow may occur. To overcome the problem, the sample can be dried under vacuum in the presence of 5 g of adsorbent and placed on a 25-g silica-gel column. This approach usually improves the flow rate without affecting component resolution.

2. Florisil Column Chromatography

Kiribuchi *et al.* (1966) reported the complete separation of ASG from SG with a 1.0-cm i.d. column packed with 12 g of Florisil. To elute the SE and FS, a linear gradient of diethyl ether from 0 to 50% in *n*-hexane was used, for a total volume of 304 ml. Collected were 8-ml fractions, and the SE (fractions 5 through 9) and the FS (fractions 11 through 20) were completely separated. However, since the esters were eluted within the first ten fractions, they were contaminated with pigments. A 20-g Florisil column decreases pigment contamination. The ASG and SG were eluted with a linear gradient of methanol from 0–30% in diethyl ether, for a total volume of 480 ml. The ASG were eluted in fractions 50 to 60, and the SG in fractions 65 to 88. Recovery of SG was 95–105%; however, the peak was quite broad with a long trailing portion. The trailing effect is characteristic for fully activated Florisil because adsorption chromatography dominates. Deactivating Florisil with water reduces trailing but causes phospholipid contamination. One difficulty with Florisil is that even trace amounts of water in the adsorbent or solvent result in the elution of phosphatides along with the glycolipids; the more water present, the more phospholipids elute. Elimination of water during sample preparation can be difficult, particularly if the lipid sample to be separated is large and hard to dry completely. Complete retention of phosphatides is possible with very dry Florisil (heat activated) and dry solvents, which can be obtained by adding 2,2-dimethoxypropane.

If preliminary fractionation is required to reduce the phospholipid content, very good results can be obtained with a Florisil (10–30 g). The lipid fraction is loaded in *n*-hexane, and the sterols are eluted with 30% methanol in diethyl ether. The exact volume of solvent needed to elute the glycosides depends to some degree upon the column diameter, but a good working approximation is 25 ml of solvent per gram of Florisil.

C. High-Performance Liquid Chromatography

HPLC has a number of advantages over the other methods of chromatography. Like TLC and CC, HPLC is nondestructive. The advantage of HPLC is that separation is very rapid; unlike CC, HPLC does not require large volumes of eluent. The most important advantage of HPLC, however, is that one can separate the various glycoside species (Kesselmeier *et al.*, 1985). HPLC finds an important application in the separation of labile steryl glycoside-species such as Δ^7- and Δ^5-avenasteryl glycosides. ASG, however, are not as readily separated because of their fatty acid moiety, which influences adsorption kinetics.

Separation of SG from free sterol is accomplished with a reversed-phase (RP) HPLC system, in which the solvent is 4% aqueous methanol. Unfortunately, the SG elutes as a "bulk" fraction, $\alpha_c \sim 0.5$, so that the individual steryl glycosides are not resolved (Nes *et al.*, 1982). However, separation of the sterols derivatized with sugar has recently been accomplished on a reversed-phase column (Spherisorb Hexyl, 5 μm, 125 × 4.6 mm, Bischoff, FRG) using a 30-min gradient elution from 50–100% acetonitrile in water at a flow rate of 1 ml/min (Kesselmeier *et al.*, 1985). Detection was by UV at 200 nm. The elution sequence of the SG species followed exactly that of the FS (cholesterol and Δ^7-avenasterol, Δ^5-avenasterol, campesterol, stigmasterol and Δ^7-stigmastenol, and sitosterol), thus showing that the carbohydrate residue had no effect on separation except for elution velocity.

D. Gas–Liquid Chromatography

Gas–liquid chromatography (GLC) is not generally used in the analysis of glycosterols because retention times are quite long, up to 50 min with a 3% SE-30 column at a carrier-gas flow rate of 60 ml/min and a temperature of 265°C (Elbein and Forsee, 1975). However, GLC is an excellent approach if it is used in conjunction with mass spectrometry (MS). Laine and Elbein (1971) and Elbein and Forsee (1975) subjected the purified glycosterol fraction, as the trimethylsilyl derivative, to GLC/MS using a column containing 1% SE-30 on Chromosorb W and a column temperature of 220–280°C with excellent success.

GLC is the method most often used to analyze SG and ASG for sterol moieties. This analysis requires hydrolysis of the glycosides and is usually accomplished by refluxing the sample for 18 to 22 h in 95% ethanol or methanol containing 0.5% H_2SO_4. Stronger acidic conditions have also been used, such as boiling the sample for 3 h in 10% H_2SO_4 (80% methanol) or in 6% HCl (50% methanol) for 2 h. Hydrolysis with strong acids can, however, cause a significant loss of sterols, as has been shown for the Δ^7- and Δ^5-avenasteryl glycosides (Kesselmeier *et al.*, 1985). The liberated sterols can be extracted from the alcohol phase after neutralization, with either *n*-hexane or petroleum ether. For the analysis of sterols, see the chapter by W. R. Nes.

IV. MASS SPECTROMETRY

The SG, as trimethylsilyl ethers, have been subjected to mass spectrometry (MS) (Laine and Elbein, 1971; Elbein and Forsee, 1975; Fujino and Ohnishi, 1979). The trimethylsilyl ether can be formed with either bis(trimethylsilyl)trifluoroacetamide at 110°C for 60 min (Elbein and Forsee, 1975) or with trimethylsilylimidazole at 60°C for 30 min (Fujino and Ohnishi, 1979). Although the mass spectra showed no ions that suggested the molecular weight, characteristic ion patterns were observed. Although ion M-15 was not clear in the spectra, ion M-90-15 (sterol-trimethylsilanol-CH_3) and M-90-90-15 were observed. For example, ions at *m/z* 757 and 667 were observed for stigmasteryl glucoside. Cleavage of the sterol-3-(C-O) bond with charge retention on the steroid produced an ion corresponding to the sterol in question; with stigmasteryl glucoside this ion had a *m/z* value of 395. Charge retention on the sugar portion (tetratrimethylsilyl) and cleavage of the sugar C-O-glycoside gave characteristic ions of hexose at *m/z* 451, 361, 217, 204, and 147. The *m/z* 204 ion was very prominent and is an indication of the hexose pyranoside configuration. The sterol moieties of the glycosides campesterol, stigmasterol, and sitosterol show ions at 383, 395, and 397, respectively.

The oligoglycosylsterols gave similar mass spectra below *m/z* 500, as did the monoglycosylsterols (Fujino and Ohnishi, 1979). All spectra exhibited ions due to the carbohydrate chain (e.g., for hexoses at *m/z* 451, 361, 217, 204 and 147). The spectra also showed ions for the sterol-3-(C-O) cleavage at *m/z* 383, 395, and 397, respectively, for campesterol, stigmasterol, and sitosterol. Ions of M-105 and M-90-105 for diglycosylsterols at *m/z* 1137 and 1047 and for monoglycosylsterols at *m/z* 759 and 669 can be used to conjecture molecular weights.

Heinz *et al.* (1975) examined the ASG (hydrogenated before acylation) and found that the spectra exhibited molecular ions, for example, for 2,3,4-tri-*O*-acetyl-6-*O*-palmitoyl-*β*-D-glucopyranosyl sitosterol at *m/z* 940. They reported that fragments characteristic of the carbohydrate, acylated carbohydrate, and sterol moieties were evident.

V. BIOSYNTHESIS

A. Steryl Glycoside Synthesis

Meystre and Miescher (1944) described a simple method to synthesize a number of steroid glycosides. In general, the same procedure can be used to produce any desired SG. A 43% yield was reported in the synthesis of cholesteryl glucoside, and it can be anticipated that the use of any other sterol and carbohydrate would result in similar yields. The most important aspect of this procedure is that only dry solvents can be used because even small amounts of water can reduce yield significantly.

Meystre and Miescher (1944) dissolved 5 g of silver nitrate and 6 g of sterol in 200 ml of dry benzene, brought the mixture to a boil, and under continuous stirring added, drop by drop, 13.3 g of acetobrome-D-sugar dissolved in 300 ml dry benzene to form the tetraacetate steryl glycosides. The reaction mixture was extensively washed with water to remove the silver salts. The benzene fraction was filtered and reduced to dryness under vacuum. The tetraacetate glycoside residue was dissolved in 200 ml of methanol and placed in an ice bath; sodium methanolate (about 1.2 volume) was added until the solution became clearly alkaline. The mixture was allowed to stand for 3 h at 20°C, during which time the SG precipitated spontaneously. The mixture was neutralized with either acetic acid or dilute HCl, and the precipitated SG were collected by filtration, washed with alcohol and ether, boiled in water, cooled and filtered, and again washed with water. The residue was dissolved in hot pyridine and filtered; water was added until a precipitate formed. The collected SG were washed with alcohol and ether. The SG can be further purified by CC (Grunwald, 1971). Kiribuchi *et al.* (1967) described a modified procedure; however, the yield was somewhat less.

B. Acylsteryl Glycoside Synthesis

The ASG can be synthesized according to the method of Kiribuchi *et al.* (1967). To produce 6-*O*-palmitoyl-β-D-glucosyl sitosterol, they dissolved 826 mg of sitosteryl glycoside in dry pyridine and added, drop by drop, 400 mg of palmitoyl chloride dissolved in 5 ml of dry benzene. The mixture was allowed to stand for 3 h at room temperature, acidified with dilute H_2SO_4, and extracted with chloroform. The chloroform fraction was washed with water and dried *in vacuo*. The residue is a mixture of mono-, di-, and tetrapalmitoyl steryl glycoside. The ASG can be separated either by alumina CC or by silica-gel TLC. The TLC R_f values with chloroform/methanol/acidic acid/water (90:8:1:1, v/v) as eluent were 0.16, 0.79, and 0.93, respectively, for the mono-, di-, and tetrapalmitate steryl glucoside. With the same solvent system, SG had an R_f value of 0.10.

REFERENCES

Aneja, R., and Harries, P. C. (1974). Sitosteryl-β-D-(6-*O*-fatty acyl)-glucopyranosides from the crude phosphatides of maize. *Chem. Phys. Lipids* **12**, 351–362.

Duperon, R., Thiersault, M., and Duperon, P. (1983). Occurrence of steryl glycosides and acylated steryl glycosides in some marine algae. *Phytochemistry* **22**, 535–538.

Duperon, R., Thiersault, M., and Duperon, P. (1984). High level of glycosylated sterols in species of *Solanum* and sterol changes during the development of the tomato. *Phytochemistry* **23**, 743-746.

Eichenberger, W., and Grob, E. C. (1969). Enzymatic formation of steryl glycosides by homogenates and chloroplast preparations from lettuce and spinach leaves. *Prog. Photosynth. Res.* **1**, 338–344.

Eichenberger, W., and Grob, E. C. (1970). Über die quantitative Bestimmung von Sterinderivaten in Pflanzen und die intrazellulare Verteilung der Steringlycoside in Blättern. *FEBS Lett.* **11**, 177–180.

Eichenberger, W., and Menke, W. (1966). Sterole in Blättern und Chloroplasten. *Z. Naturforsch., B: Anorg Chem., Org. Chem., Biochem., Biophys., Biol.* **21B**, 859–867.

Eichenberger, W., and Newman, D. W. (1968). Hexose transfer from UDP-hexose in the formation of steryl glycoside and esterified steryl glycoside in leaves. *Biochem. Biophys. Res. Commun.* **32**, 366–374.

Elbein, A. D., and Forsee, W. T. (1975). Biosynthesis and structure of glycosyl diglycerides, steryl glucosides, and acylated steryl glucosides. *Lipids* **10**, 427–436.

Esders, T. W., and Light, R. J. (1972). Occurrence of a uridine diphosphate glucose:sterol glucosyltransferase in *Candida bogoriensis. J. Biol. Chem.* **247**, 7494–7497.

Folch, J., Lees, M., and Sloane-Stanley, G. H. (1957). A simple method for the isolation and purification of total lipids from animal tissues. *J. Biol. Chem.* **226**, 497–509.

Forsee, W. T., Valkovich, G., and Elbein, A. D. (1976). Acylation of steryl glucosides by phospholipids. *Arch. Biochem. Biophys.* **172**, 410–418.

Fujino, Y., and Ohnishi, M. (1979). Isolation and structure of diglycosylsterols and triglycosylsterols. *Biochim. Biophys. Acta* **574**, 94–102.

Ghosal, S. (1985). Steryl glycosides and acyl steryl glycosides from *Musa paradisiaca. Phytochemistry* **24**, 1807–1810.

Grunwald, C. (1970). Sterol distribution in intracellular organelles isolated from tobacco leaves. *Plant Physiol.* **45**, 663–666.

Grunwald, C. (1971). Effects of free sterols, steryl ester, and steryl glycoside on membrane permeability. *Plant Physiol.* **48**, 653–655.

Grunwald, C. (1978). Steryl glycoside biosynthesis. *Lipids* **13**, 697–703.

Grunwald, C. (1980). Steroids. *Encycl. Plant Physiol.*, new. ser. **8**, 221–256.

Gupta, O. C. D., Rizvi, S. A. I., and Gupta, P. C. (1971). Chemical examination of a phytosterolin from the seeds of *Ipomoea fistulosa. Planta Med.* **20**, 172–177.

Hartmann, M. A., Fonteneau, P., and Benveniste, P. (1977). Subcellular localization of sterol synthesizing enzymes in maize coleoptile. *Plant Sci. Lett.* **8**, 45–51.

Heinz, E., Dieler, H. P., and Rullkotter, J. (1975). Enzymatic acylation of steryl glycoside. *Z. Pflanzenphysiol.* **75**, 78–87.

Hou, C. T., Umemura, Y., Nakamura, M., and Funahashi, S. (1967). Enzymatic synthesis of steryl glucoside by a particulate preparation from immature soybean seeds. *J. Biochem. (Tokyo)* **62**, 389–391.

Iribarren, A. M., and Pomilio, A. P. (1984). Sitosterol 3-*O*-β-D-xylopyranoside from *Bauhinia candicans. Phytochemistry* **23**, 2087–2088.

Izzo, R., and Navari-Izzo, F. (1981). Sterol composition and accumulation in *Glycine max* (L.) Merr. leaves under different filtered sunlight conditions. *Plant Physiol.* **67**, 1073–1077.

Jacin, H., and Mishkin, A. R. (1965). Separation of carbolydrates on borate-impregnated silica gel plates. *J. Chromatogr.* **18**, 170–173.

Kesselmeier, J., Eichenberger, W., and Urban, B. (1985). High performance liquid chromatography of molecular species from free sterols and sterylglycosides isolated from oat leaves and seeds. *Plant Cell Physiol.* **26**, 463–471.

Khanna, I., Seshadri, R., and Seshadri, T. R. (1974). Sterol and lipid components of green *Thea sinensis. Phytochemistry* **13**, 199–202.

Kiribuchi, T., Mizunaga, T., and Funahashi, S. (1966). Separation of soybean sterols by florisil chromatography and characterization of acylated steryl glucoside. *Agric. Biol. Chem.* **30**, 770–778.

Kiribuchi, T., Yasimatsu, N., and Funahashi, S. (1967). Synthesis of 6-*O*-palmitoyl-β-D-glucosyl-β-sitosterol. *Agric. Biol. Chem.* **31**, 1244–1246.

Köstens, J., and Willuhn, G. (1973). Steringlyoside und Acyl-Steringlycoside in Blätten on *Solanum dulcamara. Planta Med.* **24**, 278–285.

Laine, R. A., and Elbein, A. D. (1971). Steryl glucosides in *Phaseolus aureus.* Use of gas-liquid chromatography and mass spectrometry for structural identification. *Biochemistry* **10**, 2547–2553.

Lepage, M. (1964). Isolation and characterization of an esterified form of steryl glucoside. *J. Lipid Res.* **5**, 587–592.

Mackie, A. M., and Turner, A. B. (1970). Partial characterization of a biologically active steroid glycoside isolated from the starfish *Marthasterias glacialis. Biochem. J.* **117**, 543–550.

McMorris, T. C., and White, R. H. (1977). Cholesterol β-D-glucoside-6′-*O*-palmitate, a metabolite of *Pythium sylvaticum. Biochim. Biophys. Acta* **486**, 308–312.

Meystre, C., and Miescher, K. (1944). Über Steroide. Zur Darstellung von Saccharidderivaten der Steroide. *Helv. Chim. Acta* **27**, 231–236.

Mudd, J. B. (1980). Sterol interconversions. *In* "The Biochemistry of Plants: A Comprehensive Treatise" (P. K. Stumpf, ed.), Vol. 4, pp. 509–534. Academic Press, New York.

Nes, W. D., Yoniv, Z., and Heftmann, E. (1982). Translocation of cholesterol from leaves to ripening fruits of *Solanum Khasianum. Phytochemistry* **21**, 581–583.

Newman, H. A. I., Liu, C.-T., and Zilversmit, D. B. (1961). Evidence for the physiological occurrence of lysolecithin in rat plasma. *J. Lipid Res.* **2**, 403–411.

Ohnishi, M., and Fujino, Y. (1981). Mono- and triglycosylsterols from the leafy stem of rice. *Phytochemistry* **20**, 1357–1358.

Ongun, A., and Mudd, J. B. (1970). The biosynthesis of steryl glucosides in plants. *Plant Physiol.* **45**, 255–262.

Power, F. B., and Salway, A. H. (1913). The identification of ipuranol and some allied compounds as phytosterol glucosides. *J. Chem. Soc.* **159**, 399–406.

Rothblat, G. H., and Smith, P. F. (1961). Nonsaponifiable lipids of representative pleuropneumonia-like organisms. *J. Bacteriol.* **82**, 479–491.

Smith, P. F., and Mayberry, W. R. (1968). Identification of the major glycolipids from *Mycoplasma* sp. strain J as 3,4,6-triacyl-β-glucopyranose. *Biochemistry* **7**, 2706–2710.

Sucrow, W. (1966). $^{\Delta 5,25}$Stigmastadienol-(3β) und sein β-D-Glucosid. *Chem. Ber.* **99**, 2765–2777.

Thompson, C., Henson, R. C., Gueldner, R. C., and Hedin, P. A. (1970). Sterol galactosides and sterol esters of the cotton bud. *Lipids* **5**, 283–284.

Tin-Wa, M., Farnsworth, N. R., Fon, H. H. S., Blomster, R. J., Trojanek, J., Abraham, D. J., Peersinos, D. J., and Dokosi, O. B. (1971). Biological and phytochemical evaluation of plants. IX. Antitumor activity of *Maytenus senegalensis* (Celastraceae) and a preliminary phytochemical investigation. *Lloydia* **34**, 79–87.

Tiwari, K. P., and Choudhary, R. N. (1979). Two new steryl glycosides from *Lindenbergia indica. Phytochemistry* **18**, 2044–2045.

Tunmann, P., and Frank, W. (1972). Steringlucosidfettsäureester in der Frucht von *Cucumis sativus* L. *Arch. Pharm. (Weinheim, Ger.)* **305**, 469–471.

Wojciechowski, Z. A., and Zimowski, J. (1975). Acyl composition and biosynthesis of acylated steryl glucosides in *Calendula officinalis. Biochim. Biophys. Acta* **398**, 111–117.

Wojciechowski, Z. A., Zimowski, J., and Tyski, S. (1977). Enzymatic synthesis of steryl 3β-D-monoglucosides in the slime mold *Physarum polycephalum. Phytochemistry* **16**, 911–914.

4

Analysis of Brassinosteroids, Antheridiol, and Oogoniols

Trevor C. McMorris
Department of Chemistry
University of California, San Diego
La Jolla, California

I. INTRODUCTION

The steroids treated in this chapter were discovered as a result of intensive efforts to identify the substances responsible for specific biological effects, sexual reproduction or cell elongation and division, in certain fungi and plants. As is the case with other hormones, pheromones, and growth factors, these steroids occur in minute amounts in the organisms, and their isolation depended on the use of sensitive bioassays. After the pure compounds were available and their spectral and chemical properties determined, methods for analysis could be developed that are more precise and as sensitive in some instances as the bioassays.

We shall discuss the biological and chemical properties and the analysis of brassinolide, the plant-growth hormone first isolated from the rape plant *Brassica napus*, as well as other brassinosteroids. This will be followed by a similar treatment of antheridiol, the male-activating hormone, and of oogoniols, female-activating hormones, of the water mold *Achlya*. These hormones have been known longer than brassinolide, and their specific functions in the organism are much better defined.

II. BRASSINOLIDE

Determination of the structure of brassinolide, first reported in 1979, was the result of many years of effort by John W. Mitchell and other scientists at the USDA laboratories in Beltsville, Philadelphia, and Peoria to identify the substance in pollen of the rape plant *Brassica napus* responsible for abnormal growth of the pinto bean plant (Grove *et al.*, 1979). They employed the so-called bean second-internode assay, which had been developed for detecting gibberellins. At a concentration of 0.1 μg per plant, brassinolide causes the unique effect of splitting of the bean stem above the second pair of leaves.

Workers at Nagoya University in Japan reported in 1968 the presence of substances in leaves of *Distylium racemosum* that were active in the rice lamina-inclination assay (Marumo *et al.*, 1968). This assay developed by Maeda is specific for brassinolide, which is active at a concentration of 5×10^{-3} μg/ml, and other closely related steriods (brassinosteroids). Indole acetic acid (IAA) and gibberellin are almost completely inactive. By means of the assay, brassinosteroids have been detected in a wide variety of plants and are now well established as a new class of plant hormones.

A. Isolation and Structure of Brassinosteroids

Brassinolide was isolated from rape pollen, in which it is estimated to be present in the very low concentration of 100 μg per kg of pollen. Pollen was studied because it is involved in sexual reproduction and might, it was felt, contain substances affecting plant development. Two batches of pollen (2 × 250 lb) were extracted with isopropanol. The extract was partitioned between carbon tetrachloride-methanol-water, and the aqueous methanol fraction was chromatographed repeatedly on silica gel, first with chloroform-methanol 9:1 and then with toluene-absolute ethanol 9:1 as eluant. This was followed by high-performance liquid chromatography (HPLC) on a μ-Bondapak C-18 column (methanol:water 65:35 eluant). The bean second-internode assay was used to guide the fractionation. In this way, pure brassinolide was obtained which, after recrystallization from methanol, weighed 10 mg and melted at 274°–275°C. The stucture was determined by X-ray analysis as (22R,23R,24S)-2α,3α,22,23-tetrahydroxy-24-methyl-B-homo-7-oxa-5α-cholestan-6-one, and the structure of the hormone has been confirmed by synthesis by several groups.

An intermediate in the synthesis (22R,23R,24S)-2α,3α,22,23-tetrahydroxy-24-methyl-5α-cholestan-6-one (castasterone) with a ketone rather than lactone in ring B has been isolated from chestnut insect gall by similar chromatographic procedures including HPLC (Yokota *et al.*, 1982a; Arima *et al.*, 1984). The isolation was guided by the lamina-inclination test. At the present time, more than a dozen analogs of brassinolide have been identified from a variety of sources including rice, tea, Chinese cabbage, and beans, as well as *Pinus thunbergi* and *Pica sitchensis.* They are listed in Fig. 1. An important point is that the Brassinosteroids were found in young, actively growing and differentiating plant tissues, and it is such tissues that respond best to the application of brassinolide and related steroids.

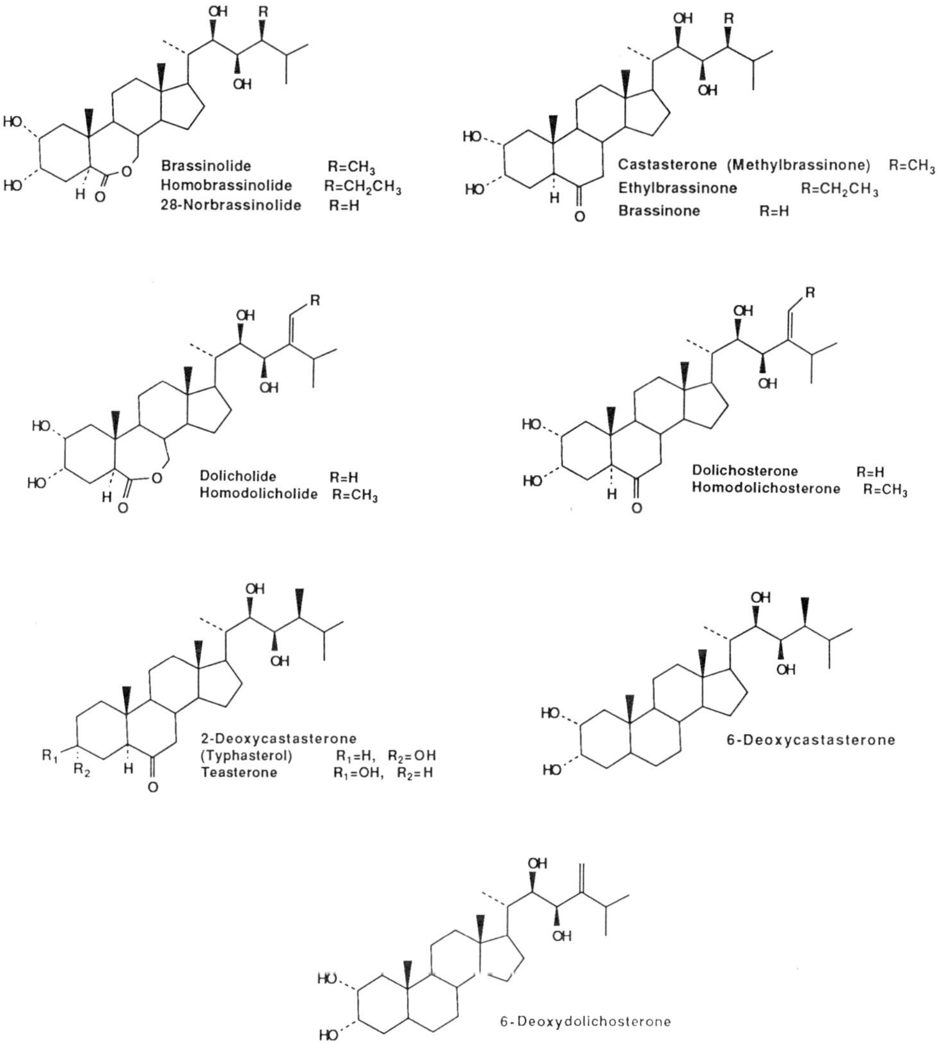

Figure 1 Structures of natural brassinosteroids.

All naturally occurring brassinosteroids possess carbon skeletons that are derived from or are identical to those of common plant sterols: cholesterol, 24-methylene cholesterol, campesterol, sitosterol, and 28-isofucosterol. It is possible that these sterols are intermediates in the biosynthesis of the various brassinosteroids, which are formed by hydroxylation and further oxidative reactions. This would be analogous to the biosynthesis of other steroid hormones [see, for example, biosynthetic studies of ecdysteroids (Rees *et al.*, 1981) and of antheridiol and oogoniol (Section II.B)]. The immediate precursor of the dihydroxy side chain might perhaps be naturally occurring

Δ^{22}-unsaturated sterols such as stigmasterol and 22-dehydrocampesterol. However, no biosynthetic studies on brassinolide havebeen reported, and the above proposals are only speculative.

B. Bioassay for Brassinolide

Although the mechanism of action of brassinolide in plant development has not been established, a number of assays indicate that brassinolide is involved in cell elongation and cell division and that it is active in bioassays that have been developed for other plant hormones: gibberellins, auxins, and cytokinins.

In the bean second-internode bioassay (Thompson *et al.*, 1981), plants were grown at 25°–27°C with light 7.5 kilolux in 12-h periods. The test compound was dispersed in lanolin, and the mixture (250 μg) was applied to the second internode of each 6-day-old bean seedling (*Phaseolus vulgaris* L., pinto variety). The internode was no more than 2-mm-long to ensure the optimum effect. Control plants were treated with lanolin only. After four days the increase in internode length of the treated plants compared with the controls was recorded. Test plants showed not only elongation but also curvature, swelling, and splitting of the internodes, depending on the amount of brassinolide. Both natural and synthetic brassinolide gave elongation with curvature and swelling at 0.01 μg and splitting of the internodes at 0.1 μg, as indicated in Table 1. Synthetic isomers of brassinolide were also found to be active but at a higher concentration than the natural compound.

Brassinolide and its isomers were evaluated in the bean first-internode curvature bioassay (Thompson *et al.*, 1982). This assay is sensitive to indole acetic acid (IAA) and other auxins at picomolar concentrations. Brassinosteroids had little effect on the

Table 1 Effect of brassinolide and its isomers on the elongation and growth response of internodes in the bean second-internode bioassay

	Elongation over Controls and Growth Responses (%)[a]			
Brassinosteroid	10 μg	1 μg	0.1 μg	0.01 μg
Natural brassinolide	271 (5)	187 (5)	200 (5)	163 (4)
Synthetic brassinolide	136 (5)	136 (5)	156 (5)	183 (4)
22R23R24R brassinolide	237 (5)	178 (5)	228 (4)	224 (3)
22S23S24R brassinolide	163 (5)	136 (5)	152 (3)	140 (2)
22S23S24S brassinolide	257 (5)	129 (4)	116 (2)	80 (1)

[a] Growth response of the treated internodes was rated arbitrarily on a 0-to-5 scale (see numbers in parentheses): 0, no elongation; 1, elongation only; 2, elongation with slight curvature and swelling; 3, elongation with good curvature and swelling; 4, elongation with excellent curvature and swelling; and 5, elongation with split internodes.

Table 2 Effect of brassinolide and its isomers on the elongation of internodes in the bean first-internode bioassay

Brassinosteroid	Growth Rate (mm/h)[a]			Total Growth (mm)
	After 1 h[b]	After 2 h[b]	After 3 h[b]	
Control (IAA)	1.69 ± 0.26a	1.13 ± 0.16a	0.57 ± 0.16a	3.40
Brassinolide	2.48 ± 0.23b	1.76 ± 0.28bc	1.04 ± 0.13b	5.28
22R23R24R Brassinolide	2.19 ± 0.31ab	1.68 ± 0.17b	1.17 ± 0.15bc	5.04
22S23S24R Brassinolide	3.22 ± 0.31c	2.24 ± 0.32c	1.36 ± 0.15c	6.82
22S23S24S Brassinolide	1.96 ± 0.22a	1.60 ± 0.19b	1.24 ± 0.20bc	4.80

[a] Means followed by the same letter are not significantly different at the 5% level by Duncan's multiple range test.

[b] Hours after treatment.

internodes by themselves but produced a synergistic effect when applied shortly before the auxins. Etiolated bean seedlings (*P. vulgaris* L. cv. Bush Burpee Stringless) 6 days old were used for excision of the first internodes (4.0–5.0 cm long). The test compound (0.1 μg) dissolved in ethanol was applied to the base of the excised internode 1 h prior to application of 0.1 nM of auxin. The control plant was treated with auxin alone. The growth of the sections was measured 1, 2, and 3 h after application of the auxin. Brassinolide and its (24R)- and (22S, 23S, 24R)-isomers caused a rapid growth response within 1 h in the presence of exogeneous auxin, and the internodes continued to grow at a high rate during the second and third hour (Table 2).

The mung bean epicotyl bioassay, which is responsive to gibberellic acid but not to auxins, has also been used for brassinolide. Mung bean cuttings responded to brassinosteroids at much lower concentrations (10^{-6} to 10^{-10} M) and at a faster rate than bean cuttings in the second-internode assay (Gregory and Mandava, 1982). The latter required four days to fully show the biological acivity whereas the former showed a very good response in 24 h. Treated mung bean epicotyls showed elongation, curvature, and swelling, and the epinastic response extended to the primary leaves, which tended to droop. Mature hypocotyls did not respond, but the growing epicotyls were very sensitive in this bioassay. Gibberellic acid also elicited epicotyl elongation but was completely inhibited by ancymidol whereas brassinolide was not.

The rice lamina-inclination assay has been developed mainly by Shingo Marumo and co-workers at Nagoya University in Japan (Wada *et al.*, 1984). It can be used as a microquantitative assay for brassinolide and castasterone in the concentration range of 5×10^{-5} to 5×10^{-3} μg/ml. Etiolated seedlings of the rice cultivars Arborio J-1 and Nihonbare were grown for seven days, and uniform seedlings were then selected. Leaf segments, which consisted of the second leaf lamina (0.7 cm long) and the second lamina joint and sheath (0.7 cm long), were excised. These segments were floated on

Table 3 Comparative effects of brassinolide and castasterone on the lamina inclination of excised segments of rice cultivars

		Angle between Lamina and Sheath (deg)[a]						
			Brassinolide Concentration (μg/ml)			Castasterone Concentration (μg/ml)		
Rice Variety	Seedlings Length (cm)	Control	0.005	0.01	0.025	0.01	0.025	0.05
Arborio J-1	14.0 cm	78	162	168	174	158	170	172
Nihonbare	9.0	48	108	111	119	98	101	114

[a] The angles are means of values for eight segments per treatment.

distilled water for 24 h, after which uniformly bent segments were selected. Eight of these segments werre incubated in 1 ml of 2.5-mM aqueous dipotassium maleate solution containing the brassinosteroid. After the segments had incubated for 48 h at 29°C in darkness, the magnitude of the angle induced between the leaf and sheath was measured. Table 3 gives values found for various concentrations of brassinolide and castasterone.

In the tests with both cultivars, a linear correlation was obtained between 5×10^{-3} and 5×10^{-5} μg/ml for the two brassinosteroids. The induced angles leveled off at higher concentrations. IAA was tested and was found to produce only a weak effect, five orders of magnitude less than brassinolide. Cytokinins were inactive and actually counteracted the effect of brassinolide. Abscisic acid also counteracted the effect of brassinolide. This assay is thus highly specific for brassinosteroids and is also the most sensitive, concentrations as low as 0.05 ng/ml of brassinolide being readily detected.

A wheat leaf unrolling test has been developed recently, in which brassinosteroids showed strong activity (Wada *et al.*, 1985). Wheat seedlings (*Triticum aestivum* L. cv. Norin No. 61) were grown in darkness at 26°C for six days, and leaf segments (1.5 cm long) were excised from the region1.5–3.0 cm from the leaf tip under a dim green safelight. Ten of these segments were incubated in 1 ml of 2.5 mM dipotassium maleate solution containing the test sample for 24 h at 30°C in the dark. The unrolling of the leaf segment was determined by measuring their width with calipers.

Brassinolide and castasterone dramatically stimulated leaf unrolling, their activities being dose dependent. At 0.5 ng/ml both compounds markedly stimulated unrolling, and at 0.01 μg/ml or higher, brassinolide produced complete unrolling of the leaf segments to about 3.6 cm. This assay is about one-tenth as sensitive as the rice lamina-inclination test, but it is simpler to carry out. Gibberellin A3 produced only slight unrolling at 0.1 to 10 μg/ml, as did the cytokinin 6-(3-methyl-2-butenyl)-aminopurine. However, zeatin, 6-(4-hydroxy-3-methyl-2-butenyl)aminopurine, caused complete unrolling at 1 μg/ml and had a measurable effect at 0.001 μg/ml. Abscisic acid, indole acetic acid, and indole acetonitrile inhibited unrolling of leaf segments.

A method that holds promise for routine analysis of brassinolide in plant tissues involves the use of monoclonal antibodies to brassinolide. In experiments reported by Horgen *et al.* (1984), synthetic C-24 epimer of brassinolide was the hapten that was noncovalently bound to fetal calf serum. Hybridoma clones were generated from CAF_1 mice and employed in an enzyme-linked immunosorbent assay (ELISA) for examination of brassinolide distribution in *Brassica napus* tissues. Pollen-producing parts gave the highest ELISA values, extracts of pistils also gave high values, roots gave moderately high values, and leaves and petals gave low values. It should be noted that the assay did not exhibit complete specificity for brassinolide or its C-24 epimer, although the latter gave the most positive ELISA values. Natural brassinolide gave values 25% lower than the antigen whereas ecdysone, a naturally occurring plant steroid and sitosterol (a very common plant sterol), gave values 50% lower, Ergosterol and stigmasterol reacted considerably less effectively.

C. Analysis of Brassinosteroids by Mass Spectrometry

Of the various physical techniques for analysis of brassinosteroids, mass spectrometry (ms) in combination with gas-liquid chromatography (GLC) has been used almost exclusively. Brassinolide itself is highly polar and involatile, and no molecular ion is observed on electron-impact mass spectrometry (EI-MS). Chemical-ionization mass spectrometry (CI-MS) is more sensitive (about 100 times) than EI-MS, and the Cl-MS of brassinolide ($C_{28}H_{48}O_6$, MW 480.35) has been reported to give the following ions: *m/z* 481 $(M + 1)^+$, 463 (M + 1-H_2O), 445 (M + 1-2H_2O), 427 (M + 1-3H_2O), 409, 379, 361, 349, 343, 321, 303, 279. The formation of these ions can be accounted for by successive loss of H_2O molecules and fragmentation of the side chain (Fig. 2). The mass spectrum of brassinolide has also been obtained by field desorption (FD) and fast-atom bombardment (FAB) methods, which yield good M + 1 signals.

The FAB-MS of castasterone (Yokota *et al.*, 1982a) gave the molecular ion (M + 1, *m/z* 465) as base peak and ions at *m/z* 447 and 429. The molecular formula $C_{28}H_{48}O_5$ was deduced from the compositions of the fragment ions, such as *m/z* 393 $C_{23}H_{37}O_5$ and 364 $C_{22}H_{36}O_4$ (base peak), determined in the high-resolution EIMS. The former results from fission at C_{23}-C_{24} and the latter from fission at C_{22}-C_{23} with gain of a hydrogen. Similarly, the FAB-MS of dolicholide (Yokota *et al.*, 1982b) showed prominent peaks at *m/z* 479 (M + 1) and *m/z* 571 [M + 1 + 92 (glycerin)]. In the high-resolution EI-MS strong ions at *m/z* 379.2431 (relative intensity 47%, $C_{22}H_{35}O_5$) and 100.0878 (base peak, $C_6H_{12}O$) are derived from C_{22}-C_{23} bond fission.

The pollen of *Typha latifolia* (cattail) is reported to contain 2-deoxycastasterone (1.7 mg from 25 kg pollen; Schneider *et al.*, 1983). FAB-MS gave as base peak an ion at *m/z* 471 (M + Na). High-resolution EI-MS gave M^+ *m/z* 448.3548, $C_{28}H_{48}O_4$, and base peak at *m/z* 348.2630, $C_{22}H_{36}O_3$ (C_{22}-C_{23} fission and transfer of a hydrogen).

a

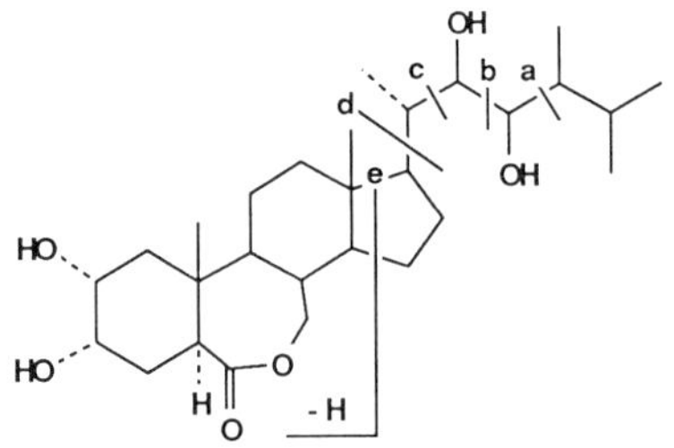

	m/z
a	409, 71
b	379, 101, 361, 343
c	349, 131
d	321, 303
e	279

b

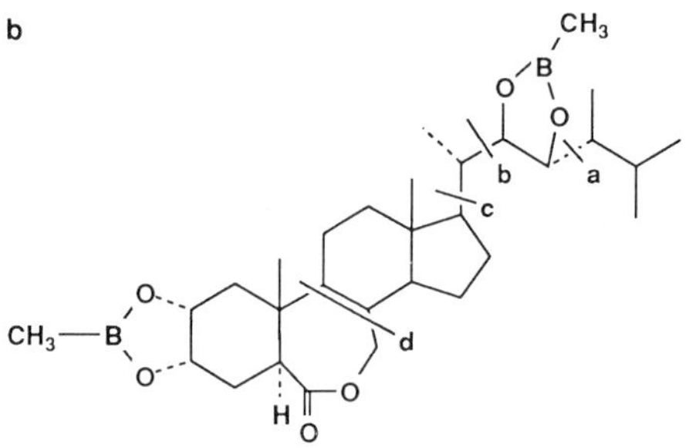

	m/z
M⁺	528
a	457, 71
b	374, 155
c	345
d	332

Figure 2 Mass spectral fragmentation of (a) brassinolide and (b) its bismethaneboronate.

Use has been made of the presence of two pairs of vicinal hydroxyl groups to prepare the bismethaneboronate derivative of brassinolide. This derivative is suitable for analysis by gas chromatography/mass spectrometry (Ikekawa *et al.*, 1984). It was made in the following way: Methaneboronic acid (CH_3-$B(OH)_2$, 100 μg) was dissolved in 50 μg of dry pyridine, the solution was added to 100 μg of brassinolide, and the mixture was heated at 60°C for 30 min and then injected directly into the gas chromatograph. For GC/EI-MS a column packed with 2% OV-17 on Chromosorb W (80–100 mesh, 0.5 m × 2 mm i.d.) was used at 290°C; the carrier gas (helium) flow rate was 30 ml/min; electron energy, 20 eV; electron current, 60 μA; acceleration high voltage, 3.5 kV; ion source temperature, 290°C. For GC/CI-MS the same packed column was used; the reagent gas was isobutane, the carrier gas (helium) flow rate was 30 ml/min; electron energy, 150 eV; box current, 150 μA; acceleration high voltage, 3.5 kV; ion source temperature, 250°C.

The bismethaneboronate of brassinolide and its analogs homobrassinolide and norbrassinolide were well separated on GC and gave sharp peaks. A weak molecular ion ($M^+ = 528$) was obtained and stronger peaks at *m/z* 457 (C_{23}-C_{24} fission), 374 (C_{20}-C_{22} fission), 345 (C_{17}-C_{20} fission), and 332 (B-ring fission). The base peak was at *m/z* 155 (C_{20}-C_{22} fission). In the CI mass spectrum the M + 1 ion (529) was the base peak. The presence of this peak could be used to detect brassinolide at a level of 1 ng or less. By the technique of selected ion monitoring, brassinolide (detected as its bismethaneboronate, *m/z* 529) and castasterone or (24S)-24-methylbrassinone (bismethaneboronate, *m/z* 513) were found (3 μg and 0.5 μg) in extensively purified fractions from extracts of the immature seeds and sheaths of the Chinese cabbage, *Brassica campestris* var. pekinensis (320 kg). Similarly, an active fraction from extracts of the leaves of green tea, *Thea sinensis* (65 kg) yielded 0.3 μg brassinolide and 7.2 μg (24S)-24-methylbrassinone. Chestnut galls (70 g) contained 0.08 μg brassinolide and 0.8 μg (24S)-24-methylbrassinone.

In another report (Abe *et al.*, 1983), Chinese cabbage (320 kg) was also found to contain 250 ng brassinone, 40 ng (24 S)-24-ethylbrassinone, and 400 ng 28-norbrassinolide. Green tea (65 kg) contained 130 ng brassinone and 30 ng (24 S)-24-ethylbrassinone, and chestnut insect gall (3.5 kg) contained 40 ng brassinone.

However, using the same technique of selected ion monitoring, Arima and coworkers (1984) did not detect brassinone (molecular weight of bismethaneboronate, 498) in chestnut insect gall. Instead they identified 6-deoxycastasterone, whose bismethaneboronate has the same molecular weight as that of brassinone bismethaneboronate but differs in retention time.

D. Analysis of Brassinosteroids by NMR Spectroscopy

Analysis of naturally occurring brassinosteroids by NMR spectroscopy has been reported in only a few cases because the steroids have been isolated in amounts that are too small for spectral determination. The ^{1}H NMR data (400 MHz, $CDCl_3$) for brassinolide, castasterone, dolicholide, and 2-deoxycastasterone (typhasterol) are given in Table 4 (Yokota *et al.*, 1982a,b; Schneider *et al.*, 1983). The partial ^{13}C-NMR spectrum (CD_2Cl_2-CD_3OD, 9:1) of brassinolide has the following signals: δ 10.3, 11.9, 12.1, 15.6, 20.8, 21.0, 68.3, 68.4, 71.0, 73.7, 74.8, 177.6 ppm (Grove *et al.*, 1979).

Table 4 ^{1}H-NMR data for brassinolide, (24S)-24-methyl brassinone, dolicholide, and 2-deoxycastasterone

H position	Brassinolide	24 Methyl Brassinone	Dolicholide	2-Deoxycastasterone
18	0.72	0.69	—	0.69
19	0.93	0.76	0.92	0.76
28	0.85 (d)	0.85	—	0.85
26 (or 27)	0.91 (d)	0.91	1.08	0.92
27 (or 26)	0.95 (d)	0.95	1.11	0.95
21	0.97 (d)	0.97	0.96	0.97
5	3.12 (dd,5,12Hz)	2.69 (dd,4,13Hz)	3.11 (dd,5,12Hz)	2.76
22 (or 23)	3.54 (d,9Hz)	3.56 (d,9Hz)	3.62 (d,8Hz)	3.56 (d,9Hz)
23 (or 22)	3.72 (dd,2,9Hz)	3.72 (d,9Hz)	4.03 (d,8Hz)	3.72 (d,9Hz)
2	3.72 (br)	3.77 (bs,s,$w_{1/2}$23Hz)	3.72 (br)	—
3	4.03 (bs.s,$w_{1/2}$10Hz)	4.06 (br,s,$w_{1/2}$8Hz)	4.02 (br,s)	4.17 (br.s)
7	4.09 (m)		4.09 (m)	—

Note: The chemical shifts are in ppm downfield from TMS.

Synthesis of brassinolide and other brassinosteroids has been the subject of many studies; however, discussion of this work is beyond the scope of this chapter. The reader is referred to original papers (Ishigura *et al.*, 1980; Fung and Siddall, 1980; Takatsuto *et al.*, 1984; Thompson *et al.*, 1981;Sakakibara *et al.*, 1982; Mori *et al.*, 1984; Hayami *et al.*, 1983; Donaubauer *et al.*, 1984; Takahashi *et al.*, 1985) and the excellent review by Adam and Marquardt (1986) for information on various syntheses of brassinolide.

III. ANTHERIDIOL AND OOGONIOLS

The path to the discovery of the hormones of *Achlya* differs somewhat from that of brassinolide because it involved a well-studied phenomenon of cell differentiation that appeared to be caused by specific substances. The sexual reproductive process in *Achlya* had been thoroughly investigated by John Raper, who established that the process is controlled by diffusible compounds secreted by the sexual partners into their aqueous milieu (Raper, 1939, 1940). Raper attempted to isolate the substances responsible for specific biological functions. Continuation of this work by Barksdale and McMorris at the New York Botanical Garden led to the isolation of antheridiol, the male-activating steroid, in 1965 (McMorris and Barksdale, 1967) and later to identification of oogoniols, the female-activating hormones (McMorris *et al.*, 1975; Preus and McMorris, 1979). The isolation of these hormones was guided by assays developed by Raper and Barksdale, which remain the most sensitive means of detecting the steroids.

A. Sexual Reproductive Process in Achlya

Achlya is a genus of the aquatic fungi that inhabit fresh-water ponds, lakes, or rivers and are worldwide in distribution. These fungi are composed of filaments that grow in length by apical extension. The filaments and their branches lack cross walls except for those that delimit the reproductive organs, sexual and asexual. The sex organs, which are morphologically distinct, consist of a tubular or lobed male organ, the antheridium, and a spherical female organ, the oogonium.

Sexual reproduction is initiated by the steroid antheridiol (Fig. 3), which is secreted continuously by the female into the surrounding water. In response to antheridiol, the male hyphae produce specialized branches that later bear the antheridia. The antheridial branch is sinuous and narrower than the vegetative hypha and is easily distinguished. The sexually activated male then secretes oogoniol, to which the female reacts by producing branches on which oogonia are borne. Oogonial initials are believed to secrete relatively large amounts of antheridiol, which acts as a chemotropic agent and directs the growth of the antheridial hyphae to the developing oogonioum, leading to conjugation of the sex organs.

Antheridiol has other functions. At concentrations appreciably higher than those required to initiate antheridial branches, it causes the terminal part of the antheridial branch to become enlarged and lobed; and 8–12 h postinduction, a cross wall forms

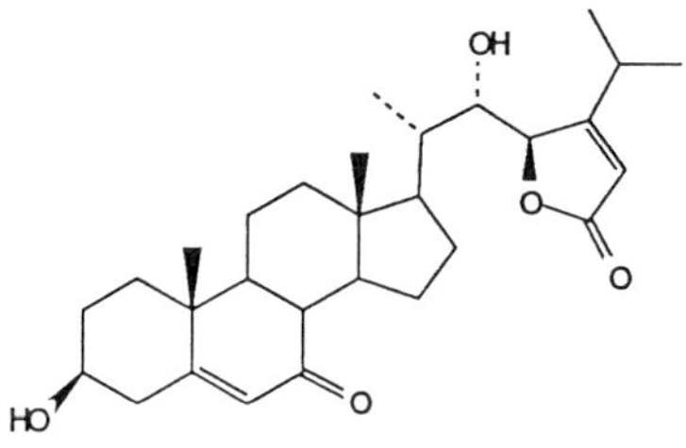

Antheridiol

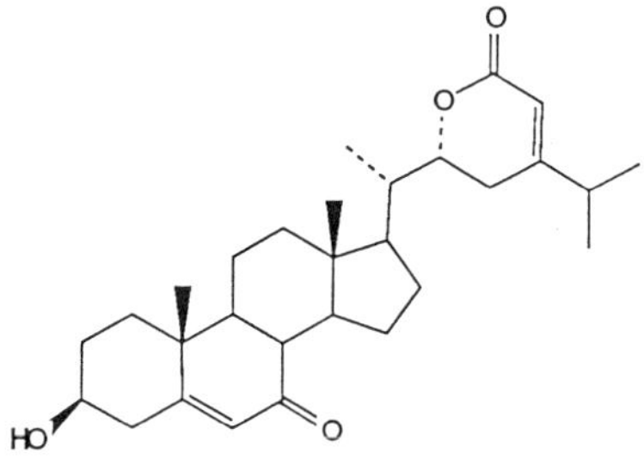

23-Deoxyantheridiol

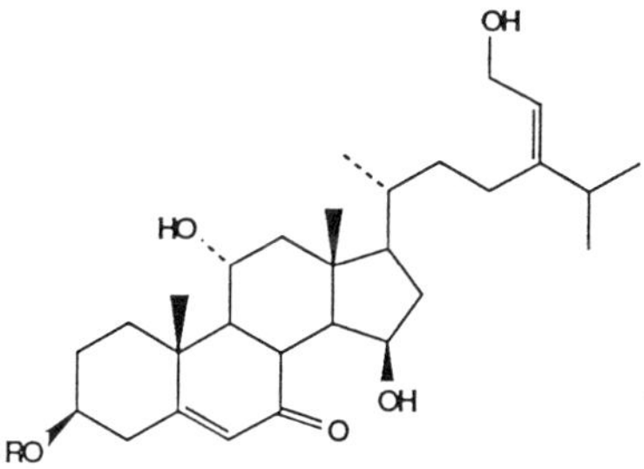

Dehydrooogoniol	R = H
Dehydrooogoniol-1	R = $(CH_3)_2CHCO$
Dehydrooogoniol-2	R = CH_3CH_2CO
Dehydrooogoniol-3	R = CH_3CO

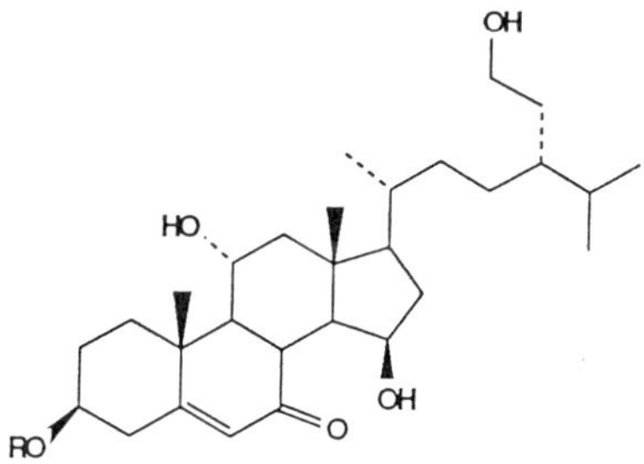

Oogoniol	R = H
Oogoniol-1	R = $(CH_3)_2CHCO$
Oogoniol-2	R = CH_3CH_2CO
Oogoniol-3	R = CH_3CO

Figure 3 Structures of hormones of *Achlya*.

that delimits the antheridium. At about the same time, a cross wall is formed at the base of the oogonium. Within the oogonium, protoplasm reorganizes to form between 1 and 20 mononucleate eggs. Fertilization is accomplished by passage of male nuclei through tiny tubes that extend from the antheridium to each egg. Meiosis is believed to take place in the antheridium and oogonium, and the fertilized egg or oospore is thus diploid. On germination, the thick-walled resistant oospore develops into the hypha of a new plant.

Asexual reproduction in *Achlya* is accomplished by the formation of spore sacs at the tips of hyphae. Each spore sac produces about a thousand uninucleate, biflagellate cells (zoospores), each of which is capable of developing into a new plant.

Most species of *Achlya* are hermaphroditic, each plant bearing functional male and female sexual organs. A few species are heterosexual, each plant bearing organs of only one sexual type, and sexual reproduction occurs only when two compatible plants grow together. The tendency to produce antheridial or oogoniol initials differs from one strain to another, and so does the ability for self-conjugation. For instance, strains of *A. bisexualis* and *A. ambisexualis* seldom self-conjugate, but within species they readily conjugate with one another. They can be arranged on a scale between the two extremes of "male" and "female." The expression of a male or female character is not constant but depends on the mating partner and also on the environmental conditions (Barksdale 1967). Thus, *A. ambisexualis* strain C5 behaves as a female when combined with the male E87 but serves as a male with the female strain 734.

Not surprisingly, females differ in their ability to secrete antheridiol. Females of *A. bisexualis* secrete about 2×10^{-8} g/ml, which is 3 to 10 times as much hormone as secreted by females of *A. ambisexualis*. Also, males of *A. bisexualis* secrete about one-tenth as much antheridiol as the female of this species whereas males of *A. ambisexualis* secrete little or no antheridiol. The latter are very sensitive to antheridiol, responding by branching to concentrations as low as 6×10^{-12} g/ml. The males of *A. bisexualis*, however, are relatively insensitive to antheridiol, a concentration of 6×10^{-9} g/ml being insufficient to induce branching (Barksdale, 1967).

Recent experiments have confirmed an observation of Raper that strong females, when juxtaposed with homothallic strains, can suppress the production of oogonia in the latter. In fact, antheridiol inhibited both oogoniogenesis and asexual sporangiogenesis in a homothallic *A. heterosexualis* isolate (Thomas and McMorris, 1987).

Wheras the growing female mycelium secretes antheridiol continuously, the male secretes oogoniols only at the end of the growth phase and only after it has responded to antheridiol. An hermaphroditic strain *A. heterosexualis*, however, has been found to secrete up to about 5×10^{-8} g/ml of hormone (which is a mixture of oogoniol-1, -2, and -3 and their C-24(28)-dehydro analogs) without prior stimulation by exogenous antheridiol.

B. Isolation and Structure of Antheridiol and Oogoniols

For isolation of antheridiol, culture liquids of *A. bisexualis* were extracted with dichloromethane, and the extract was chromatographed on silica gel with ethyl acetate-hexanes 1:1 to give crystalline antheridiol and 23-deoxyantheridiol. The yield of antheridiol was 1 mg from 85 liters of culture liquid; the 23-deoxyantheridiol yield was similar (Green *et al.*, 1971).

The structure of antheridiol (Fig. 3) was determined by spectroscopic analysis of the hormone and its derivatives and confirmed by synthesis (Edwards *et al.*, 1969, 1972; McMorris *et al.*, 1974). It proved to be an oxygenated derivative of the common plant sterol fucosterol. The structure of 23-deoxyantheridiol was also established by spectroscopic analysis and later confirmed by synthesis (Weihe and McMorris, 1978).

A. heterosexualis was used for investigation of oogoniol structures. About 10 mg of a mixture of closely related compounds was obtained from 200 liters of culture liquid. This mixture was separated by slica-gel chromatography followed by reversed-phase HPLC on a μ-Bondapak C18 column, with 70% MeOH in water as solvent, into several steriods: oogoniol, 24(28)-dehydrooogoniol; oogoniol-1, -2, and -3 and their 24(28)-dehydroanalogs. The structures were determined by spectroscopic evidence;

and, in the case of dehydrooogoniol, the structure was later confirmed by synthesis (McMorris *et al.*, 1983). Like antheridiol, dehydrooogoniol is an oxygenated derivative of fucosterol and oogoniol possesses the skeleton of clionasterol, a sterol found in several algae.

All of the hormones of *Achlya* are derived from fucosterol, which is the major sterol in the fungus. The postulated pathway for the biosynthesis of antheridiol (Fig. 4)

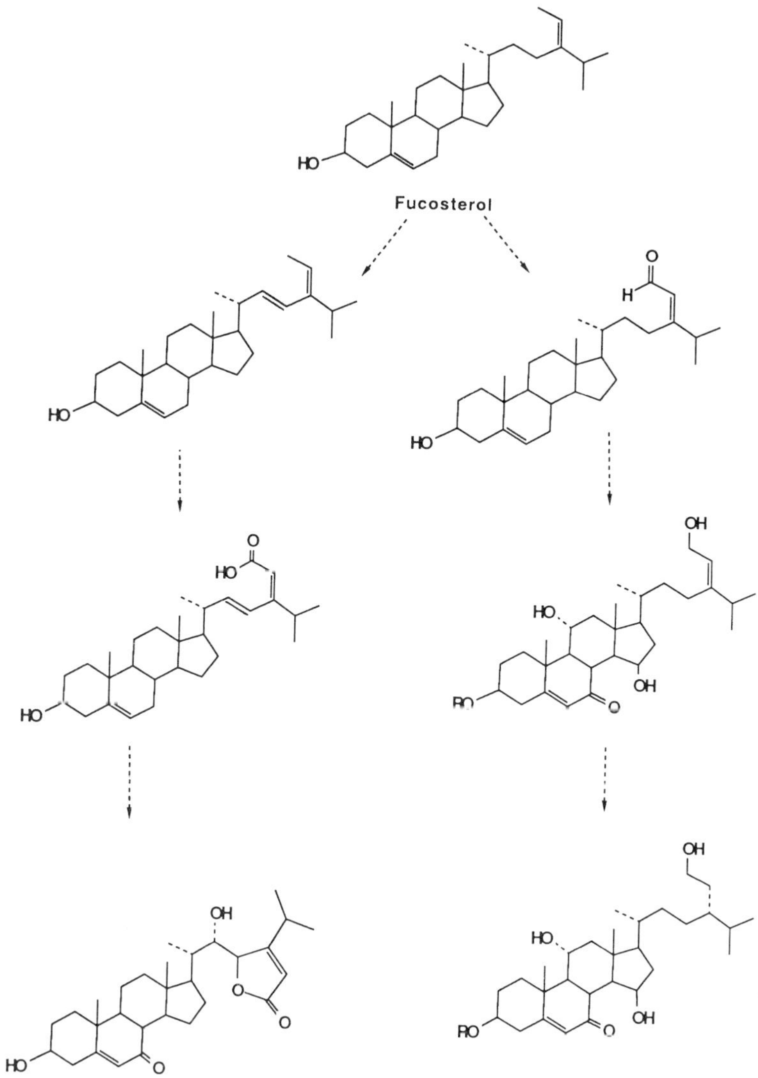

Figure 4 Proposed biosynthetic pathways to the sex hormones of *Achlya*.

involves dehydrogenation of fucosterol at C_{22}-C_{23} followed by oxidation at C_{29} to the level of carboxyl, hydroxylation of the C_{22}-C_{23} double bond, and lactonization leading to the hydroxybutenolide side chain (Popplestone and Unrau, 1974). For the oogoniols, oxidation of fucosterol at C_{29} to the level of aldehyde is believed to be the first step. This is followed by hydroxylation in the steroid nucleus. Reduction of the C_{24}-C_{28} double bond may take place after all the functional groups have been introduced, at C_7, C_{11} and C_{15}. (White and McMorris, 1978; Barrow and McMorris, 1982).

C. Bioassay for Antheridiol

The following very sensitive assay for antheridiol was developed by Barksdale *et al.* (1974) and modified by Thomas. To obtain sexual spores, about half a dozen agar plugs with mycelium of the strong male *A. ambisexualis* E87 were cut aseptically with a cork borer, from a culture grown on agar medium in a standard Petri dish. The medium was either

- PYG: peptone, 1.25 g; yeast extract, 1.25 g; glucose, 3.20 g; agar 15 g; distilled H_2O, 1.0 liter (Cantino and Lovett, 1960), or
- M: sodium glutamate 0.4 g; glucose, 2.8 g; tris-(hydroxymethyl)-amino-methane, 1.2 g; L-methionine 15 mg/ml in 1 N HCl, 1 ml; KCl 14.9 g/100 ml H_2O, 1 ml; $MgSO_4 \cdot 7H_2O$, 12.32 g/100 ml, 1 ml; $CaCl_2$ 5.55 g/100 ml, 1 ml; EDTA disodium salt, 1 g/100 ml, 2 ml; KH_2PO_4, 13.6 g/100 ml, 1.5 ml; $Fe(NH_4)_2(SO_4)_2 \cdot 6H_2O$, 1.44 g + $ZnSO_4 \cdot 7H_2O$, 0.44 g + $MnSO_4 \cdot H_2O$, 0.15 g/100 ml, 10 ml; agar 15 g; distilled H_2O, 1 liter (Mullins and Barksdale, 1965).

The plugs were transferred to a 250-ml Erlenmeyer flask containing 100 ml PYG (without agar), which was then placed on a shaker for 18 to 24 h. Sporulation was induced by decanting the residual PYG medium from the spherical colonies that had formed and replacing it with 100-ml $CaCl_2$ solution (5.55 mg/100 ml). A trace of charcoal added to this first rinse usually promoted sporulation. The flask was placed on the shaker for 30 min, and then the $CaCl_2$ solutiuon was poured off and replaced with fresh $CaCl_2$ solution (but without charcoal). The flask was placed on the shaker overnight, then the spore suspension was decanted into a sterile flask and stored at 4°C.

Antheridiol (or other steroid to be tested) was dissolved either in methanol or acetone, but this solution had to be diluted with distilled water to give a final concentration of methanol or acetone no greater than 1%. Higher concentrations of organic solvent inhibited development of antheridia. An aliquot of this solution was added to the mycelial mat grown from spores for 24 h at 25°C in liquid PYG medium (1 ml spore suspension, from above, in 100 ml medium) or for 72 h in liquid M medium. Mycelia grown on PYG medium was rinsed in and transferred to M medium for bioassays. The treated mycelium was kept for about 3 h and then examined for antheridial branches. If branching had occurred on 25% or more of the hyphae nearest the surface, the bioassay was positive.

The lowest concentration of antheridiol to cause branching was about 10×10^{-12} g/ml of solution. The concentration of antheridiol determined both the number of branches initiated and the time that elapsed between the addition of hormone and the appearance of branches. The number of branches increased with increasing concentration of hormone until an upper limit was attained. The length of time before branches appeared was found to decrease with increasing concentration until a minimum of 40–50 min was reached. Branching could be enhanced by adding edamin and glucose. It should be noted that vegetative branching is induced by amino acids (Fischer and Weiner, 1955).

Besides antheridiol, only a few closely related steroids gave a positive test in the bioassay. The structure lacking the C-7 ketone, 7-DA, had about 10% of the activity of antheridiol. Structures with a different configuration at C-22 or C-23 had activities that were 0.1% or less that of antheridiol. 23-Deoxyantheridiol and the trienoic acid, believed to be an intermediate in the biosynthesis of antheridiol, each possessed about 0.1% of the activity of antheridiol. A number of other steroids including mammalian sex hormones were inactive in the biossay.

These results compare well with the results of recent radioligand-binding studies with [1,2-^{3}H]7-DA. The cytosol of male cells has been found to contain a specific binding protein that may represent the endogenous receptor for antheridiol (Riehl and Toft, 1984; Riehl *et al.*, 1984). Competition for specific [^{3}H]7-DA binding to this protein by various streroids is shown in Table 5. Aliquots of the cytosol (1 ml = 234 μg protein) containing [^{3}H]-7DA at a final concentration of 1.0 nM (88,800 dpm/ml) and unlabeled steroids at the concentration indicated were incubated for 1 h at 0°C. The amount of [^{3}H]-7DA specifically bound was determined by subtraction of the amount of nonspecific binding measured in the presence of 50 nM antheridiol (approx. 7500 dpm/ml) from the total amount bound (approx. 30,000 dpm/ml) in the absence

Table 5 Competition for specific [^{3}H]7-DA binding in *Achlya* cytosol by various steroids

Steroid	Conc. (nM)	Specific Binding (*f* mol/mg protein)	Control (%)
[^{3}H]7-DA	1	1047	100
Antheridiol	5	129	12
7-DA	5	371	35
	50	92	9
Progesterone	50	1008	96
Estradiol	50	1098	105
Testosterone	50	1112	106
Cortisol	50	1087	104
Cholesterol	50	1117	107
Pregnenolone	50	1249	119

of antheridiol. Values for specifically bound [^{3}H]-7DA (*f* mol/mg protein) represent the mean value from two separate experiments. It is clear that apart from antheridiol and 7-DA there was no binding of the various steroids tested. This kind of binding experiment can be adapted for assay of the receptor of antheridiol in cytosols of various strains of *Achlya*.

D. Bioassay for Oogoniols

Mycelium of the female *A. ambisexualis* 734 was prepared, and the test solution was added in the same way as described for the E87 strain and for antheridiol. Oogonial initials were visible after about 12 h and reached a maximum number in 24–48 h. Like antheridial hyphae, the number of oogoniol initials increased with increasing oogoniol concentration. They had a distinct spherical shape and were easily counted. In a strongly positive reaction, there were well over 50 in any field near the edge of the mycelial mat when viewed through a microscope at a magnification of ×40. The protoplasm in the oogoniol initial was often quite dense compared with that in the hyphae. However, protoplasm did not differentiate to form oospheres, as was observed when male and female strains were grown together and conjugation of antheridial hyphae and oogoniol initials occurred. The most active of the oogoniols was 24(28)-dehydrooogoniol-1, which elicited a response at concentrations as low as 5×10^{-8} g/ml. Dehydrooogoniol possessed similar activity whereas oogoniol-1 and oogoniol were about 100 times less active. The activities of oogoniol and its analogs have not been thoroughly compared because the compounds are not readily available either by fermentation or synthesis.

E. Analysis of Antheridiol and Oogoniols by Mass Spectrometry

Mass spectral evidence was important for elucidation of the structure of antheridiol. The high-resolution EI-MS gave a very weak molecular ion (*m/z* 470), $C_{29}H_{42}O_5$, and a base peak (*m/z* 344) for $C_{22}H_{32}O_3$. The latter is formed by McLafferty rearrangement involving cleavage at C_{22}-C_{23} and loss of one hydrogen atom. The other cleavage fragment $C_7H_{10}O_2$ also gave an intense ion (*m/z* 126). Other important fragment ions correspond to $C_{22}H_{30}O_2$, $C_{21}H_{30}O$, $C_{19}H_{27}O_2$, and $C_{19}H_{25}O$ resulting from loss of H_2O from the ion $C_{22}H_{32}O_3$ and from cleavage of the C_{17}-C_{20} bond and further loss of H_2O. Catalytic hydrogenation of antheridiol gave a tetrahydroderivative that exhibited a more intense M^+ (*m/z* 474) than antheridiol and also gave an abundant ion (*m/z* 347), $C_{22}H_{35}O_3$, resulting simply from cleavage of the C_{22}-C_{23} bond.

The mass spectrum of 23-deoxyantheridiol showed the abundant molecular ion at *m/z* 454, $C_{29}H_{42}O_4$, an ion at *m/z* 436, and important fragment ions resulting from cleavage of C_{21}-C_{22} and gain of one hydrogen (*m/z* 316) and cleavage of C_{13}-C_{17}, C_{14}-C_{15} and further loss of one hydrogen (*m/z* 245), base peak, $C_{16}H_{21}O_2$.

Mass spectral data also contributed greatly in elucidation of the structures of the oogoniols. Thus, the EI-MS of oogoniol-1 gave the molecular ion *m/z* 546·3908

($C_{33}H_{54}O_6$) and a fragment ion at *m/z* 458 (base peak, $C_{29}H_{46}O_4$), resulting from loss of isobutyric acid. Similarly, oogoniol-2 gave molecular ion *m/z* 532·3762 ($C_{32}H_{52}O_6$) and 458, oogoniol-3 gave molecular ion *m/z* 518·3588 ($C_{31}H_{50}O_6$) and 458, and oogoniol gave M^+ 476 ($C_{29}H_{48}O_5$) and 458. Other important ions in the spectra of these compounds were *m/z* 440, 425, 422, 301 (relative intensity 6 %, from cleavage at C_{17}-C_{20}), 283 (37 %), and 265 (14 %).

Dehydrooogoniol-1 showed no M^+ in the EI-MS. The largest fragment ion was *m/z* 456·3250 ($C_{29}H_{44}O_4$, 14%), and there were ions at *m/z* 438 (91 %), 423 (36 %), 342, and 299·1647 (100%, $C_{19}H_{23}O_3$). This last fragment resulted from cleavage of the C_{17}-C_{20} bond with further loss of two hydrogen atoms from the tetracyclic nucleus. Such fragmentations are typical for sterols containing a side-chain double bond (Wyllie and Djerassi, 1968).

F. Analysis of Antheridiol and Oogoniols by NMR Spectroscopy

The ^1H NMR spectral data provided much structural information of the steroids of *Achlya* (Table 6). Of particular interest were the vicinal coupling contents for H-22 and H-23 in antheridiol, which indicate a preferred conformation for the side chain in which these protons are antiparallel. It has been proposed on the basis of X-ray crystallographic analysis and NMR data (Nakane and Ikekawa, 1977) that the stable conformation of the steroidal side chain is that which avoids parallel 1,3-interaction between C-22 substituents and the C-16 methylene group. This enables one to predict the stable conformation of the entire side chain.

Another point of interest is that the chiral center at C-23 results in different chemical shifts for the C-26 and C-27 protons. The chiral center at C-24 in oogoniol likewise leads to two doublets for the methyls of the isopropyl group.

Table 6 ^1H-NMR data for antheridiol, 23-deoxyantheridiol, oogoniol, and 24(28)-dehydrooogoniol

H position	Antheridiol	23-Deoxyantheridiol	Oogoniol	24(28)-Dehydrooogoniol
18	0.72	0.72	0.99	0.99
19	1.23	1.20	1.36	1.34
21	—	1.03(d,6Hz)	—	—
26(or 27)	1.17(d,7Hz)	1.10(d,7Hz)	0.828(d7Hz)	1.02(d,6.5Hz)
27(or 26)	1.23(d,7Hz)	1.10(d,7Hz)	0.850(d,7Hz)	1.02(d,6.5Hz)
3	—	3.6(m)	—	3.65
22	3.6(d,8Hz)	4.38(dt,12,4.5Hz)	—	—
11	—	—	4.15(m)	4.16(m)
29	—	—	3.63(t,7Hz)	4.16(m)
15	—	—	4.69(m)	4.69(m)
23	4.98(d,8Hz)	—	—	—
6	5.70	5.67	5.83	5.82
28	5.79	5.73	—	5.36(m)

Note: The chemical shifts are in ppm downfield form TMS.

Antheridiol and 23-deoxyantheridiol gave characteristic infrared absorption peaks at 1675 and 1672 cm^{-1} for the conjugated ketone and at 1742 and 1705 cm^{-1} for the conjugated γ-lactone and δ-lactone, respectively. In the case of oogoniols, the conjugated ketone absorption peak appeared at the slightly lower value of 1660 cm^{-1} because of hydrogen bonding of the ketone with the 15β-hydroxyl group. The ultraviolet (UV) spectra in the oogoniols gave a characteristic absorption band at λ_{max} 235 nm (ε 14,000). However, with antheridiol the presence of the conjugated ketone and conjugated lactone chromophores resulted in an absorption band at λ_{max} 220 nm (ε 17,000). Similarly, 23-deoxyantheridiol gave an absorption band at λ_{max} 226 nm (ε 18,800).

IV. CONCLUSION

The biochemical events that are brought by antheridiol in *Achlya* closely parallel what is known to take place in mammalian target tissue in response to steroid sex hormones. However, discussion of this is beyond the scope of this chapter, and only brief mention can be made of stimulation of RNA, protein synthesis, and the induction of a cellulase enzyme by antheridiol. This enzyme is believed to cause a localized softening of the hyphal wall, which produces weak spots that are blown out into lateral blebs, by turgor pressure, thus leading to formation of the antheridial branches. (Thomas and Mullins, 1967; Mullins and Ellis, 1974). For more information on these topics, the reader is referred to recent papers by Horgen (1981) and Horgen *et al.* (1983).

REFERENCES

Abe, H., Morishita, T., Uchiyama, M., Takatsuto, S., Ikekawa, N., Ikeda, M., Sassa, T., Kitsuwa, T., and Marumo, S. (1983). *Experimenta* **39**, 351.

Adam, G., and Marquardt, V. (1986). *Phytochemistry* **25**, 1787.

Arima, M., Yokota, T., and Takahashi, N. (1984). *Phytochemistry* **23**, 1587.

Barksdale, A. W. (1967). *Ann. N.Y. Acad. Sci.* **144**, 313.

Barksdale, A. W., McMorris, T. C., Seshadri, R., Arunachalam, T., Edwards, J. A., Sundeen, J., and Green, D. M. (1974). *J. Gen. Microbiol.* **82**, 295.

Barrow, S. E., and McMorris, T. C. (1982). *Lipids* **17**, 383.

Cantino, E. C., and Lovett, J. S. (1960). *Physiol. Plant* **13**, 450.

Donaubauer, J. R., Greaves, A. M., and McMorris, T. C. (1984). *J. Org. Chem.* **49**, 2833.

Edwards, J. A., Mills, J. S., Sundeen, J., and Fried, J. H. (1969). *J. Am. Chem. Soc.* **91**, 1248.

Edwards, J. A., Sundeen, J., Salmond, W., Iwadare, T., and Fried, J. H. (1972). *Tetrahedron Lett.* 791.

Fischer, F. G., and Weiner, G. (1955). *Z. Physiol. Chem. Hoppe-Seyler's* **300**, 211.

Fung, S., and Siddall, J. B. (1980) *J. Am. Chem. Soc.* **102**, 6581.

Green, D. M., Edwards, J. A., Barksdale, A. W., and McMorris, T. C. (1971). *Tetrahedron* **27**, 1199.

Gregory, L. E., and Mandava, N. B. (1982). *Physiol. Plant*, **54**, 239.

Grove, M. D., Spencer, G. F., Rohwedder, W. K., Mandava. N., Worley, J. F., Warthen, J. D., Jr., Steffens, G. L., Flippen-Anderson, J. L., and Cook, J. C., Jr. (1979). *Nature* **281**, 216.

Hayami, H., Sato, M., Kanemoto, S., Morizawa, Y., Oshima, K., and Nozaki, H. (1983). *J. Am. Chem. Soc.* **105**, 4491.

Horgen, P. A. (1981). *In* "Sexual Interactions in Eukaryotic Microbes" (D. H. O'Day and P. A. Horgen, eds.), p. 155. Academic Press, New York.

Horgen, P. A., Iwanochko, M., and Bettiol, M. F. (1983). *Arch. Microbiol.* **134**, 314.

Horgen, P. A., Nakagawa, C. H., and Irvin, R. T. (1984). *Can. J. Biochem. Cell Biol.* **62**, 715.

Ikekawa, N., Takatsuto, S., Kitsuwa, T., Saito, H., Morishita, T., and Abe, H. (1984). *J. Chromatography* **290**, 289.

Ishiguro, M., Takatsuto, S., Morisaki, M., and Ikekawa, N. (1980). *Chem. Commun.* **20**, 962.

McMorris, T. C., and Barksdale, A. W. (1967). *Nature (London)* **215**, 320.

McMorris, T. C., Seshadri, R., and Arunachalam, T. (1974). *J. Org. Chem.* **39**, 669.

McMorris, T. C., Seshadri, R., Weihe, G. R., Arsenault, G. P., and Barksdale, A. W. (1975). *J. Am. Chem. Soc.* **97**, 2544.

McMorris, T. C., Le, P. H., Preus, M. W., Schow, S. R., and Weihe, G. R. (1983). *J. Org. Chem.* **48**, 3370.

Marumo, S., Hatori, H., Abe, H., Nonoyama, Y., and Munakata, K. (1968). *Agric. Biol. Chem.* **32**, 528.

Mori, K., Sakakibara, M., and Okada, K. (1984). *Tetrahedron* **40**, 1767.

Mullins, J. T., and Barksdale, A. W. (1965). *Mycologia* **57**, 352.

Mullins, J. T., and Ellis, E. A. (1974). *Proc. Natl. Acad. Sci. U.S.A.* **71**, 1347.

Nakane, M., and Ikekawa, N. (1977). *J. Chem. Soc. Perkin Trans. 1*, p. 1426.

Popplestone, C. R., and Unrau, A. M. (1974). *Can. J. Chem.* **52**, 462.

Preus, M. W., and McMorris, T. C. (1979). *J. Am. Chem. Soc.* **101**, 3066.

Raper, J. R. (1939). *Am. J. Bot.* **26**, 639.

Raper, J. R. (1940). *Am. J. Biol.* **27**, 162.

Rees, H. H. (1983). *In* "Biosynthesis of Isoprenoid Compounds" (J. W. Porter and S. L. Spurgeon, eds.), Vol. 2, p. 463, Wiley, New York,

Riehl, R. M., and Toft, D. O. (1984). *J. Biol. Chem.* **259**, 15324.

Riehl, R. M., Toft, D. O., Meyer, M. D., Carlson, G. L., and McMorris, T. C. (1984). *Exp. Cell. Res.* **1543**, 544.

Sakakibara, M., Okada, K., Ichikawa, Y., and Mori, K. (1982). *Heterocycles* **17**, 301.

Schneider, J. A., Yoshihara, K., Nakanishi, K., and Kato, N. (1983). *Tetrahedron Lett.* **24**, 3859.

Takahashi, T., Ootake, A., Yamada, H., and Tsuji, J. (1985). *Tetrahedron Lett.* **26**, 69.

Takatsuto, S., Yazawa, N., Ishiguro, M., Morisaki, M., and Ikekawa, N. (1984). *J. Chem. Soc., Perkin Trans.* **1**, 139.

Thomas, D. des S., and McMorris, T. C. (1987). *J. Chem. Ecol.* **13**, 1131.

Thomas, D. des S., and Mullins, J. T. (1967). *Science* **156**, 84.

Thompson, M. J., Mandava, N. B., Meudt, W. J., Lusby, W. R., and Spaulding, D. W. (1981). *Steroids* **38**, 567.

Thompson, M. J., Meudt, W. J., Mandava, N. B., Dutky, S. R., Lusby, W. R., and Spaulding, D. W. (1982). *Steroids* **39**, 2894.

Wada, K., Marumo, S., Abe, H. Morishita, T., Nakamura, K., Uchiyama, M., and Mori, K. (1984). *Agric. Biol. Chem.* **48**, 719.

Wada, K., Hiroaki, K., and Marumo, S. (1985). *Agric. Biol. Chem.* **49**, 2249.

Weihe, G. R., and McMorris, T. C. (1978). *J. Org. Chem.* **43**, 3942.

White, R. H., and McMorris, T. C. (1978). *Phytochemistry* **17**, 1800.

Wyllie, S. G., and Djerassi, C. (1968). *J. Org. Chem.* **33**, 305.

Yokota, T., Arima, M., and Takahashi, N. (1982a). *Tetrahedron Lett.* **23**, 1275.

Yokota, T., Baba, J., and Takahashi, N. (1982b). *Tetrahedron Lett.* **23**, 4965.

5

Analysis of Free and Conjugated Ecdysteroids and Polar Metabolites of Insects

Malcolm J. Thompson, James A. Svoboda, and Mark F. Feldlaufer
Insect and Nematode Hormone Laboratory
U.S. Department of Agriculture
Agricultural Research Service
Beltsville, Maryland

I. INTRODUCTION

In the initial isolation of the first crystalline molting hormone, ecdysone was extracted from silkworm pupae with methanol, and the methanolic extractives were purified by a series of partition systems, chromatography, and counter-current distribution (Butenandt and Karlson, 1954). Throughout the purification process, activity was monitored by the *Calliphora* bioassay (Becker and Plagge, 1939). After the structural elucidation of ecdysone 11 years later and the discovery of other ecdysteroids in insects, faster methods of analysis and quantification were sought. Many variations of analyses for the numerous free ecdysteroids of insects have since been developed, and the reader is referred to several extensive reviews (Horn, 1971; Morgan and Wilson, 1980; Lafont *et al.*, 1980, 1981; Horn and Bergamasco, 1985).

Analytical methods for ecdysteroid conjugates, however, have only been recently developed (Rees and Isaac, 1985; Hetru *et al.*, 1985). Ecdysteroid conjugates, which have major metabolic roles in certain insect stages, often account for $>95\%$ of the total ecdysteroids in adult ovaries. These ovarian ecdysteroid conjugates are apparently storage forms of the more biologically active free ecdysteroids, which can be released from the conjugates during embryogenesis. During embryonic development, as well as in other stages, new and different conjugates are formed that may function as inactivation or storage products. One of the major difficulties encountered in analyzing and identifying ecdysteroid conjugates is that the conjugates are often water-soluble and are accompanied by large quantities of other water-soluble material from insect tissue, and therefore are not easily purified by the procedures developed for the chromatography of the more organosoluble free ecdysteroids. Most analyses, therefore, have been conducted on ecdysteroids that are released after enzymatic hydrolysis of the conjugate, but the quantity, nature, or position of conjugation could not be unequivocally determined. It is only recently that new techniques and methodologies have been developed to isolate and analyze directly for intact ecdysteroid conjugates. If we are to understand the interrelationships of free and conjugated ecdysteroids and other polar metabolites, as well as their role and fate in insect development, we need to identify and quantitatively determine these ecdysteroids in the various developmental periods of an insect's life cycle.

In this chapter, we discuss the use of radiolabeled precursors in ecdysteroid isolation; the isolation and purification of free and conjugated ecdysteroids; high-performance liquid chromatography (HPLC) of free ecdysteroids, intact ecdysteroid conjugates, and polar metabolites; and the use of Fourier transform nuclear magnetic resonance spectroscopy (FT-NMR) and mass spectrometry (MS) to identify ecdysteroid conjugates.

II. USE OF RADIOLABELED PRECURSORS IN ECDYSTEROID RESEARCH

The reports that injected [^{3}H]cholesterol was converted to radiolabled ecdysone (Karlson and Hoffmeister, 1963) and subsequently to 20-hydroxyecdysone (Willig *et al.*, 1971) by larval *Calliphora erythrocephala* (= *vicina*) demonstrated that cholesterol was indeed the primary sterol precursor for the C_{27} ecdysteroids and therefore offered a means for studying ecdysteroid biosynthesis and metabolism in insects.

More recently, the incorporation of labeled cholesterol into the ovarian ecdysteroids of adult female insects, and ultimately into eggs, has been particularly useful in studying ecdysteroid conjugates because ovaries and eggs contain large quantities of these conjugates compared with the relatively small amounts of free ecdysteroids in these tissues (Hsiao and Hsiao, 1979; Dinan and Rees, 1981a; Lagueux *et al.*, 1981). In fact, the conversion of [^{14}C]cholesterol by *Schistocerca gregaria* adult females to several labeled ovarian and egg products afforded the first isolation of ecdysteroid phosphate conjugates (Dinan and Rees, 1981b) and led to their subsequent identification by Isaac *et al.* (1982, 1983b) as the 22-phosphates of ecdysone, 20-hydroxyecdysone, 2-deoxyecdysone, and 2-deoxy-20-hydroxyecdysone. The efficient incorporation (0.5–1.0%) of the injected label into these conjugated ecdysteroids made it possible not only to detect and identify them but also to follow their metabolic fate during embryogenesis, resulting in a postulated scheme of events by which molting hormone levels were regulated (Isaac and Rees, 1985). The corresponding structural formulas of the free ecdysteroids and polar metabolites mentioned in this review are given in Fig. 1.

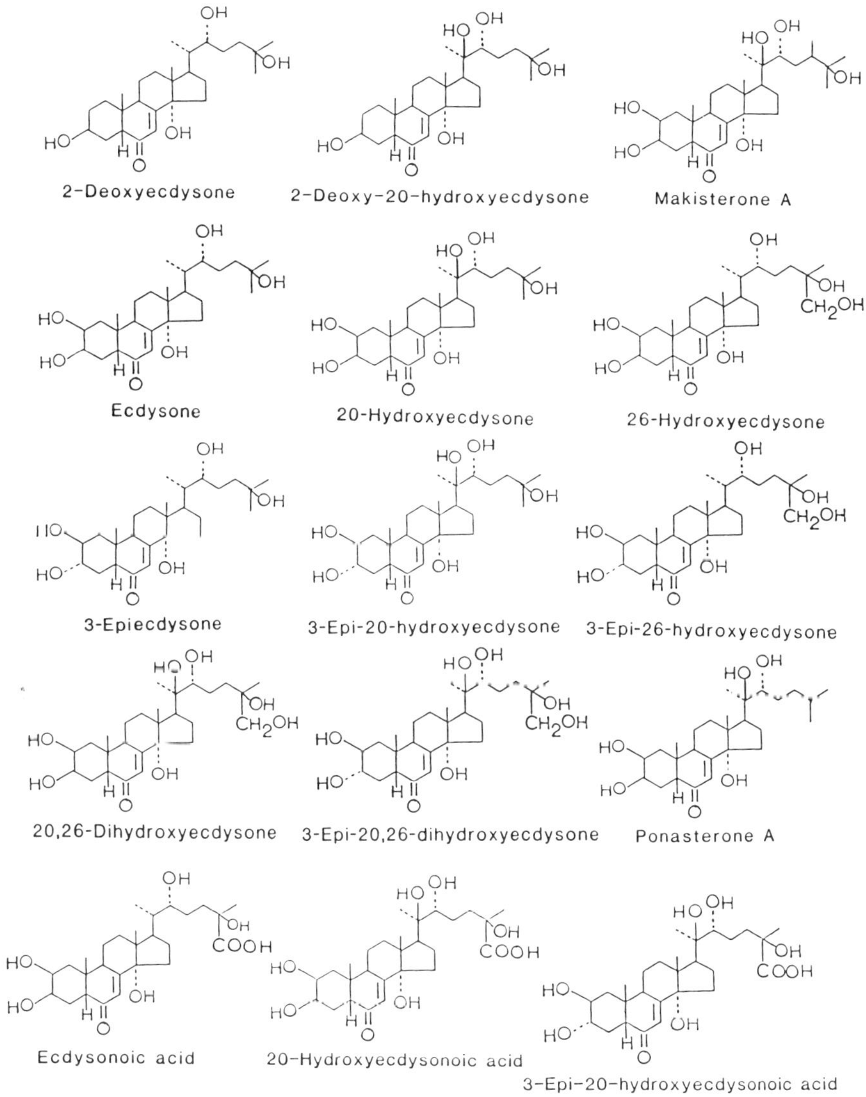

Figure 1 Structures of ecdysteroids and polar metabolites.

The fates of maternal ecdysteroid conjugates were also examined during embryogenesis in *Locusta migratoria* and compared by both a radioimmunoassay (RIA) and a radioassay of labeled conjugates isolated from females injected with [^{3}H]cholesterol (Sall *et al.*, 1983). The radioassay had a distinct advantage over the RIA because quantification of the various conjugates encountered, especially the AMP-2-deoxoyecdysone, could be made without having to account for relative cross-reactivity of immunoreactive compounds toward the antisera used in the RIA, though results, for the most part, indicated that the two methods are comparable.

The occurrence of highly polar [^{3}H]ecdysone metabolites that are not susceptible to enzymatic hydrolysis has led to the identification of the ecdysonoic and 20-hydroxyecdysonoic acids in several insect species (Lafont *et al.*, 1980, 1983; Isaac *et al.*, 1983a). In addition to these acids, analysis of labeled metabolites enabled Gibson *et al.* (1984) to identify ecdysone 3-acetate, 3-acetylecdysone 2-phosphate, and 3-acetyl-20-hydroxyecdysone 2-phosphate from larval *S. gregaria*.

Our laboratory has successfully employed labeled cholesterol to determine and study ecdysteroid conjugates in the tobacco hornworm, *Manduca sexta*. Following injection of [^{14}C]cholesterol into female pupae, more than 0.6% of the labeled precursor was converted to ovarian ecdysteroid conjugates, enabling us to detect even small quantities of these compounds and to determine their fate during embryonic development. As a result of these studies, we have been able to identify at least three different conjugates of 26-hydroxyecdysone, as well as a unique triglucoside conjugate of the C_{21} vertebrate steroid, 5-pregnen-3β,20β-diol (Thompson *et al.*, 1985a,b, 1987a,b). The details of our isolation, purification, and identification of these compounds are included as examples in this chapter.

III. ISOLATION AND PURIFICATION OF FREE AND CONJUGATED ECDYSTEROIDS

The early incorporation of a radiochemical precursor into the biosynthetic pathway of ecdysone is ideally suited to the development of isolation and purification techniques. To this end, [^{14}C]cholesterol has served well, enabling us and others to isolate and identify free and conjugated ecdysteroids and determine their metabolic fate at various developmental periods of an insect's life cycle. A detailed outline beginning with the extraction of 72–88-h-old tobacco hornworm eggs and proceeding through the purification of material suitable for HPLC analyses of both free and conjugated ecdysteroids and polar metabolites are presented in Figs. 2 and 3.

A. Partition Systems

Extracts of insect tissue require the removal of numerous nonecdysteroid contaminants prior to HPLC. Although purification procedures using solvent partition systems are considered time-consuming and tedious, the overall result of having cleaner samples containing compounds of similar polarity more than compensates for the time spent. In fact, the time required to partially purify a sample by solvent partitions can

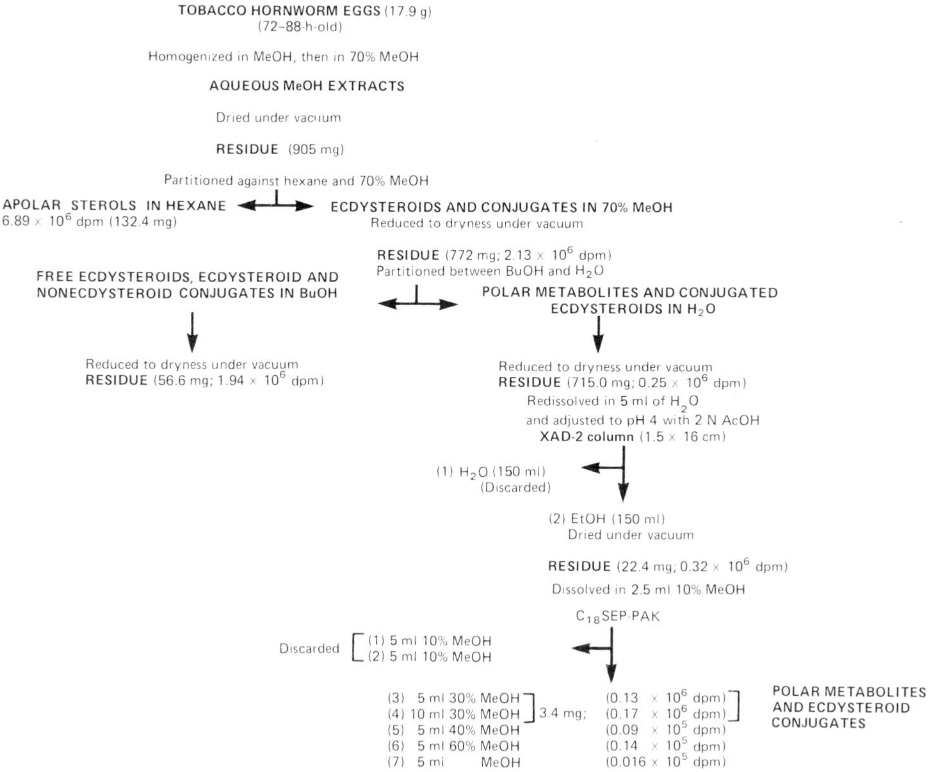

Figure 2 Procedure used for the isolation and purification of ecdysteroid conjugates from the aqueous phase of a butanol/water partition system.

be shortened if centrifugation to remove insoluble particulates from the extract is employed immediately after initial homogenization of the insect tissue. To this end, the solvent partitions of the extractives can also be conducted in centrifuge tubes, should centrifugation be needed to separate emulsions of the solvent phases.

The partitioning of the extractives of tobacco hornworm eggs (Fig.2) between hexane and 70% methanol (countersaturated) results in apolar lipids, including unmetabolized [^{14}C]cholesterol, its esters and apolar metabolites being partitioned into the hexane phase. After removal of solvent, the free ecdysteroids, nonecdysteroid and ecdysteroid conjugates, and other polar metabolites can be recovered from the 70% methanol phase. This methanolic residue can then be partitioned between butanol and water by five transfers of the upper phase (butanol) over three tubes containing lower phase. By this procedure the free ecdysteroids, including the very polar 20, 26-dihydroxyecdysone, and the 5-pregnen-3β,20β-diol di- and triglucosides are totally partitioned into the butanol phase. Approximately 50% of the 26-hydroxyecdysone

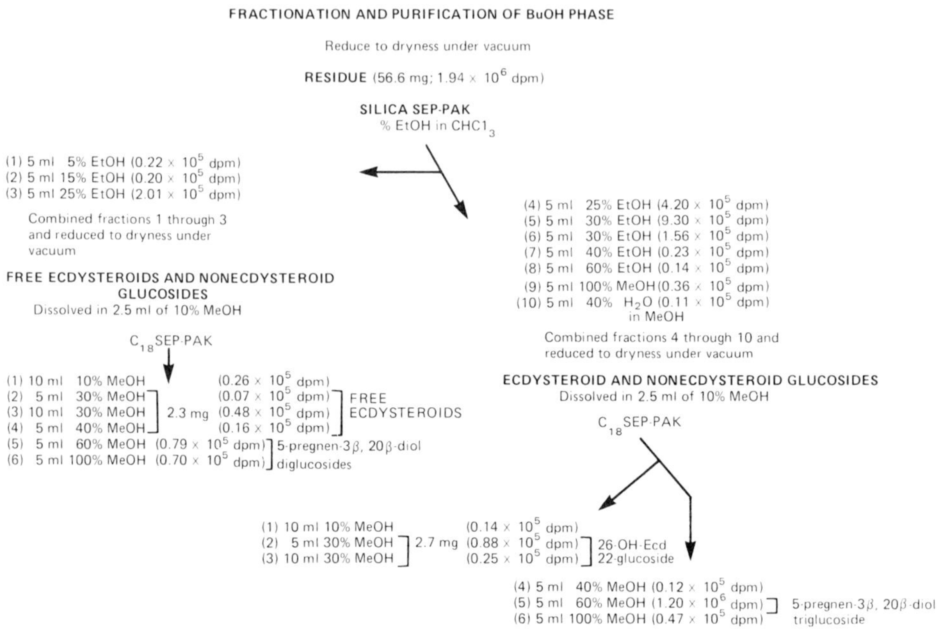

Figure 3 Procedure used for the isolation and purification of free ecdysteroids, ecdysteroid, and nonecdysteroid conjugates from the butanol phase of a butanol/water partition system.

22-glucoside conjugate is also partitioned into the butanol phase. On the other hand, the 2- and 26-phosphate conjugates of 26-hydroxyecdysone (Thompson *et al.*, 1987a,b) and better than 95% of 20-hydroxyecdysonoic acid and its 3α-epimer partition into the aqueous phase of the water/butanol partition system. In this system, however, less polar ecdysteroid phosphates, such as ecdysone and 20-hydroxyecdysone 22-phosphates, are distributed into the butanolic and aqueous phases (Dinan and Rees, 1981a). Thus, it must be emphasized that the ideal solvent system, which would completely separate the free ecdysteroids from ecdysteroid conjugates, does not exist. Certainly, though, the butanol/water partition system has been most useful in separating the free ecdysteroids from the large quantity of water-soluble polar material also extracted from insect tissues. Of the partition systems cited by Horn (1971), the partition coefficients of free ecdysteroids are highest in a butanol/water system, and this is the system of choice for partitioning free ecdysteroids. In fact, less than 10% of the mass present in the methanol phase from the hexane/70% methanol partition system partitions into the butanol phase of the butanol/water solvent system. For example, only about 57 mg is present in the butanol phase from the butanol/water partitioning from a starting residue of 772 mg (Fig. 2). Obviously, it is far easier to isolate the free ecdysteroids from 57 mg than from 772 mg.

Other solvent partition systems that have enabled removal of more apolar material are hexane/acetonitrile (Holman and Meola, 1978) and chloroform/water (Koolman, 1980). The chloroform/water system enables recovery of 99% of ecdysone in the aqueous phase, which would also contain the ecdysteroid conjugates if present. This system has been successfully used in the isolation and identification of ecdysonoic and 20-hydroxyecdysonoic acids from the aqueous phase (Lafont *et al.*, 1983). The ecdysteroid, ponasterone A (25-deoxy-20-hydroxyecdysone), however, partitions equally into both phases (Lafonte *et al.*, 1982); so a disadvantage of the chloroform/water system is that ecdysteroids that are less polar than ecdysone would not be completely extracted into the aqueous phase. Another disadvantage of this system is that a considerable quantity of material is not soluble in either the chloroform or the aqueous phase and thus could entrap free ecdysteroids. Yet this aqueous phase from the chloroform/water partition should still lend itself to further purification via an Amberlite XAD-2 resin column (Fig. 2; see Section III.B), which we have successfully used in purifying ecdysteroid conjugates to remove as much as 97% of the impurities (Thompson *et al.*, 1985a).

B. Purification with an XAD-2 Column and Sep-Pak Cartridges

As mentioned earlier, one of the major difficulties encountered in isolating and identifying ecdysteroid conjugates is that the conjugates are water-soluble and are therefore often accompanied by large quantities of other water-soluble material from insect tissue. The Amberlite resins, XAD-2 and XAD-16, which have been used in columns or in batch operations to adsorb soluble organic compounds from aqueous streams, have also been used in ecdysteroid research. The resin, Amberlite XAD-2, was first used as the stationary phase to separate ecdysteroids by reversed-phase HPLC, and even crude methanol extracts from plants could be analyzed by this method (Imai *et al.*, 1968; Hori, 1969). In an HPLC analysis of ecdysteroids using Amberlite XAD-2 and a linear gradient of 20 to 70% ethanol, a series of ecdysteroids were separated in 6–11 h (Nakanishi, 1971a). The author speculated that elution times could be shortened greatly by improved instrumentation and packing materials. XAD-2 resin was also used in a medium-scale separation of the plant ecdysteroids, ponasterone A and C (Nakanishi, 1971b).

We have used XAD-2 resin with excellent results to adsorb ecdysteroid conjugates obtained from the aqueous phase of our butanol/water partition system for eggs and pupae of the tobacco hornworm (Thompson *et al.*, 1985a, 1987a,c). As indicated in Fig. 2, as much as 97% of the impurities were removed from an XAD-2 column with water, followed by the elution of the partially purified ecdysteroid conjugates with (95%) ethanol. Radioassay revealed that all of the radioactive material eluted in the ethanol eluate.

A great advantage of XAD-2 resin is that it can be used again and again without any apparent loss of efficiency. Simply, after removal of the adsorbed conjugates with ethanol, the column can be reconditioned with water or with 5% sodium chloride solution, followed by back-flushing with water to remove colloidal particles; it is then ready for reuse.

Sep-Pak chromatography is a quick, simple, and effective method for cleaning biological samples prior to analysis of free and conjugated ecdysteroids by HPLC (Watson and Spaziani, 1982; Lafont *et al.*, 1982; Isaac *et al.*, 1982). Evaluation of this procedure for ecdysteroid analysis has been presented for a C_{18} Sep-Pak (Lafont *et al.*, 1982). In our hands, a C_{18} Sep-Pak fractionation of the XAD-2 ethanol eluant removed 85% of the remaining impurities; the polar metabolites (20-hydroxyecdysonoic acid and its 3α-epimer) and the ecdysteroid conjugates (26-hydroxyecdysone 2- and 26-phosphates, and 26-hydroxyecdysone 22-glucoside) were eluted in fractions 3 and 4 with 30% MeOH (Fig. 2).

The butanol phase, from the butanol/water partitioning, is also amenable to purification by Sep-Pak fractionation. Free ecdysteroids, including the very polar

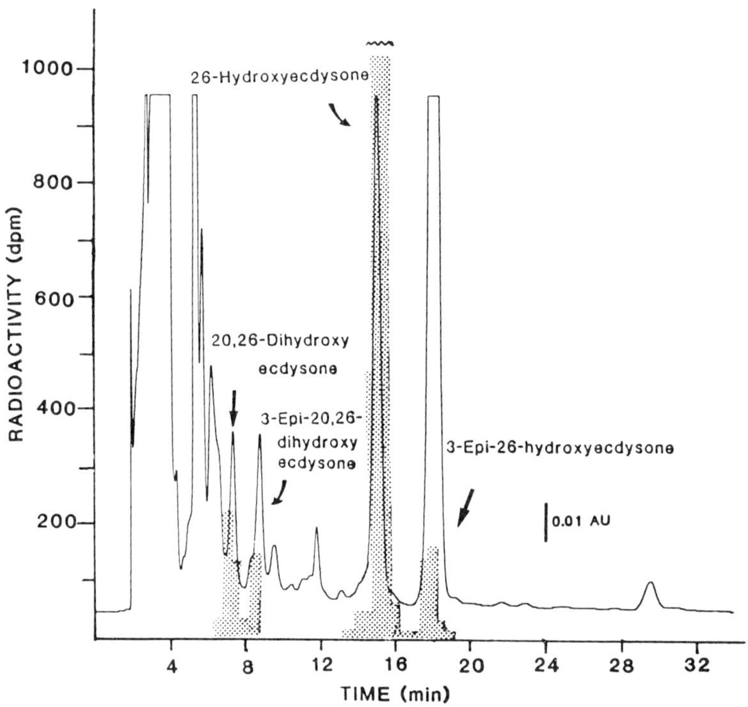

Figure 4 Reversed-phase HPLC trace (UV) and radioassay analysis of partially purified free ecdysteroids from 72–88-h-old tobacco hornworm eggs. Column conditions: Shandon ODS-Hypersil column (250 mm × 4.6 mm i.d., 5-μm particle size); eluted isocratically with methanol/water (38:62) at a flow rate 1.0 ml/min; column temperature 33°C; detection, UV at 254 nm. Shaded areas indicate radioactivity; 0.5-ml fractions were collected for monitoring radioactivity.

20,26-dihydroxyecdysone, 26-hydroxyecdysone 22-glucoside, and 5-pregnen-3β,20β-diol di- and triglucosides, were chromatographed over a silica Sep-Pak, and ten fractions were collected as shown in Fig. 3. Following thin-layer chromatography (TLC) analysis and radioassay (Thompson *et al.*, 1987a), fractions 1–3 and 4–10 (Fig. 3) were combined and each group refractionated via C_{18} Sep-Pak. After TLC analysis and radioassay of the fractions, the free and conjugated ecdysteroid fractions were further analyzed by reversed-phase high-performance liquid chromatography (RP-HPLC) and ion-suppression reversed-phase high-performance liquid chromatography (IS-RP-HPLC), respectively. The radioassay and RP-HPLC analysis of 2% of combined fractions 3 and 4 gave the free ecdysteroid profile shown in Fig. 4. Similarly, the radioassay and IS-RP-HPLC analysis of 2% of the combined C_{18} Sep-Pak fractions 3 and 4 (Fig. 2) and fractions 2 and 3 (Fig. 3) gave the polar metabolite and ecdysteroid conjugate profile of 72–88-h-old tobacco hornworm eggs (Fig. 5). Both profiles attest to the efficiency of Sep-Pak in the overall purification procedure (Figs. 2 and 3).

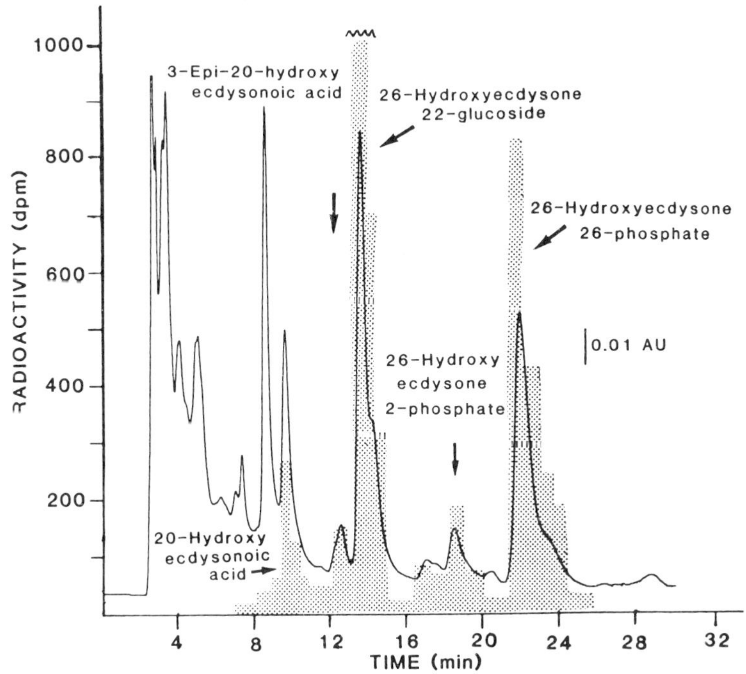

Figure 5 Ion-suppression-RP-HPLC trace (UV) and radioassay analysis of partially purified ecdysteroid acids and conjugates from 72–88-h-old tobacco hornworm eggs. Column conditions: Shandon MOS-Hypersil column (250 mm × 4.6 mm i.d., 5-μm particle size); eluted isocratically with 26% methanol in 30-mM aqueous NaH_2PO_4 solution (pH5) at a flow rate of 1.0 ml/min; column temperature 33°C; detection, UV at 254 nm. Shaded areas indicate radioactivity; 0.5-ml fractions were collected for monitoring radioactivity.

Fractionation of free and conjugated ecdysteroids using C_{18} Sep-Pak, however, does not always give reproducible results. When the solvent system for the C_{18} Sep-Pak in Fig. 3 is used, 26-hydroxyecdysone and 20,26-dihydroxyecdysone may be eluted completely with 30% methanol, or some of the material may be eluted with 40% methanol. When ecdysone and 20-hydroxyecdysone are applied to a C_{18} Sep-Pak and then eluted with 5 ml each of 30, 60, and 100% methanol, the ecdysteroids are eluted with 60% methanol (Thompson *et al.*, 1985c; Weirich, 1985; Weirich *et al.*, 1986). The 26-hydroxyecdysone 2- and 26-phosphates are also eluted from the C_{18} Sep-Pak in 30 and 40% methanol fractions (Fig. 2). The use of a C_{18} Sep-Pak, however, may be manipulated according to one's need. For example, to purify the ecdysteroids released by enzymatic hydrolyis of conjugates from impurities present in the incubation medium, the sample was applied to a C_{18} Sep-Pak and eluted successively with 5 ml of 20% methanol and 7 ml of 80% methanol. The 80% methanol fraction contained all of the ecdysteroids and could be directly analyzed by RP-HPLC (Scalia and Morgan, 1982). Interestingly, the 26-hydroxyecdysone 22-glucoside is consistently eluted from a C_{18} Sep-Pak with 30% methanol and 5-pregnen-3β,20β-diol triglucoside with 60% methanol. Thus, the C_{18} Sep-Pak fractionation should be monitored by high-performance TLC, as well as by HPLC, rather than assuming that the free or conjugated ecdysteroid will be eluted in a specific fraction. Our work included both radiolabled ecdysteroids and a greater quantity of labeled 5-pregnen-3β,20β-diol di- and triglucoside, which did create somewhat of a purification problem. However, high-performance TLC enabled the detection and development of a method for the removal of these polar nonecdysteroids.

IV. HIGH-PERFORMANCE LIQUID CHROMATOGRAPHY

In the initial development of analytical methods for ecdysteroids, both normal-phase and reversed-phase HPLC were conducted. As more efficient HPLC column packings were developed, RP-HPLC became more widely used, and several excellent reviews and book chapters encompassing the HPLC methods have been written (Morgan and Wilson, 1980; Lafont *et al.*, 1980, 1981; Horn and Bergamasco, 1985; Rees and Isaac, 1985; Hetru *et al.*, 1985).

A. Free Ecdysteroids

The screening of insect extracts for free ecdysteroids in our work has presented several problems. First, samples of hemolymph or insect tissue may contain only picogram quantities of ecdysteroids, far below the detection limit of UV detectors. Second, nonecdysteroid, UV-absorbing material in the sample can obscure peaks of interest, regardless of how rigorously samples are purified prior to HPLC. Therefore, identifications that rely solely on the comparison of retention times of UV-absorbing compounds with those of known standards are usually inadequate and unreliable because nonecdysteroid compounds may co-elute or elute near the compounds of

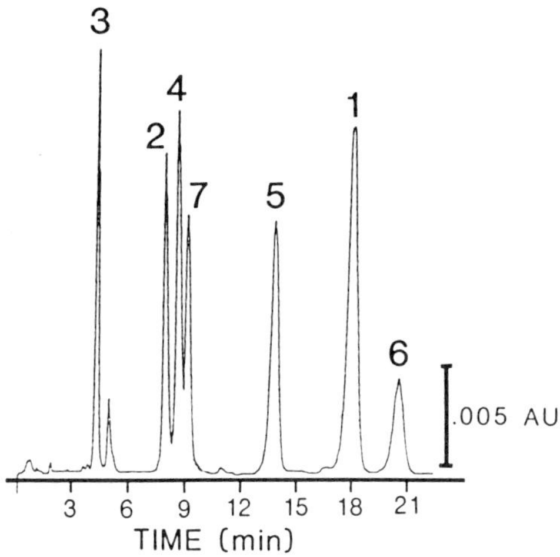

Figure 6 Separation of free ecdysteroids on an octyl (C_8) column (IBM; 150 mm × 4.6 mm i.d., 5-μm particle size). Mobile phase: methanol/water (35:65); flow rate of 1 ml/min; column temperature 33°C; detection, UV at 254 nm. Peaks: 3, 20.26-dihydroxyecdysone (4.26 mon); 2, 20-hydroxyecdysone (7.93 min); 4, 26-hydroxyecdysone (8.63 min); 7, 3-epi-20-hydroxyecdysone (9.13 min); 5, makisterone A (13.70 min); 1, ecdysone (17.93 min); 6, 3-epiecdysone (20.46 min). Numbers in parentheses represent actual retention times.

interest. These problems can be circumvented, to a large extent, by off-line sample analysis after HPLC by RIA with ecdysteroid-specific antisera (Borst and O'Connor, 1972, 1974; Horn *et al.*, 1976; Spindler *et al.*, 1978; Reum *et al.*, 1981; Soumoff *et al.*, 1981). Essential to using RIA to quantify picogram quantities of ecdysteroid and to distinguish immunoreactive areas of interest in a chromatogram is the clear resolution of individual ecdysteroid peaks on at least two different supports and solvent systems.

Reversed-phase HPLC, employing one of the better octyl (C_8) stationary phases and an unbuffered methanol/water solvent system, can be used to separate seven insect ecdysteroids ranging in polarity from 20,26-dihydroxyecdysone to 3-epiecdysone (Fig. 6). Total analysis time is usually less than 22 min. This particular chromatographic system is able to separate ecdysone and 20-hydroxyecdysone from their corresponding 3-epimers by about 2.5 and 1.2 min, respectively. This column, however, could not separate 3-dehydroecdysone and 3-epiecdysone in the solvent system of methanol and water. Normal-phase HPLC, however, on an amino propyl silica column employing the solvent system of dicholoroethane/methanol (96:6) provides good separation of ecdysone, 3-epiecdysone, and 3-dehydroecdysone (Dinan *et al.*, 1981). Since 3α-ecdysteroids have only marginal molting hormone activity and were first isolated from an *in vitro* enzyme system and from insect meconium, a known depot of metabolic waste, the 3α-epimers of certain ecdysteroids may actually represent deactivation products (Nigg *et al.*, 1974; Thompson *et al.*,

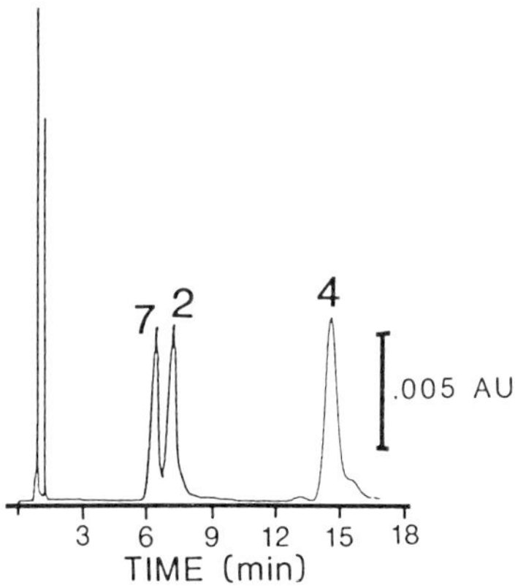

Figure 7 Separation of selected free ecdysteroids on a silica column (Rainin Microsorb; 150 mm × 4.6 mm i.d., 5-μm particle size). Mobile phase: methylene chloride/2-propanol/water (125:30:2); flow rate of 2 ml/min; column temperature 33°C; detection, UV at 254 nm. Peaks: 7, 3-epi-20-hydroxyecdysone (6.67 min); 2, 20-hydroxyecdysone (7.29 min); 4, 26-hydroxyecdysone (14.37 min). Numbers in parentheses represent actual retention times.

1974). Their adequate resolution by HPLC, therefore, is of utmost importance in any studies directed at ecdysteroid biosynthesis and metabolism.

The presence of 26-hydroxyecdysone in a sample, usually encountered in certain stages of *M. sexta*, can complicate reversed-phase fractionation of ecdysteroids due to the similarity of its chromatographic behavior to that of 20-hydroxyecdysone and 3-epi-20-hydroxyecdysone. This problem can be resolved by a subsequent HPLC fractionation on silica (Fig. 7) using a solvent system modified from Lafont *et al.* (1979) as 20-hydroxyecdysone elutes at 7.3 min and 26-hydroxyecdysone elutes at 14.4 min. Interestingly, 26-hydroxyecdysone elutes after 20-hydroxyecdysone on both reversed-phase and normal-phase supports.

Another problem is in obtaining RP-HPLC columns from manufacturers that all give similar good separations of ecdysteroids. Although a column supplied initially adequately separated the ecdysteroids (Fig. 8a), subsequent columns gave poor resolution and peak shape for some of the compounds tested (Fig. 8b). The separation of the pentahydroxy ecdysteroids, ecdysone, and 3-epiecdysone was essentially unchanged, but the peak shapes of the hexahydroxy compounds, 20-hydroxyecdysone, and makisterone A were noticeably altered. We can offer no explanation for this phenomenon. Solvents for all fractionations were from the same batch, and all conditions (temperature, flow rate, etc.) were identical. Furthermore, we found that the difference between the columns could not be attributed to the degree of endcapping. Thus, an investigator must exercise caution by testing individual manufacturer's octyl columns for their ability to resolve specific ecdysteroids, and not rely solely on the declared stationary support, because columns of supposedly identical specifications from a single source differed widely in their ability to separate four test ecdysteroids.

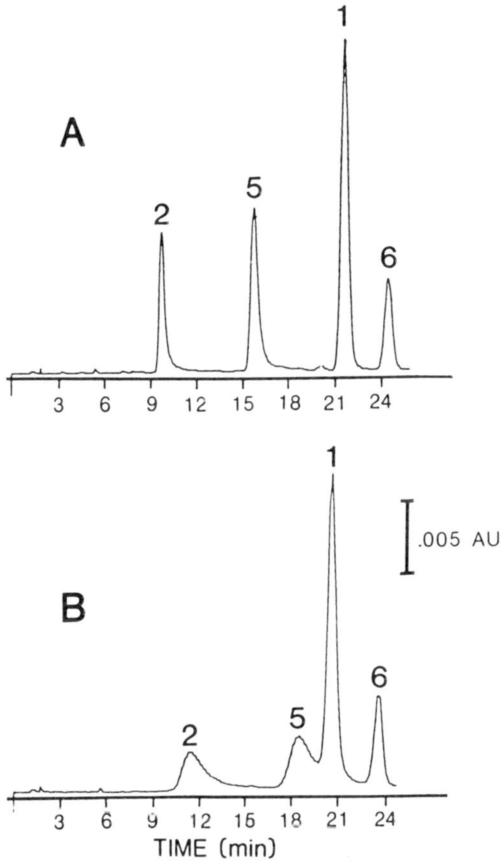

Figure 8 Chromatograms of selected free ecdysteroids fractionated on octyl (C_8) columns of different batch numbers from the same manufacturer. (a) Column conditions identical to Fig. 6., Initial column tested; (b) column type currently available.

In summary, we have employed two different chromatographic systems to separate free ecdysteroids of insects sufficiently so that subsequent analysis by RIA yields unambiguous results. The benefits of this reversed-phase system lie in its use of an unbuffered isocratic solvent system with an analysis time of less than 22 min. The use of an unbuffered mobile phase is particularly useful when samples are subjected to RIA because it eliminates a desalting step. Additionally, the extra time required for subsequent fractionation of certain ecdysteroids on silica is definitely offset by the ability to clearly resolve 20-hydroxyecdysone or 3-epi-20-hydroxyecdysone from 26-hydroxyecdysone. This subsequent fractionation on silica can also serve as an additional purification step prior to mass spectral analysis (Feldlaufer *et al.*, 1984).

B. Intact Ecdysteroid Conjugates and Polar Metabolites

The techniques of RP-HPLC are by far the most widely used techniques for the direct analysis and purification of the more polar ecdysteroid metabolites and ecdysteroid conjugates. To separate these ionic compounds by a reversed-phase system, one must make them behave as nonionic species with some lipophilic characteristics at acid pH (Waters Associates, 1976) or as ionic species paired with a strongly ionic counterion (neutral pH). These techniques are referred to as ion-suppression (IS) and ion-paired or paired-ion (PI) chromatography (PIC), respectively. Several PIC reagents are available, and the PIC reagent with a pH of about 3.5 in the mobile phase enables separation of weakly acidic compounds by ion suppression.

1. Paired-Ion Reversed-Phase HPLC

Perhaps one of the first applications of paired-ion reversed-phase HPLC (PI-RP-HPLC) to ecdysteroid research was the demonstration that certain polar metabolites of ecdysone in *Pieris brassicae* pupae exhibited different retention times in three different buffered solvent systems at pHs of 8.5, 5.7, and 2.0. Lowering the pH increased the retention times of the polar metabolites, yet the retention times of ecdysone and 20-hydroxyecdysone remained unchanged, and they eluted after the polar metabolites. By PI-RP-HPLC with cetylmethylammonium bromide as the counterion in the mobile phase, the retention times of polar metabolites are increased to the extent that they are eluted after ecdysone (Lafont *et al.*, 1980). These polar ecdysteroid metabolites were later identified as ecdysonoic and 20-hydroxyecdysonoic acid (Lafont *et al.*, 1983). Both acids were also isolated and purified from eggs of the locust *S. gregaria* and pupae of *Spodoptera littoralis*, by RP-HPLC with a linear gradient of methanol in 0.02 M sodium citrate buffer, pH 6.5, (1:9 v/v) changing to methanol in the same buffer (7:3 v/v) (Isaac *et al.*, 1983a).

A rapid and direct method for the determination of ecdysteroid conjugates by PI-RP-HPLC was demonstrated for 1- and 11-day-old eggs of *S. gregaria* using a gradient solvent system of methanol-water containing 0.4 M ammonium acetate and tetra-*n*-butylammonium acetate (Scalia and Morgan, 1982). The limit of detection was equivalent to approximately 10 ng of the conjugate at a sensitivity of 0.005 absorbance units. Following enzymatic hydrolysis, the aglycone moieties of the conjugates were identified as ecdysone, 2-deoxyecdysone, and 20-hydroxyecdysone. More recently the conjugated ecdysteroids from the yolk fraction of *S. gregaria* eggs at stages 5–7 were separated by PI-RP-HPLC (Scalia *et al.*, 1987).

PI-RP-HPLC on a radial compression C_{18} column has also been used to resolve five different conjugates from *M. sexta* midgut supernatant incubated with [^{3}H]ecdysone (Weirich *et al.*, 1986).

2. Ion-Suppression Reversed-Phase HPLC

Most of our studies of ecdysteroid conjugates have relied upon ion-suppression reversed-phase HPLC (IS-RP-HPLC). These analyses have been conducted on C_{18} μBondapak, IBM C_8, and Shandon MOS columns eluted isocratically with 26 to 30%

methanol in 0.025 or 0.03 M aqueous NaH_2PO_4 solution (pH 5). A typical IS-RP-HPLC trace (UV) and radioassay analysis of partially purified ecdysteroid conjugates and polar metabolites from 72–88-h-old eggs is shown in Fig. 5. In this chromatogram we have separated the 2- and 26-phosphates of 26-hydroxyecdysone, 20-hydroxyecdysonoic acid, and its 3α-epimer, and 26-hydroxyecdysone 22-glucoside. We have observed that the retention of the ecdysteroid conjugates increased with length of the bonded hydrocarbon chain and perhaps gives better resolution of conjugates that are difficult to separate, such as the 25R and 25S isomers of the ecdysteroid conjugates as indicated by the shoulders on the downside of the 26-hydroxyecdysone 22-glucoside and 26-phosphate peaks. We have found that after collection from IS-RP-HPLC, followed by removal of the Na_2HPO_4 by desalting on a C_{18} Sep-Pak, the conjugates could be directly analyzed by fast-atom bombardment (FAB) mass spectrometry and proton magnetic resonance (PMR) spectroscopy. For that reason we prefer IS-RP-HPLC to PI-RP-HPLC; furthermore, IS-RP-HPLC is less expensive and is less harsh on acidic conjugates. It should be mentioned that phosphate esters are rather unstable in the presence of amines. Because many RP-HPLC analyses are carried out in buffered solutions including Tris, and because tris (hydroxymethyl)aminomethane was identified as the cation associated with an ecdysteroid conjugate (Tsoupras *et al.*, 1982), we would suggest caution in using this buffer in isolation procedures and in HPLC analyses of ecdysteroid conjugates above room temperature. Although RP-HPLC could analyze for the ecdysteroid glucoside, the phosphates and acids exhibited variation in retention times and unsymmetrical peaks.

Two ecdysteroid mononucleotides, namely the 22-AMP ester of 2-deoxyecdysone and the 22-N^6-(isopentenyl)-AMP ester of ecdysone are easily isolated by RP-HPLC (Tsoupras *et al.*, 1982, 1983), yet the 22-phosphate of 2-deoxyecdysone is not separated from the 22-AMP of 2-deoxyecdysone by RP-HPLC (Sall *et al.*, 1983). It would be interesting to examine these two compounds by IS-RP-HPLC and PI-RP-HPLC.

In an impressive study with as little as 250 mg of eggs, the combination of IS-RP-HPLC and radioimmunoassay (RIA) employing two relatively nonspecific complementary antisera was used to identify and quantify both free and conjugated ecdysteroids and other polar metabolites during embryogenesis in the tobacco hornworm (Warren *et al.*, 1986). Although the method did not permit the authors to identify the 3α-ecdysteroids, they observed a new glucoside conjugate of 26-hydroxyecdysone in the developing eggs, which they subsequently isolated from 80 g of newly hatched larvae. This conjugate was also isolated and unequivocally identified from newly hatched larvae as 26-hydroxyecdysone 22-glucoside by Thompson *et al.* (1987a).

The combination of IS-RP-HPLC and an ion-exchange HPLC has afforded the isolation and identification of several conjugates and polar metabolites from eggs of *S. gregaria* including 3-acetylecdysone 2-phosphate and the 22-phosphate esters of ecdysone, 2-deoxyecdysone, 20-hydroxyecdysone, and 2-deoxy-20-hydroxyecdysone (Isaac *et al.*, 1983b, 1984).

V. PHYSICOCHEMICAL METHODS OF CHARACTERIZATION

A. Fourier Transform Nuclear Magnetic Resonance

The proton magnetic resonance (PMR) spectra of sterols are usually complex because of the presence of a large number of aliphatic and alicyclic methylene groups. Nevertheless, studies of PMR spectra of steroids have shown that the three proton signals of the methyl groups, resulting from the equivalence of the protons, were the most pronounced and sharpest peaks in the spectra, being above the background of methylene and methine protons in the regions of 0.5–1.5 ppm (Shoolery and Rogers, 1958). Similarly, the PMR spectra of free ecdysteroids, usually obtained in deuteropyridine, are complex, but the methyl groups of ecdysteroids appear as sharp peaks in the spectra and provide valuable information concerning their structures, especially with respect to the position of various hydroxyl groups. Since the ecdysteroids of insects, as well as those of many plants, differ from each other by only the number and/or position of hydroxyl groups, all of the insect ecdysteroids and a large number of plant ecdysteroid structures could be derived simply by mass spectral analyses and a comparison of the chemical shifts of the methyl signals in their PMR spectra (Horn, 1971; Horn and Bergamasco, 1985) with those of ecdysone, the structure of which has been established by X-ray diffraction (Huber and Hoppe, 1965).

With the advent of newer Fourier transform instruments, which operate at or above 250 MHz, it is possible even to obtain good spectra with microgram quantities of ecdysteroids in deutero solvents, in which the ecdysteroid is only sparingly soluble, and to observe chemical shifts of methyl resonances of less than 0.01 ppm. The —CH—OH signals at C-2, C-3, C-22 and the —CH_2—OH signal at C-26 can readily be assigned in spectra recorded with these instruments. This has enabled assignment of substitutents at any of these positions and has thus enhanced the structural elucidation of ecdysteroid conjugates. The ^{13}C-NMR spectra can also be obtained; however, the quantity of sample required is usually larger.

In the first identification of two ecdysteroid phosphate conjugates to be isolated, the PMR spectrum of one of the conjugates recorded at 250 MHz and obtained in CD_3OD was compared with the spectrum of ecdysone. This spectrum was similar to that of ecdysone except the 22-H (4.20 ppm) and 21-methyl signals (1.18 and 1.19 ppm) were shifted downfield from that of ecdysone in the conjugate. For ecdysone, the corresponding signals were at 3.61 ppm (22-H) and at 0.94 and 0.97 ppm (d, 21-3H). These data, together with mass spectral data, which will be discussed later, indicated that the phosphate moiety was at C-22 and that the conjugate is ecdysone 22-phosphate (Isaac *et al.*, 1982). The spectrum of the second conjugate recorded at 360 MHz was compared with that of 2-deoxyecdysone, and it differed significantly only in that the 22-H and 21-3H signals in the conjugates were shifted downfield as in the case of ecdysone conjugate. The data indicated that the second conjugate was 2-deoxyecdysone 22-phosphate (Isaac *et al.*, 1982).

The structures of 22-phosphate esters of 20-hydroxyecdysone and 2-deoxy-20-hydroxyecdysone were derived in a similar manner (Isaac *et al.*, 1983b). The chemical shifts (ppm) of the characteristic protons of these four ecdysteroid phosphates and their corresponding free ecdysteroids were compiled and compared. The ^{13}C-NMR chemical shifts are also reported for C-2, C-3, C-14, C-20, C-22, and C-25 of these compounds.

The location of the conjugate moiety of the major ecdysteroid conjugate in young eggs and embryos of *L. migratoria* was determined by ^{13}C-NMR. All of the signals of 2-deoxyecdysone except that of C-22, which was shifted downfield by 5 ppm, were identical. These data, including the fact that C-20 and C-23 signals were shifted 2 ppm up field, placed the conjugate moiety at C-22. The conjugate was identified as the 22-adenosine monophosphoric ester of 2-deoxyecdysone (Tsoupras *et al.*, 1982). Similarly, the 22-N^6-(isopentenyl)-adenosine monophosphoric ester of ecdysone was identified as a maternal conjugate in newly laid eggs of *L. migratoria* by mass spectrometry and PMR, ^{13}C and ^{31}P NMR (Tsoupras *et al.*, 1983). The use of PMR spectroscopy enhanced the identification of the following conjugates from developing eggs of *S. gregaria*: 3-acetyl-20-hydroxyecdysone 2-phosphate, 3-epi-2-deoxyecdysone 3-phosphate, 3-acetylecdysone 22-phosphate, and 2-acetylecdysone 22-phosphate (Isaac and Rees, 1984).

The PMR spectra of three ecdysteroid conjugates, isolated from developing *M. sexta* eggs and 0–1-h-old larvae, and 26-hydroxyecdysone recorded at 400 MHz in D_2O are compared (Figs. 9 and 10). There are certain obvious differences in each conjugate spectrum in the —CH—OH or —CH_2—OH region when compared with that of 26-hydroxcyecdysone. The multiplicity of peaks in the region of 3.25 to 3.91 ppm in the spectrum of 26-hydroxyecdysone 22-glucoside (which are absent in the spectrum of 26-hydroxyecdysone; see Fig. 9) is due to protons of the glucose unit. We had suggested that the two doublets centered at 3.905 and 3.872 ppm in the spectrum of the conjugate could be the C-22 proton signal (Thompson *et al.*, 1987a). We now, however, have evidence that the C-22 proton of the glucoside conjugate is in a region similar to that of the C-22 proton of 26-hydroxyecdysone. Comparisons of the spectra of the conjugate and 26-hydroxyecdysone indicate that, of all the methyl resonances, only the C-21, which occurred as a doublet at 0.953 and 0.938 ppm in the spectrum of 26-hydroxyecdysone, was shifted farther downfield to 0.962 and 0.947 ppm, respectively, whereas the resonances for the C-2, C-3, and C-26 protons were not appreciably shifted in the conjugate. The PMR spectrum indicates that the glucose moiety of the ecdysteroid conjugate is at C-22 and the conjugate is 26-hydroxyecdysone 22-glucoside (Thompson *et al.*, 1987a).

The major differences between the PMR spectra of 26-hydroxyecdysone 2-phosphate and of 26-hydroxyecdysone is that the C-2 signal in the ecdysteroid conjugate appears as a broad peak centered at 4.30 ppm and is thus 0.31 ppm farther downfield than in the spectrum of 26-hydroxyecdysone, where it occurred as a doublet at 4.01 and 3.98 ppm, centered at 3.995 ppm (Fig. 10). Similarly, the C-3 proton signal in the ecdysteroid conjugate also appeared 0.16 ppm farther downfield than in the spectrum of 26-hydroxyecdysone. Thus, the PMR spectrum indicates that

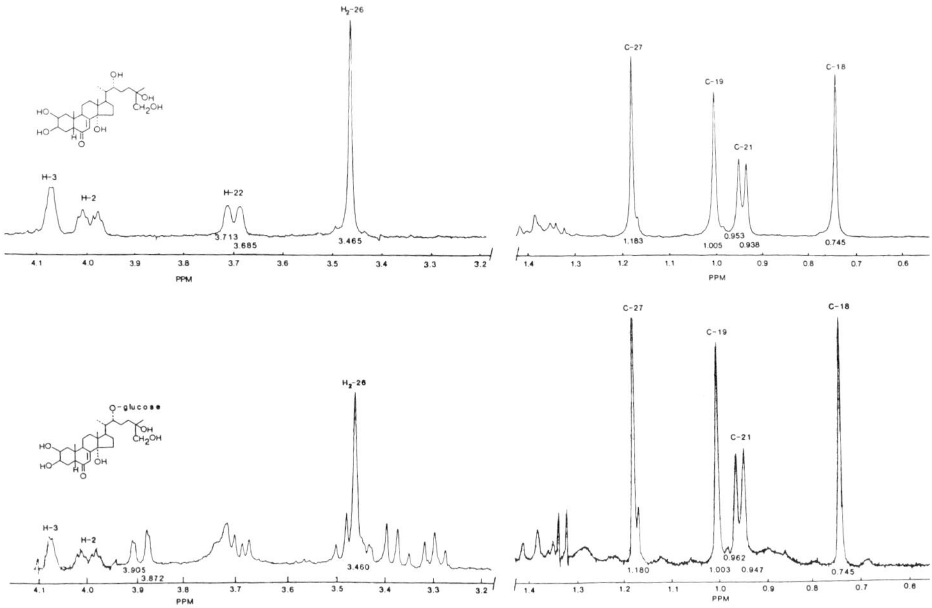

Figure 9 Partial PMR spectra of 26-hydroxyecdysone and 26-hydroxyecdysone 22-glucoside taken in D_2O with a Bruker 400 MHz instrument. Spectra were referenced to 3-trimethylsilyl-2,2,3,3-tetradeuteropropionic acid.

the phosphate group of the ecdysteroid conjugate is at C-2 (Thompson *et al.*, 1987b). Comparisons of spectra of ecdysone and ecdysone 2-phosphate taken in CD_3OD show that the C-2 and C-3 protons of the conjugate had similarly shifted downfield by 0.52 and 0.22 ppm, respectively (Isaac *et al.*, 1984).

In the identification of the first ecdysteroid conjugate to be isolated from tobacco hornworm eggs, 26-hydroxyecdysone 26-phosphate, it was obvious from the PMR spectrum that the phosphate moeity was at C-26. The C-26 proton signal of $—CH_2—OH$ in the ecdysteroid conjugate appeared as a doublet at 3.710 and 3.698, which is centered at 3.70 ppm and is thus 0.24 ppm farther downfield than in the spectrum of 26-hydroxyecdysone, where it occurred at 3.468 ppm (Fig. 10). It is apparent that the phosphate moiety affects the resonances at or close to C-26 as indicated by the slight, though very obvious, chemical shift for the C-27 methyl, which is 0.03 ppm farther downfield in the spectrum of the conjugate than in that of 26-hydroxyecdysone (Thompson *et al.*, 1985a).

The unequivocal identification of ecdysonoic and 20-hydroxyecdysonoic acids from developing eggs of *S. gregaria* and pupae of *S. littoralis* was determined by PMR and mass spectrometry. The major difference between the PMR spectra of ecdysone and ecdysonoic acid is that the 26-methyl signal is not observed in the acid and the 27-methyl signal has shifted downfield to 1.33 ppm from that of 1.20 ppm in ecdysone

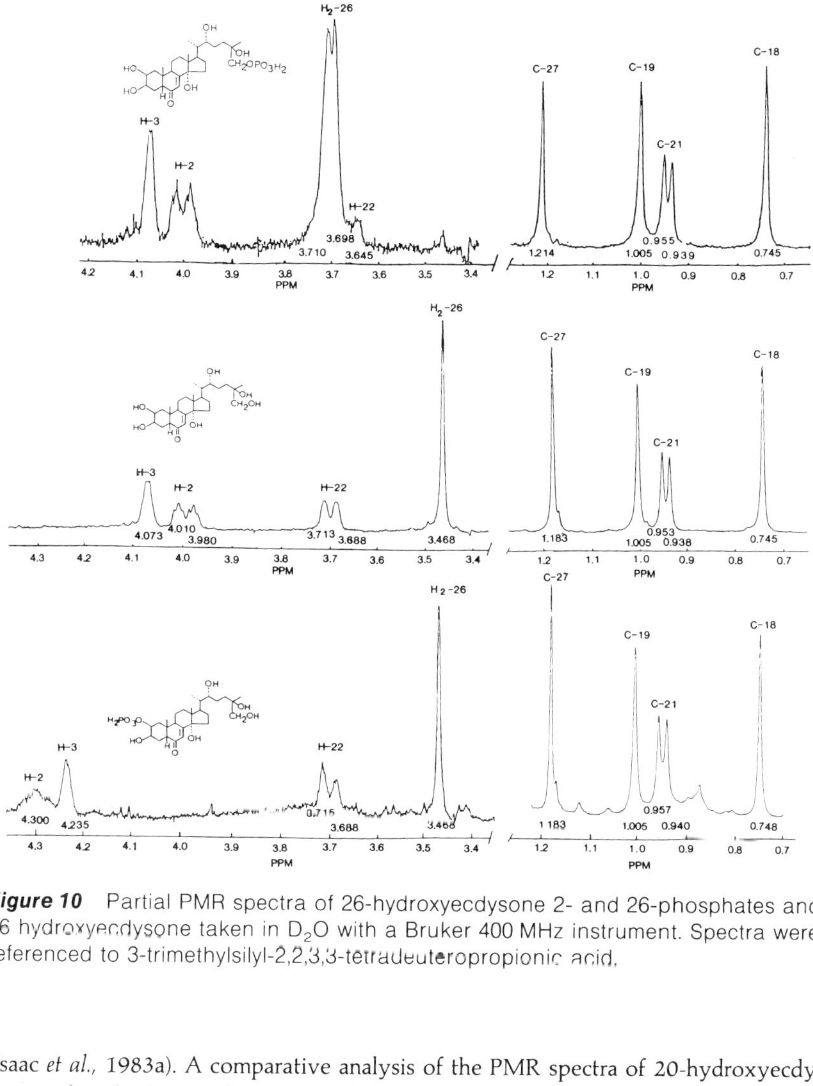

Figure 10 Partial PMR spectra of 26-hydroxyecdysone 2- and 26-phosphates and 26 hydroxyecdysone taken in D_2O with a Bruker 400 MHz instrument. Spectra were referenced to 3-trimethylsilyl-2,2,3,3-tetradeuteropropionic acid.

(Isaac *et al.,* 1983a). A comparative analysis of the PMR spectra of 20-hydroxyecdysone and 20-hydroxyecdysonoic acid showed similar results (Isaac *et al.,* 1983b).

From these examples it is obvious that if the ecdysteroid conjugates can be isolated, the location of the conjugate moiety can readily be determined by PMR spectroscopy.

B. Mass Spectrometry

Mass spectral analyses can reveal considerable information about side-chain and molecular structure. Electron-ionization (EI) mass spectra of the ecdysteroids are characterized by numerous ions, 18 mass units apart, that result from successive losses of water from the molecule. Initially it was often difficult to obtain the molecular ions; nevertheless, the mass spectra provided valuable information about the molecular weights and the number of hydroxyl groups in the molecule. In ecdysteroids, such as 26-hydroxyecdysone, that contain a 20,22-vicinal diol function, side-chain cleavage generally occurs at this location, as indicated in the spectrum by prominent peaks at *m/z* 363 (M-117) and 345 (M-117-18). These side-chain fragments are further indicated by major peaks at *m/z* 99 and 81 (Hampshire and Horn, 1966) and have been tabulated for a number of ecdysteroids (Nakanishi, 1971a).

Ammonia and methane chemical-ionization (CI) or desorption-chemical-ionization (DCI) mass spectral analyses of ecdysteroids provide not only a means for unambiguous determination of molecular weight but also information about the nature of the steroid nucleus and the side-chain portions of the molecule (Lusby *et al.*, 1987). Although DCI mass spectrometry of ecdysteroid conjugates give ions characteristic of the respective ecdysteroids, it does not give ions indicative of intact molecules or of the inorganic conjugate moiety. On the other hand, ammonia DCI of 26-hydroxyecdysone 22-glucoside, the major conjugate of 0–1-h-old tobacco hornworm larvae, confirmed its identity by exhibiting major peaks at *m/z* 660 (13%, $M + NH_4$), 642 (84%, $M + NH_4\text{-}H_2O$), 625 (100%, $M + H\text{-}H_2O$), 480 (91%, $M\text{-}C_6H_{10}O_5$), 464 (65%) and 446 (56%). The peaks at *m/z* 642 and 480 are conicidentally equivalent to the molecular ions of the ecdysteroid conjugate and ecdysteroid, respectively (Thompson *et al.*, 1987a).

The ecdysteroid conjugates that contain an inorganic conjugate moiety do not give an ion characteristic of the intact molecule by EI or DCI mass spectrometry due to their thermal lability. However, when analyzed by fast-atom bombardment (FAB) mass spectrometry, which is particularly suitable for relatively nonvolatile and thermally labile compounds (Barber *et al.*, 1981), the negative-ion mass spectrum of the conjugate will show a $[M\text{-}H]^-$ ion (Rees and Isaac, 1985). Thus, negative-ion FAB mass spectra of 22-phosphates of ecdysone and 2-deoxyecdysone, the first ecdysteroid phosphate conjugates to be isolated from an insect, gave major ions at *m/z* 543 and 527, respectively. These [M-H] ions indicate molecular weights of 544 for ecdysone 22-phosphate and 528 for 2-deoxyecdysone 22-phosphate (Isaac *et al.*, 1982). Small $[M\text{-}H]^-$ peaks for the monosodium salts, which are commonly observed in negative-ion FAB mass spectra, were also observed in the spectra of the 22-phosphates of ecdysone and 2-deoxyecdysone at *m/z* 565 and 549, respectively.

The negative-ion FAB mass spectra of the 22-phosphate esters of ecdysone, 2-deoxyecdysone, 20-hydroxyecdysone, and 2-deoxy-20-hydroxyecdysone, in addition to the distinct $[M\text{-}H]^-$ ions, all showed major peaks at *m/z* 79 and 97 that correspond to PO_3^- and $H_2PO_4^-$ ions, respectively (Isaac *et al.*, 1983b). In contrast, sulfate esters of sterols yield large peaks at *m/z* 80 (SO_3^-) and 97 (HSO_4^-) (Rose *et al.*, 1983). These very large peaks in negative-ion FAB mass spectra are therefore highly diagnostic of the conjugate moiety.

Similarly, negative-ion FAB mass spectra of the 2- and 26-phosphates of 26-hydroxyecdysone show $[M\text{-}H]^-$ ion peaks at *m/z* 559 and base peaks at *m/z*

79 (PO_3^-) and the $H_2PO_4^-$ ions at *m/z* 97 (Thompson *et al.*, 1985a, 1987b). Even negative-ion FAB mass spectra of the 3-acetylecdysone 2-phosphate, which is unstable when stored at $-20°C$, and ecdysone 2-phosphate show distinct $[M\text{-}H]^-$ ions at *m/z* 585 and 543, respectively, and large peaks at *m/z* 79 and 97 (Isaac *et al.*, 1984).

Ammonia DCI mass spectrometry was successfully used in the first identification of 20-hydroxyecdysonoic acid as its methyl ester (Lafont *et al.*, 1983). The mass spectrum showed major ions at *m/z* 525 (MH^+), 510 ($MH^+ + NH_3$-MeOH), base peak at *m/z* 493 (MH^+-MeOH), and other peaks, as well as peaks indicating side-chain cleavage at C-20 and C-22 and loss of one molecule of water at *m/z* 363 and 345, respectively. Negative-ion FAB mass spectra of 20-hydroxyecdysonoic acid and ecdysonoic acids showed abundant $[M\text{-}H]^-$ ions at *m/z* 509 and 493, respectively, indicating their molecular weights of 510 and 494 (Isaac *et al.*, 1983a). The negative-ion FAB mass spectrum of the methyl esters of 20-hydroxyecdysonoic acid and ecdysonoic acid gave prominent ions at *m/z* 491 $[M\text{-}H\text{-}MeOH]^-$ and 475 $[M\text{-}H\text{-}MeOH]^-$, respectively. Less abundant ions indicative of $[M\text{-}H]^-$ ions were observed for both compounds at *m/z* 523 and 507, respectively.

Thus, although NMR spectroscopy can readily determine the location of the conjugate moiety and often the nature of the conjugate, mass spectrometry confirms the nature of the conjugate and gives valuable information about the molecular weight as well as structural features of the ecdysteroid conjugates. The combination of NMR and mass spectrometry can most often lead to the unequivocal identification of free ecdysteroids, polar metabolites, and ecdysteroid conjugates.

VI. CONCLUSIONS

Methods of extraction, separation, and isolation of free and conjugated ecdysteroids from insect tissues have evolved to a stage in which it is not overly difficult to analyze, isolate, and identify them. Better methods of IS-RP-HPLC or PI-RP-HPLC, however, are needed to separate the 25R and 25S isomers of the ecdysonoic and 20-hydroxyecdysonoic acids and of the conjugates of 26-hydroxyecdysone, even though one isomer usually predominates. In the isolation and analyses of ecdysteroids, we have progressed from working with quantities of a few kilograms of insect tissue to just a few grams. Also, bioassay methods of analyses have been replaced by other methods that are often more sensitive. With present-day instrumentation and techniques, both free and conjugated ecdysteroids are routinely isolated and characterized from 10–20 g of insect tissues. The combination of RP-HPLC/RIA and IS-RP-HPLC/RIA permits the quantitation of free ecdysteroids and of both free and conjugated ecdysteroids, respectively, with less than 1 g of embryonic tissues. Although RP-HPLC/RIA, PI-RP-HPLC/RIA, and IS-RP-HPLC/RIA have proven to be very valuable tools, each is useful only to the point of analyzing for compounds of known cross-reactivity or for detecting new compounds (and perhaps, eventually, for identification or characterization). A tremendous amount of effort may be required to isolate and identify new ecdysteroid conjugates by RP-HPLC/RIA to the point of purification, at which time they can be analyzed directly or monitored by RP-HPLC. However, having labeled cholesterol or campesterol converted to labeled free and conjugated C_{27} and C_{28} ecdysteroids (known ecdysteroids of insects), respectively, has afforded us the opportunity to isolate ecdysteroids and follow their fate at any period of an insect's life cycle. Normal-phase and reversed-phase HPLC have also enabled excellent purification of these compounds so that their final characterization can be achieved by NMR and mass spectrometry, as described in this review. Thus, with present-day instrumentation and techniques, the characterization or structural elucidation of new, free and conjugated ecdysteroids is limited only by the effort and ingenuity we put into isolating these biologically important compounds from insects. Yet, instrumentation and techniques will continue to be improved because we, as scientists, are continuously searching for faster and better ways of expediting our research.

REFERENCES

Barber, M., Bordoli, R. S., Sedgwick, R. D., and Tyler, A. N. (1981). Fast atom bombardment of solids as an ion source in mass spectrometry. *Nature (London)* **293**, 270–275.

Becker, E., and Plagge, E. (1939). Uber das pupariumbildung auslosende hormon der fliegen. *Biol. Zentralbl.* **59**, 326–341.

Borst, D. W., and O'Connor, J. D. (1972). Arthropod molting hormone radioimmune assay. *Science* **178**, 418–419.

Borst, D. W., and O'Connor, J. D. (1974). Trace analysis of ecdysones by gas-liquid chromatography, radioimmunoassay and bioassay. *Steroids* **24**, 637–657.

Butenandt, A., and Karlson, P. (1954). Uber die isolierung eines metamorphose-hormone der insekten in kristallisierten form. Z. *Naturforsch., B: Anorg. Chem., Org. Chem., Brochem., Brophys., Biol.* **9B**, 389–391.

Dinan, L. N., and Rees, H. H. (1981a). The identification and titres of conjugated and free ecdysteroids in developing ovaries and newly-laid eggs of *Schistercerca gregaria. J. Insect Physiol.* **27**, 51–58.

Dinan, L. N., and Rees, H. H. (1981b). Incorporation *in vivo* of [4-^{14}C]cholesterol into the conjugated ecdysteroids in ovaries and eggs of *Schistocerca gregaria. Insect Biochem.* **11**, 255–265.

Dinan, L. N., Donnahey, P. L., Rees, H. H., and Goodwin, T. (1981). High-performance liquid chromatography of ecdysteroids and their 3-epi, 3-dehydro and 26-hydroxy derivatives. *J. Chromatogr.* **205**, 139–145.

Feldlaufer, M. F., Lusby, W. R., Svoboda, J. A., and Thompson, M. J. (1984). Identification of 20-hydroxyecdysone and ecdysone from the pupa of the gypsy moth, *Lymantria dispar. Arch. Insect Biochem. Physiol.* **1**, 323–330.

Gibson, J. M., Isaac, R. E., Dinan, L. N., and Rees, H. H. (1984). Metabolism of [^{3}H]ecdysone in *Schistocerca gregaria*: Formation of ecdysteroid acids together with free and phosphorylated ecdysteroid acetates. *Arch. Insect Biochem. Physiol.* **1**, 385–407.

Hampshire, F., and Horn, D. H. S. (1966). Structure of crustecdysone, a crustacean moulting hormone. *J. Chem. Soc., Chem. Commun.* pp. 37–38.

Hetru, C., Luu, B., and Hoffmann, J. A. (1985). Ecdysone conjugates: Isolation and identification. *In* "Methods in Enzymology" (J. H. Law and H. C. Rilling, eds.), Vol. 111, pp. 411–419. Academic Press, Orlando, Florida.

Holman, G. M., and Meola, R. W. (1978). A high performance liquid chromatography method for the purification and analysis of insect ecdysones: Application to measurement of ecdysone titres during pupal-adult development of *Heliothis zea*. *Insect Biochem.* **8**, 275–278.

Hori, M. (1969). Automatic column chromatographic method for insect-moulting steroids. *Steroids* **14**, 33–46.

Horn, D. H. S. (1971). The ecdysones. *In* "Naturally Occurring Insecticides" (M. Jacobson and D. G. Crosby, eds.), pp. 333–459. Dekker, New York.

Horn, D. H. S., and Bergamasco, R. (1985). Chemistry of ecdysteroids. *In* "Comprehensive Insect Physiology, Biochemistry and Pharmacology" (G. A. Kerkut and L. I. Gilbert, eds.), Vol. 7, pp. 185–248. Pergamon, Oxford.

Horn, D. H. S. Wilkie, J. S., Sage, B. A., and O'Connor, J. D. (1976). A high affinity antiserium specific for the ecdysone nucleus. *J. Insect Physiol.* **22**, 901–905.

Hsiao, T. H., and Hsiao, C. (1979). Ecdysteroids in the ovary and the egg of the greater wax moth. *J. Insect Physiol.* **25**, 45–52.

Huber, R., and Hoppe, W. (1965). Zur chemie des ecdysons. VII. Die kristall-und molekulstrukturanalyse des insektenverpuppungs hormons ecdyson mit der automatisierten faltmolkulmethode. *Chem. Ber.* **98**, 2403–2424.

Imai, S. Hori, M., Fujioka, S., Murata, E., Goto, M., and Nakanishi, K. (1968). Insect hormones. VIII. Isolation of four new phytoecdysones, makisterone A, B, C, D and the structure of makisterone A, a C_{28} steroid. *Tetrahedron Lett.* **36**, 3883–3886.

Isaac, R. E., and Rees, H. H. (1984). Isolation and identification of ecdysteroid phosphates and acetylecdysteroid phosphates from developing eggs of the locust, *Schistocerca gregaria*. *Biochem. J.* **221**, 459–464.

Isaac, R. E., and Rees, H. H. (1985). Metabolism of maternal ecdysteroid-22-phosphates in developing embryos of the desert locust, *Schistocerca gregaria*. *Insect Biochem.* **15**, 65–72.

Isaac, R. E., Rose, M. E., Rees, H. H., and Goodwin, T. W. (1982). Identification of ecdysone-22-phosphate and 2-deoxyecdysone-22-phosphate in eggs of the desert locust *Schistocerca gregaria* by fast atom bombardment mass spectrometry and N.M.R. spectroscopy. *J. Chem. Soc., Chem. Commun.* pp. 249–251.

Isaac, R. E., Milner, N. P., and Rees, H. H. (1983a). Identification of ecdysonoic acid and 20-hydroxyecdysonoic acid isolated from developing eggs of *Schistocerca gregaria* and pupae of *Spodoptera littoralis*. *Biochem. J.* **213**, 261–265.

Isaac, R. E., Rose, M. E., Rees, H. H., and Goodwin, T. W. (1983b). Identification of the 22-phosphate esters of ecdysone, 2-deoxyecdysone, 20-hydroxyecdysone and 2-deoxy-20-hydroxyecdysone from newly laid eggs of the desert locust, *Schistocerca gregaria*. *Biochem. J.* **213**, 533–541.

Isaac, R. E., Desmond, H. P., and Rees, H. H. (1984). Isolation and identification of 3-acetylecdysone 2-phosphate, a metabolite of ecdysone, from developing eggs of *Schistocerca gregaria*. *Biochem. J.* **217**, 239–243.

Karlson, P., and Hoffmeister, H. (1963). Zur biogenese des ecdysons. I. Umwandlung von cholesterin in ecdyson. *Hoppe-Seyler's Z. Physiol. Chem.* **331**, 298–300.

Koolman, J. (1980). Analysis of ecdysteroids by fluorometry. *Insect Biochem.* **10**, 381–386.

Lafont, R., Somme-Martin, G., and Chambet, J.-C. (1979). Separation of ecdysteroids by using high-pressure liquid chromatography of microparticulate supports. *J. Chromatogr.* **170**, 185–194.

Lafont, R., Somme-Martin, G., Mauchamp, B., Maume, B. F., and Delbecque, J.-P. (1980). Analysis of ecdysteroid by high-performance liquid chromatography and coupled gas-liquid chromatography-mass spectrometry. *In* "Progress in Ecdysone Research" (J. A. Hoffmann, ed.), pp. 45–68. Elsevier/North-Holland, Amsterdam.

Lafont, R., Beydon, P., Mauchamp, B., Somme-Martin, G., Andrian-Jafintrimo, M., and Krien, P. (1981). Recent progress in ecdysteroids analytical methods. *In* "Regulation of Insect Development and Behavior" (F. Sehnal, A. Zabza, J. J. Menn, and B. Cymborowski, eds.), pp. 125–144. Wroclaw Tech. Univ. Press, Wroclaw, Poland.

Lafont, R., Pennetier, J.-L., Andrianjafintrimo, M., Claret, J., Modde, J.-F., and Blais, C. (1982). Sample processing for high-performance liquid chromatography of ecdysteroids. *J. Chromatogr.* **236**, 137–149.

Lafont, R., Blais, C., Beydon, P., Modde, J.-F., Enderle, U., and Koolman, J. (1983). Conversion of ecdysone and 20-hydroxyecdysone into 26-OIC derivatives is a major pathway in larvae and pupae of species from three insect orders. *Arch. Insect Biochem. Physiol.* **1**, 41–58.

Lagueux, M., Sall, C., and Hoffmann, J. A. (1981). Ecdysteroids during embryogenesis in *Locusta migratoria. Am. Zool.* **21**, 715–726.

Lusby, W. R., Oliver, J. E., and Thompson, M. J. (1987). Application of desorption chemical ionization techniques for analysis of biologically active compounds isolated from insects. *In* "Application of New Mass Spectrometry Techniques in Pesticide Chemistry" (J. D. Rosen, ed.), pp. 99–115. Wiley, New York.

Morgan, E. D., and Wilson, I. D. (1980). Progress in the analysis of ecdysteroids. *In* "Progress in Ecdysone Research" (J. A. Hoffmann, ed.), pp. 29–43. Elsevier/North-Holland, Amsterdam.

Nakanishi, K. (1971a). The ecdysones. *Pure Appl. Chem.* **25**, 167–195.

Nakanishi, K. (1971b). Recent studies on insect hormones. *Int. Congr. Pure Appl. Chem., 23rd, 1971.* Vol. 3, pp. 27–53.

Nigg, H. N., Svoboda, J. A., Thompson, M. J., Kaplanis, J. N., Dutky, S. R., and Robbins, W. E. (1974). Ecdysone metabolism: Ecdysone dehydrogenase-isomerase. *Lipids* **9**, 971–974.

Rees, H. H., and Isaac, R. E. (1985). Biosynthesis and metabolism of ecdysteroids and methods of isolation and identification of the free and conjugated compounds. *In* "Methods in Enzymology" (J. H. Law and H. C. Rilling, eds.), Vol. 111, pp. 377–410. Academic Press, Orlando, Florida.

Reum, L., Haustein, D., and Koolman, J. (1981). Immunoadsorption as a means for purification of low molecular weight compounds: Isolation of ecdysteroids from insects. *Z. Naturforsch., C: Biosci.* **36C**, 790–797.

Rose, M. E., Veares, M. P., Lewis, I. A. S., and Goad, J. (1983). Analysis of steroid conjugates by fast atom bombardment mass spectrometry. *Biochem. Soc. Trans.* **11**, 602–603.

Sall, C., Tsoupras, G., Kappler, C., Lagueux, M., Zachary, D., Luu, B., and Hoffmann, J. A. (1983). Fate of maternal conjugated ecdysteroids during embryonic development in *Locusta migratoria. J. Insect Physiol.* **6**, 491–507.

Scalia, S., and Morgan, E. D. (1982). Rapid and direct method for the determination of ecdysteroid conjugates by liquid chromatography. *J. Chromatogr.* **238**, 457–464.

Scalia, S., Sbrenna-Micciarelli, A., Sbrenna, G., and Morgan, E. D. (1987). Ecdysteroid titres and location in developing eggs of *Schistocerca gregaria. Insect Biochem.* **17**, 227–236.

Shoolery, J. N., and Rogers, M. T. (1958). Nuclear magnetic resonance spectra of steroids. *J. Am. Chem. Soc.,* **80**, 5121–5135.

Soumoff, C., Horn, D. H. S., and O'Connor, J. D. (1981). Production of a new antiserum to arthropod molting hormone and comparison with two other antiserums. *J. Steroid Biochem.* **14**, 429–435.

Spindler, K.-D., Beckers, C., Groschel-Stewart, U., and Emmerich, H. (1978). A radioimmunoassay for arthropod moulting hormones, introducing a novel method of immunogen coupling. *Hoppe-Seyler's Z. Physiol. Chem.* **359**, 1269–1275.

Thompson, M. J., Kaplanis, J. N., Robbins, W. E., Dutky, S. R., and Nigg, H. N. (1974). 3-Epi-20-hydroxyecdysone from meconium of the tobacco hornworm. *Steroids* **24**, 359–366.

Thompson, M. J., Weirich, G. F., Rees, H. H., Svoboda, J. A., Feldlaufer, M. R., and Wilzer, K. R., Jr. (1985a). New ecdysteroid conjugate: Isolation and identification of 26-hydroxyecdysone 26-phosphate from eggs of the tobacco hornworm, *Manduca sexta* (L.). *Arch. Insect Biochem. Physiol.* **2**, 227–236.

Thompson, M. J., Svoboda, J. A., Lusby, W. R., Rees, H. H., Oliver, J. E., Weirich, G. F., and Wilzer, K. R., Jr. (1985b). Biosynthesis of a C_{21} steroid conjugate in an insect: The conversion of [^{14}C]cholesterol to 5-[^{14}C]pregnen-3β,20β-diol glucoside in the tobacco hornworm, *Manduca sexta*. *J. Biol. Chem.* **260**, 15410–15412.

Thompson, M. J., Weirich, G. F., and Svoboda, J. A. (1985c). Ecdysone 3-epimerase. *In* "Methods in Enzymology" (J. H. Law and H. C. Rilling, eds.), Vol. 111, pp. 437–442. Academic Press, Orlando, Florida.

Thompson, M. J., Feldlaufer, M. R., Lozano, R., Rees, H. H., Lusby, W. R., Svoboda, J. A., and Wilzer, K. R., Jr. (1987a). Metabolism of 26-[^{14}C]hydroxyecdysone 26-phosphate in the tobacco hornworm, *Manduca sexta* (L.), to a new ecdysteroid conjugate: 26-[^{14}C]hydroxyecdysone 22-glucoside. *Arch. Insect Biochem. Physiol.* **4**, 1–15.

Thompson, M. J., Svoboda, J. A., Rees, H. H., and Wilzer, K. R., Jr. (1987b). Isolation and identification of 26-hydroxyecdysone 2-phosphate: an ecdysteroid conjugate of eggs and ovaries of the tobacco hornworm, *Manduca sexta*. *Arch. Insect Biochem. Physiol.* **4**, 183–190.

Thompson, M. J., Lozano, R., Svoboda, J. A., Feldlaufer, M. R., and Weirich, G. F. (1987c). Free and conjugated ecdysteroids in the tobacco hornworm, *Manduca sexta*, at various developmental stages. *ACS Symp. Ser.* **325**, 187–199.

Tsourpras, G., Hetru, C., Luu, B., Lageux, M., Constantin, E., and Hoffmann, J. A. (1982). The major conjugates of ecdysteroids in young eggs and in embryos of *Locusta migratoria*. *Tetrahedron Lett.* **23**, 2045–2048.

Tsoupras, G., Luu, B., and Hoffmann, J. A. (1983). A cytokinin (isopentenyl-adenosyl-mononucleotide) linked to ecdysone in newly laid eggs of *Locusta migratoria*. *Science* **220**, 507–509.

Warren, J. T., Steiner, B., Dorn, A., Pak, M., and Gilbert, L. I. (1986). Metabolism of ecdysteroids during the embryogenesis of *Manduca sexta*. *J. Liq. Chromatogr.* **9**, 1759–1782.

Waters Associates (1976). "Paired-ion Chromatography, an Alternative to Ion-Exchange," Bull. D61.

Watson, R. D., and Spaziani, E. (1982). Rapid isolation of ecdysteroids from crustacean tissues and culture media using SEP–PAK C_{18} cartridges. *J. Liq. Chromatogr.* **5**, 525–535.

Weirich, G. F. (1985). Ecdysone 20-monooxygenase. *In* "Methods in Enzymology" (J. H. Law and H. C. Rilling, eds.), Vol. 111, pp. 454–458. Academic Press, Orlando, Florida.

Weirich, G. F., Thompson, M. J., and Svoboda, J. A. (1986). In vitro ecdysteroid conjugation by enzymes of *Manduca sexta* midgut cytosol. *Arch. Insect Biochem. Physiol.* **3**, 109–126.

Willig, A., Rees, H. H., and Goodwin, T. W. (1971). Biosynthesis of insect moulting hormones in isolated ring glands and whole larvae of *Calliphora*. *J. Insect Physiol.* **17**, 2317–2326.

6

Analysis of Spirostans, Spirosolanes, and Solanidanes

Stanley F. Osman
U.S. Department of Agriculture
Eastern Regional Research Center
Wyndmoor, Pennsylvania

I. INTRODUCTION

Substitution and subsequent cyclization of the side chain of cholesterol (1) is an important reaction sequence in the biosynthesis of many plant compounds. In this review we discuss three classes of compound that are formed by these reactions (Fig. 1): spirostans, which have the spiroketal structure (e.g., diosgenin,2a), spirosolanes, which have the spiroaminoketal structure (e.g., solasodine,2b), and solanidanes, which have the indolizidine structure (e.g., solanidine,3).

Spirostans, a part of the class of plant compounds referred to as *sapogenins*, can be found in *Agave* and *Dioscorea* among other plant species; the spirosolane and solanidane steroid alkaloids are found most prevalently in *Solanum* species; glycosides of spirostans (saponins), spirosolanes, and solanidanes (glycoalkaloids) are the common conjugates found in plants. These compounds are of more than academic interest because they are starting materials for the synthesis of steroidal hormones, and as constituents of edible plants, they are of some concern because of their toxic properties.

In this chapter the recent literature on the analysis of these compounds is reviewed. Initially, chromatographic separation techniques are discussed, followed by a summary of spectroscopic methods of characterization and brief discussion of immunoassay techniques. Standard extraction and purification procedures, such as solvent partitioning and precipitation, are not discussed; the reader can refer to the cited references for these details.

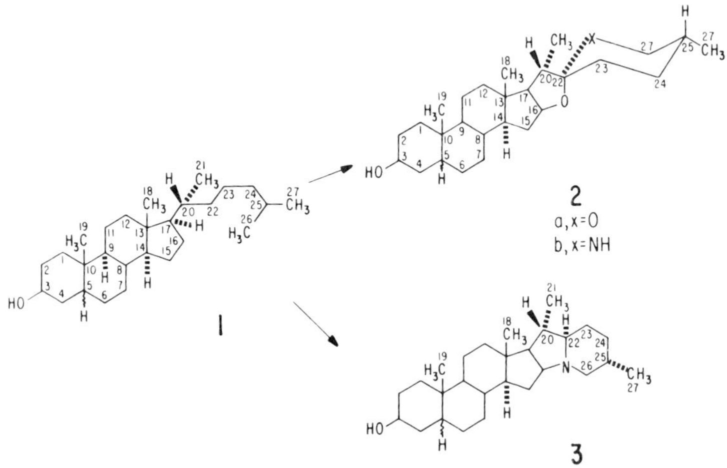

Figure 1 EF-ring carbons derived from cholesterol side chain (see text for explanation).

II. CHROMATOGRAPHIC ANALYSIS

A. Gas Chromatography

Gas chromatography (GC) is of limited value in the analysis of spirostans, spirosolanes, and solanidanes because these compounds require high column temperatures for reasonable elution times, and usually the heat decomposes them. This problem can sometimes be surmounted by the preparation of more volatile derivatives (Cripps and Blunden, 1978). Although it is possible to separate many sapogenins (VandenHeuvel and Horning, 1961) and steroidal alkaloids (VandenHeuvel *et al.*, 1961) on nonpolar packed columns, resolution is generally unsatisfactory because of peak broadening. The use of water vapor (Krohmalyuk, 1975) or dioxane (Soros and Takacs, 1969) as carrier gas does not significantly lessen this problem. One of the more difficult chromatographic problems has been the separation of Δ^5 from the saturated analog (e.g., solanidine from demissidine). To overcome this problem when analyzing mixtures containing solanidine and demissidine, the former was preferentially converted with aqueous acid to the 3,5 diene (solanthrene), which was easily separated from demissidine (Osman and Sinden, 1977). A variation of this method has been described by King (1980) in which the aglycones are converted to the trifluoroacetate derivatives and pyrolyzed, under the GC conditions of analysis (column temperature, 265°C), to solanthrene. This modification eliminates the undesireable side products that are formed with aqueous acid treatment. The use of a nitrogen-phosphorus detector significantly enhanced the sensitivity of this method. Pyrolysis of diosgenin trifluroacetate to the diene probably accounted for the separation observed in the GC of trifluoroacetate derivatives of diosogenin and its saturated analog tigogenin (Carle and Reinhard, 1980).

Demissidine, solanidine, solasodine, tomatidine (2b,22β,25R), and the dehydrodiene products of solanidine and solasodine, solanthrene and solasodiene, have been separated on a fused-silica capillary column coated with CP-Sil-5 (methyl solicone) with the column temperature programmed from 280° to 320°C (Van Gelder, 1985). Solanidine and demissidine were not completely resolved under these conditions. This method was used to determine the concentration of solanine and chaconine in potatoes by measuring the amount of solanthrene produced by aqueous HCl hydrolysis of potato extracts. GC methods for the analysis of solanine and chaconine in bovine milk (Bushway *et al.*, 1984) and potato tubers (Sinden *et al.*, 1980) by measuring solanidine in hydrolyzates have been described.

GC analyses of saponins (sapogenin glycosides) or glycoalkaloids (steroidal alkaloid glycosides) have rarely been achieved because of the nonvolatile nature of these compounds even in derivatized form. Permethylated derivatives of solanine and chaconine have been separated on OV-1 (methyl silicone) and Dexil-300 (carbonane, methyl silicone) at column temperatures above 300°C (Herb *et al.*, 1975). This method was used to study the effect of stress on the glycoalkaloid composition of potatoes.

B. High-Performance Liquid Chromatography

The disadvantages that one encounters with GC because of the heat lability of the compounds would suggest high-performance liquid chromatography (HPLC) as a preferred method of analysis. The major disadvantage in HPLC analysis is its relatively low sensitivity compared with GC. The absence of chromatographic groups with absorption maxima above 200 nm, which is often the case, dictates the use of a refractive index (RI) detector or a variable wavelength ultraviolet (UV) detector at wavelengths near 200 nm. Although the sensitivity of RI detectors has improved dramatically in recent years, their lower limit of detectability is about 25 nanograms (ng); and the low wavelength necessary for UV detection limits the solvents that can be used as the mobile phase. In both types of detection, solvent composition programming is virtually impossible when high sensitivity and reproducibility are required. Since the detection system dictates many of the other HPLC parameters, it will be used as the basis for reviewing the HPLC literature.

UV detectors have been used with considerable success in the analysis of the 3-β-*O*-glycosides, which are usually soluble in water or other protic solvents that have negligible adsorption above 200 nm. The steroid saponins from *Dioscorea* plants, collettiside I, collettiside III, collettiside IV, dioscin (C-25 epimer of collettiside III), gracillin (C-25 epimer of collettiside IV), and methylprotodioscin were separated using six different column-solvent combinations with UV detection (208 nm) in all cases (Xu and Lin, 1985). As part of this study, silica (Si), octadecyl (C18), and amino (NH2) columns were evaluated using mobile phases composed of the following solvents: water, ethanol, acetonitrile, and hexane. Although no single solvent combination was capable of separating all six compounds, the best results were obtained for the separation of the peracetylated derivatives using a Si-column and hexane (Hex)-ethanol (EtOH) as the mobile phase. The separation of spiroketal saponins that differed by the number of sugars in the glycosidic moeity could readily be achieved in all the systems tested.

Four spiroketal saponins isolated form *Avena sativa* that have the same aglycone (nuatigenin) but have glycoside residues (at both C-3 and C-26) that differ in the number of sugars were separated on an octyl (C8) column using a gradient of acetonitrile (ACN) and H_2O as the mobile phase (Kesselmeier and Strack, 1981). The effluent was monitored at 200 nm; the lower limit of detection at this wavelength was 50 ng.

Hunter *et al.* (1981) have described a system for the separation of Δ^5 from the corresponding saturated spiroketal sapogenins. Diosgenin (2a,22α,25R) and yamogenin (2a,22α,25S) acetates were separated from the saturated analogs tigogenin- and neotigogenin-acetate on a C18 column with ACN/Hex/tetrahydrofuran (THF) (17:2:1) as the eluant and monitoring at 210 nm.

A quantitative method for the determination of the commercially important compound hecogenin (2a,12oxo,22α,25S) in *Agave* species has been reported (Higgins, 1976). After hydrolysis of the glycosides, the aglycones hecogenin and tigogenin (2a,22α,25R) were converted to the benzoates and separated on a C8 column, with ACN/H_2O (80:20) as the mobile phase at a relatively high flow rate of 3.9 ml/min and detection at 235 nm.

Refractive index (RI) was the detection method of choice for HPLC analysis of spirostans when chloroform was used as a component of the mobile phase because this solvent has significant absorption above 200 nm. Hecogenin and tigogenin mixtures derived from *Agave sisalana* where quantitated using a C18 column and ACN/H_2O/methanol (MeOH)/chloroform ($CHCl_3$) (73:20:6:1) as the mobile phase (Sitton *et al.*, 1982). The HPLC-RI results compared favorably to those obtained by GC analysis. Hecogenin, tigogenin, and diosgenin were separated on a decyl (C10) column using ACN/MeOH/$CHCl_3$ (83:10:7) as the mobile phase (Tal and Goldberg, 1981).

Data for the HPLC analysis of 30 spiroketal sapogenins on both Si and C18 columns have been reported by Lin and Xu (1984). Retention volume could be correlated to compound polarity, and unique retention volumes could be obtained for all compounds except C-25 epimers using a combination of the four HPLC systems described.

HPLC methods for the analyses of solanidanes, spirosolanes, and their glycosides have been developed. Solanidine and a number of spirosolanes were separated on a Si column with Hex/MeOH/acetone (18:1:1) (Hunter *et al.*, 1980). Although the use of a UV detector was much less tedious than the previous detection method which involved collecting fractions and analyzing each by TLC (Hunter *et al.*, 1976b), there was a great difference in the response factors of the compounds that were analyzed; particularly evident was the low response of the saturated compounds compared with the Δ^5 analogs (e.g. demissidine versus solanidine).

Buffered aqueous MeOH solutions have been used for the separation of solasodine, solasodine glycosides, and Δ^3, Δ^5 solasodiene on C18 columns to minimize peak tailing of these weakly basic compounds. In this study, variables such as column temperature and solvent flow rates were optimized, and UV response and capacity factors were determined for the various HPLC conditions (Crabbe and Fryer, 1980).

As was alluded to earlier, there has been much research into developing methods for the analysis of glycoalkaloids in foods such as potatoes and tomatoes because these compounds, in sufficient quantities, can be toxic. Bushway and co-workers (1979, 1980) have developed HPLC analytical methods for the determination of potato glycoalkaloids. Best results for the analysis of solanine and chaconine were obtained on an NH2 column eluted with buffered aqueous ACN-THF and UV monitoring at 208 nm; analysis of lower glycosides of solanidine that may be present in potato tissue as the result of enzymatic glycolysis of solanine and/or chaconine was achieved by Bushway (1982a) on a carbohydrate analysis column (Waters Assoc.) using a similar solvent system. Radially compressed columns have been used for rapid glycoalkaloid analysis (Morris and Lee, 1981; Bushway, 1982b); for the analysis of solanine and chaconine, a C18 radially compressed column eluted with ACN/H_2O/ethanolamine (45:55:0.1) appears to give the best results. Prior sample cleanup by ion-pair chromatography on a C18 cartridge column has also been used to shorten analysis times (Carmen *et al.*, 1986; Bushway *et al.*, 1986).

Solasonine and solamargine (solasodine glycosides containing the trisaccharides of solanine and chaconine, respectively), the toxic components of *Solanum ptycantum* (Eastern black nightshade), have been isolated and purified using the HPLC method of Eldridge and Hockridge (1983). Milligram quantities of solanine and chaconine from *S. tuberosum* and the glycoalkaloids, demissine (a tetrasaccharide glycoside of demissidine containing xylose, glucose (2), and galactose) and commersonine (same as demissine except that the xylose has been replaced by glucose), from *S. demissum* have also been isolated by semipreparative HPLC using a Zorbax semipreparative NH2 column (Bushway and Storch, 1982).

C. Thin-Layer Chromatography

Thin-layer chromatography (TLC) has been used primarily as a qualitative method for the rapid characterization of sapogenins in plant extracts; it has also been used for the isolation of submilligram quantities of pure aglycones and glycosides. In the most comprehensive study of the TLC of sapogenins to date, the chromatographic characteristics of 20 compounds on silica gel in six different solvent systems have been determined (Takeda *et al.*, 1963). Sapogenins on TLC plates can be visualized by charring with sulfuric acid (H_2SO_4) or spraying with antimony trichloride ($SbCl_3$), which is more specific for 3-β-ol-steroids. Reliable quantitative data for *Dioscorea* sapogenins was obtained by densitometric analysis of plates sprayed with $SbCl_3$ when extreme care was taken in spotting the sample (Brain and Hardman, 1968). By use of an internal standard, problems associated with sample application could be overcome (Lockwood *et al.*, 1974). TLC has been used in conjunction with mass spectrometry for the characterization and quantitation of sapogenins in *Digitalis purpurea, D. mertonensis,*

D. Lutea, *D. ambigua*, and *D. lanata* (Evans, 1974). Sapogenins that differed by degree of hyroxylation could be readily separated and characterized.

The chromatographic behavior of 26 steroidal alkaloids, mostly of the spirosolane and solanidane type, on silica-gel plates using six different mobile phases has been reported (Hunter *et al.*, 1976a). The differential response of these compounds to H_2SO_4 charring was also described.

As with other chromatographic techniques, the separation of compounds that differ by one degree of unsaturation is difficult. This separation has been achieved for steroidal alkaloids and sapogenins using silver nitrate impregnated TLC plates with $CHCl_3$/MeOH (either 95:5 or 90:10) as the developing solvent (Roensch and Schreiber, 1967). The method was used to isolate pure saturated and Δ^5 analogs from mixtures containing both types.

The chromatographic behavior of six naturally occurring spirosolane and solanidane glycoalkaloids on silica-gel plates with either of two basic mobile phases has been reported (Böll, 1962). For increased sensitivity and specificity in detecting glycoalkaloids, Jellema *et al.* (1979) have developed TLC plates with solutions of the optical brightener Calcofluor M2R. This reagent provided a tenfold increase in sensitivity over visualization with Dragendroff's reagent (specific for nitrogen-containing compounds); however, no comparison was made with $SbCl_3$ or H_2SO_4 staining. Cadle *et al.* (1978) reported a rapid quantitative TLC procedure for the analysis of solanine and chaconine in potato tubers by densitometric analysis of $SbCl_3$ stained plates. Values were in good agreement with those obtained with paraformaldehyde-sulfuric acid staining; however, experience in our laboratory would indicate that the quantitative values are reliable only for relatively pure glycoalkaloid samples.

A novel approach to the isolation of spirosolane glycosides is the use of a centrifugally accelerated radial thin-layer chromatographic system (chromatofuge) in combination with HPLC (Hunter and Heftmann, 1983).

The advantages and disadvantages of the various chromatographic techniques are summarized in Table 1.

D. Immunoligand Analytical Methods

Immunoassay techniques appear promising for the quantitative analysis of glycoalkaloids. Antibodies have been produced for the radioimmunoassay analysis (RIA) of solanidine glycosides (Vallejo and Ercegovich, 1979). The method, which is very sensitive (as little as 150 pg of solanidine was detectable, gave comparable results to those obtained by titration (Fitzpatrick and Osman, 1974) for the determination of solanine and chaconine in potato extracts; however, the low yield of antibodies that these workers were able to isolate made the method somewhat impractical. Improvement in antibody production could result in a more cost-effective method. A more recent technique based on the same principle, known as the ELISA (enzyme-linked immunosorbent assay) method, has been applied to the analysis of solanine and chaconine in potatoes (Morgan *et al.*, 1985). Again, antibodies were prepared against an antigen containing solanidine. However, rather than depending on competitive

Table 1 Assessment of chromatographic techniques

Compound Class	Chromatographic Technique	Advantages	Disadvantages
Spirosolanes, spirostans, solanidanes	GC	Good resolution and sensitivity.	Compounds may decompose at analysis temp.; derivatization may be required.
	HPLC	Nondestructive; compound volatility not a factor; can be used preparatively.	Sensitivity and resolution generally inferior to GC.
	TLC	Rapid and cheap; can be used preparatively.	Detection may be destructive, low sensitivity, moderate resolution.
Saponins, glycoalkaloids	GC	Good resolution.	Compounds must be derivatized; decomposition a significant problem.
	HPLC	Same as for spirostans, etc.	Limited mobile phase composition with UV detection; separation depends mainly on size of carbohydrate.
	TLC	Good for sample screening.	Low sensitivity, moderate resolution.

reaction of the antibodies with radioactive and nonradioactive (the quantity being determined) solanidine-containing antigen, as is the case with the RIA method, ELISA measures the difference between antibody reaction with bound antigen and antigen in solution (the quantity being determined); detection is ultimately colorimetric, and therefore no radioisotopes are required. This method could detect as low as 2 pg of solanidine glycosides and gave comparable results to standard colorimetric procedures. The ELISA method enables the analysis of many more samples per unit time than other published methods for the measurement of potato glycoalkaloids. The development of antibodies to other glycoalkaloids should greatly expand the use of this method.

III. SPECTROSCOPIC METHODS

A. Nuclear Magnetic Resonance Spectroscopy

A review of ^{1}H and ^{13}C nuclear magnetic resonance (^{13}C-NMR) studies of the steroid nucleus appears elsewhere in this text; therefore this discussion will focus on the EF-ring system that is unique to the spirostans, spirosolanes, and solanidanes. An excellent review of ^{13}C-NMR data for sapogenins and saponins through 1983 has been published (Agrawal *et al.*, 1985). Included in this review are the unambigous assignments of carbon shifts by recent NMR developments such as the insensitive-nuclei-enhanced-by-polarization-transfer (INEPT) and the 2D-J resolved techniques. The orientation of the C-27 methyl (attached to C-25) has a significant effect on the shifts of the other carbons in the F-ring. For example, in the 22α-spirostans an axial orientation of this methyl group (i.e., 25S configuration) results in shielding of the F-ring carbons, causing an upfield shift in the resonances of carbons 23, 24, and 26 (compared with the equitorial 25R epimer) (Tori *et al.*, 1981). The reader is referred to Agrawal *et al.* (1985) for an exhaustive analysis of the spiroketal sapogenins, which includes shift data for furostans and the furospirostan, nuatigenin, as well as the spirostan ring system.

Assignments for the ^{13}C-NMR spectra of naturally occurring spirosolanes and solanidanes have been reported by Weston *et al.* (1977) and Radeglia *et al.* (1977); the assignments are in good agreement, where comparable, except for the discrepancy of 0.6 ppm for the shift of C-22 in tomatidine. A significant upfield shift for the F-ring carbon resonances of 22β versus 22α epimer [e.g., Δ^5 tomatidine (tomatidinol) versus solasodine] particularly for C-23 is most likely due to the shielding effect of C-21 in the β isomer.

B. Mass Spectrometry

Ions resulting from the fragmentation of the E- and F-rings of spirostans, spirosolanes, and solanidanes are prominant in the electron-bombardment mass spectra of these compounds and can be used as diagnostic ions for structural characterization

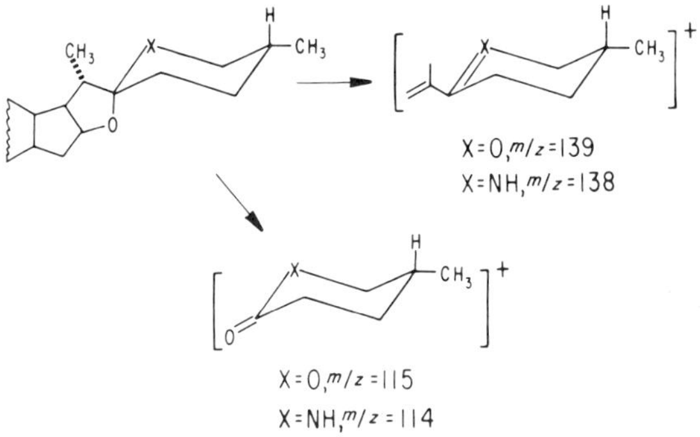

Figure 2 Characteristic MS fragment ions of spirostans and spirsolanes.

(Budzikiewicz *et al.*, 1964). The two main fragmentation pathways for spirostans and spirosolanes have been hypothesized to be those shown in Fig. 2.

For the solanidanes, the major ions resulting from fragmentation of the EF-rings are given in Fig. 3.

Since major ions in the spectra of these compounds originate from the E- and F-rings, substitution in this part of the molecule is readily discerned by mass spectrometry. For example, the spectrum of 23-hydroxysolanidine (leptinine) shows two major ions that are 16 atomic mass units (amu) higher than those found in solanidine (i.e., 166 and 220 amu), and 23-acetylsolanidine shows corresponding ions at 208 and 262, 58 amu higher than the solanidine ions (S. Osman, unpublished results).

The fast-atom bombardment mass spectra of glycoalkaloids (Price *et al.*, 1985) and the electron-impact spectra of permethylated and peracetylated saponins (Komori *et al.*, 1975) are helpful in compound characterization because molecular ions (ions corresponding to the molecular weight of the compound) and fragment ions related to cleavage at the glycosidic bonds are observed.

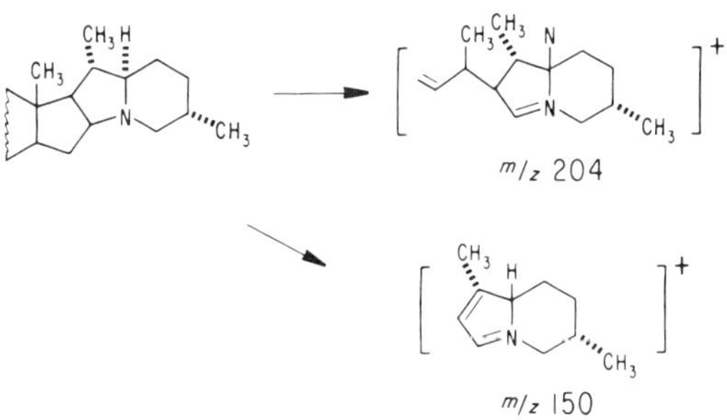

Figure 3 Characteristic MS fragment ions of solanidanes.

C. X-Ray Crystallography

The X-ray crystallographic analysis of tomatidine hydroiodide shows unambiguously that C-22 in this compound has the S configuration and that the F-ring is in a prone-chair conformation (Hoehne *et al.*, 1967). These results provide a definitive basis for NMR assignments and configurational assignments from degradation studies.

IV. SUMMARY

Modern chromatographic and spectroscopic terchniques now make it possible to purify and completely characterize sapogenins and steroidal alkaloids, and (in some cases) saponins and glycoalkaloids, starting with samples containing less than 10 mg of the compound. Unambiguous structural characterization of compounds present in nanogram quantities is also feasible, thus the analysis of plant extracts containing these substances is now, for the most part, rapid and routine.

References

Agrawal, P. K., Jain, D. C., Gupta, R. K., and Thakur, R. S. (1985). Carbon-13 NMR spectroscopy of the steroid sapogenins and steroidal saponins. *Phytochemistry* **24**, 2479–2496.

Böll, P. M. (1962). Alkaloid glycosides from *Solanum dulcumara. Acta Chem. Scand.* **16**, 1819–1830.

Brain, K. R., and Hardman, R. (1968). An improved method of densitometric thin layer chromatography as applied to the determination of sapogenin in *Dioscorea* tubers. *J. Chromatogr.* **38**, 355–363.

Budzikiewicz, H., Djerassi, C., and Williams, D. H. (1964). "Structural Elucidation of Natural Products by Mass Spectrometry," Vol. 2. Holden-Day, San Francisco, California.

Bushway, R. J. (1982a). High-performance liquid chromatographic determination of the metabolites of the potato glycoalkaloids, α-chaconine and α-solanine, in potato tubers and potato products. *J. Liq. Chromatogr.* **5**, 1313–1322.

Bushway, R. J. (1982b). High-performance liquid chromatographic separation of potato glycoalkaloids using a radially compressed amino column. *J. Chromatogr.* **247**, 180–183.

Bushway, R. J., and Storch, R. H. (1982). Semi-preparative high-performance liquid chromatographic separation of potato glycoalkaloids. *J. Liq. Chromatogr.* **5**, 731–742.

Bushway, R. J., Barden, E. S., Bushway, A. W., and Bushway, A. A. (1979). High-performance liquid chromatographic separation of potato glycoalkaloids. *J. Chromatogr.* **178**, 533–541.

Bushway, R. J., Barden, E. S., Wilson, A. M., and Bushway, A. A. (1980). Analysis of potato glycoalkaloids by high-performance liquid chromatography. *J. Food. Sci.* **45**, 1088–1089.

Bushway, R. J., McGann, D. D., and Bushway, A. A. (1984). Gas chromatographic method for the determination of solanidine and its application to a study of feed-milk transfer in the cow. *J. Agric. Food Chem.* **15**, 551–558.

Bushway, R. J., Bureau, J. L., and King, J. (1986). Modification of the rapid high-performance liquid chromatographic method for the determination of potato glycoalkaloids. *J. Agric. Food Chem.* **34**, 279–282.

Cadle, L. S., Stelzig, D. A., Harper, K. L., and Young, R. J. (1978). Thin-layer chromatographic system for the identification and quantitation of potato tuber glycoalkaloids. *J. Agric. Food Chem.* **26**, 1453–1454.

Carle, R., and Reinhard, E. (1980). Simultaneous determination of solasodine, diosgenin and tigogenin. *Plants Med.* **38**, 381–383.

Carman, A. S., Jr., Kuan, S. S., Ware, G. M., Francis, O. J., Jr., and Kirschenheuter, G. P. (1986). Rapid high performance liquid chromatographic determination of the potato glycoalkaloids α-solanine and α-chaconine. *J. Agric. Food Chem.* **34**, 272–279.

Crabbe, P. G., and Fryer, C. (1980). Rapid quantitative analysis of solasodine, solasodine glycosides and solasodiene by high-pressure liquid chromatography. *J. Chromatogr.* **187**, 87–100.

Cripps, A. L., and Blunden, G. B. (1978). A quantitative gas-liquid chromatographic method for the estimation of hecogenin and tigogenin in the leaves, juice and sapogenin concentrates of *Agave sisalana. Steroids* **31**, 661–669.

Eldridge, A. C., and Hockridge, M. E. (1983). High-performance liquid chromatographic separation of the easter black nightshade (Solanum ptycanthum) glycoalkaloids. *J. Agric. Food Chem.* **31**, 1218–1220.

Evans, F. G. (1974). Thin-layer chromatography-mass spectrometry for the identification of sapogenins from *Digitalis* species. *Biomed. Mass Spectrom.* **1**, 166–168.

Fitzpatrick, T. J., and Osman, S. F. (1974). A comprehensive method for the determination of total potato glycoalkaloids. *Am. Potato J.* **51**, 318–323.

Herb, S. F., Fitzpatrick, T. J., and Osman, S. F. (1975). Separation of potato glycoalkaloids by gas chromatography. *J. Agric. Food Chem.* **23**, 520–523.

Higgins, J. W. (1976). A high-performance liquid chromatographic analysis of benzoate esters of sapogenins isolated from *Agave. J. Chromatogr.* **121**, 329–334.

Hoehne, E., Ripperger, H., and Schreiber, K. (1967). X-ray structural analysis of tomatidine hydroiodide. Configuration of (25S)-spirosolane at C-22. *Tetrahedron* **23**, 3705–3711.

Hunter, I. R., and Heftman, E. (1983). Isolation of glycoalkaloids with the chromatotron and their determination by high-performance liquid chromatography. *J. Liq. Chromatogr.* **6**, 281–289.

Hunter, I. R., Walden, M. K., Wagner, J. R., and Heftman, E. (1976a). Thin-layer chromatography of steroidal alkaloids. *J. Chromatogr.* **118**, 259–262.

Hunter, I. R., Walden, M. K., Wagner, J. R., and Heftman, E. (1976b). High-pressure liquid chromatography of steroidal alkaloids. *J. Chromatogr.* **119**, 223–226.

Hunter, I. R., Walden, M. K., and Heftman, E. (1980). High-performance liquid chromatography of *Solanum* and *Veratrum* alkaloids. *J. Chromatogr.* **198**, 363–366.

Hunter, I. R., Walden, M. K., Bailey, G. F., and Heftman, E. (1981). High-performance liquid chromatography, infrared and raman spectra of steroidal sapogenins. *J. Nat. Prod.* **44**, 245–251.

Jellema, R., Elema, E. T., and Malingre, T. M. (1979). Optical brighteners as thin-layer chromatography detection reagents for glycoalkaloids and steroid alkaloids in Solanum species. *J. Chromatogr.* **176**, 435–439.

Kesselmeier, L., and Strack, D. (1981). High performance liquid chromatographic analysis of steroidal saponins from *Avena sativa* L. *Z. Naturforsch., C: Biosci.* **36C**, 1072–1074.

King, R. R. (1980). Analysis of potato glycoalkaloids by gas-liquid chromatography of alkaloid components. *J. Assoc. Off. Anal. Chem.* **63**, 1226–1230.

Komori, T., Mutou (nee Imatsu), Y., Miyahara, K., Nohara, T., and Kawasaki, T. (1975). Mass spectra of spirostanol and furostanol glycosides. *Biomed. Mass Spectrom.* **2**, 65–77.

Krokhamalyuk, V. V. (1975). Gas chromatography of steroid and triterpene sapogenins using water vapor as the carrier gas. *In "Issledovaniya Oblasti Farmatsi Khimii"* (V. I. Prokpishin, ed.). Kissiner. Gos. Med. Inst., Kishinev, USSR.

Lin, J-T., and Xu, C-J. (1984). High-performance liquid chromatography of steroidal sapogenins. *J. Chromatogr.* **287**, 105–112.

Lockwood, G. B., Brain, K. R., and Turner, T. D. (1974). Simultaneous estimation of sterol and steroidal sapogenins in plant extracts by densitometric thin-layer chromatography. *J. Chromatogr.* **95**, 250–253.

Morris, S. C., and Lee, T. H. (1981). Analysis of potato glycoalkaloids with radially compressed high-performance liquid chromatographic cartridges and ethanolamine in the mobile phase. *J. Chromatogr.* **219**, 403–410.

Osman, S. (1984). Steroidal glycoalkaloid biosynthesis and function in *Solanum* spp. *In* "Isopentenoids in Plants: Biochemistry and Function" (W. D. Ness, G. Fuller, and L-T. Tsai, eds.), pp. 519–530. Dekker, New York.

Osman, S. F., and Sinden, S. L. (1977). Analysis of mixtures of solanidine and demissidine glycoalkaloids containing identical carbohydrate units. *J. Agric. Food Chem.* **25**, 955–957.

Price, K. R., Mellon, F. A., Self, R., Fenwick, G. R., and Osman, S. F. (1985). Fast atom bombardment mass spectrometry of *Solanum* glyucoalkaloids and its potential for mixture analysis. *Biomed. Mass Spectrom.* **12**, 79–85.

Radeglia, R., Adam, G. and Ripperger, H. (1977). ^{13}C NMR spectroscopy of solanum steroid alkaloids. *Tetrahedron Lett.* pp. 903–906.

Roensch, H., and Schreiber, K. (1967). Solanum alkaloids. LXXXIII. Analytical and preparative thin-layer chromatographic separation of the 5α-saturated and Δ^5-unsaturated steroid alkaloids and sapogenins on silver nitrate containing adsorption layers. *J. Chromatogr.* **30**, 149–154.

Sinden, S. L., Sanford, L. L., and Osman, S. F. (1980). Glycoalkaloids and resistance to the Colorado potato beetle in *Solanum chacoense* Bitter. *Am. Potato J.* **57**, 331–344.

Sitton, D., Blunden, G., and Cripps, A. L. (1982). Quantitative high-performance liquid chromatographic method for the estimation of hecogenin and tigogenin in the leaves and saponin concentrates of *Agave sisalana. J. Chromatogr.* **245**, 138–140.

Soros, I., and Takacs, J. (1969). Gas chromatographic contribution to the chemistry of beet saponins. I. *Period Polytech. Chem. Eng.* **12**, 347–352.

Tal, B., and Goldberg, I. (1981). High-performance liquid chromatographic separation of steroidal sapogenins. *J. Nat. Prod.* **44**, 750–751.

Takeda, K., Hara, S., Wada, A., and Matsumoto, N. (1963). A systematic, simultaneous analysis of the steroid sapogenins by thin-layer chromatography. *J. Chromatogr.* **11**, 562–564.

Tori, K., Seo, S., Terui, Y., Nishikawa, J., and Yasuda, F. (1981). Carbon-13 NMR spectra of 5β-steroidal sapogenins. Reassignment of the F-ring carbon signals of (25 *S*)-spirostans. *Tetrahedron Lett.* **22**, 2405–2408.

Vallejo, R. P., and Ercegovich, C. D. (1979). Analysis of potato for glycoalkaloid content by radioimmunoassay (RIA). *NBS Spec. Publ.* (*U.S.*) **519**, 333–340.

VandenHeuvel, W. J. A., and Horning, E. C. (1961). Gas chromatographic separation of sapogenins. *J. Am. Chem. Soc.* **26**, 634–635.

VandenHeuvel, J. W. A., Horning, E. C., Sato, Y., and Ikekawa, N. (1961). Gas chromatographic separation of steroidal amines. *J. Am. Chem. Soc.* **26**, 628–629.

Van Gelder, W. J. M. (1985). Determination of the total C_{27}-steroidal alkaloid composition of *Solanum* species by high resolution gas chromatography. *J. Chromatogr.* **331**, 285–293.

Weston, R. J., Gottlieb, H. E., Hagaman, E. W., and Wenkert, E. (1977). Carbon-13 nuclear magnetic resonance spectroscopy of naturally occurring substances. LI. *Solanum* glycoalkaloids. *Aust. J. Chem.* **30**, 917–921.

Xu, C.-J., and Lin, J.-T. (1985). Comaprison of silica-, C_{18}-, and NH_2-HPLC columns for the separation of steroidal saponins from *Dioscorea* plants. *J. Liq. Chromatogr.* **8**, 361–368.

7

Analysis of Steroid Sapogenins

Toshihiro Nohara
Faculty of Pharmaceutical Sciences
Kumamoto University
Kumamoto, Japan

I. INTRODUCTION

A. Definition and Structure

The spirostanols are intramolecular-ketal derivatives of the 16,26-dihydroxy-22-keto-steroid, which consists of 27 carbons that possess a skeleton (aspirostane nucleus), in which a furan ring (E-ring) and a pyran ring (F-ring) are joined in a spiroketal form at C-22 (see Ia). Their steroid framework takes a trans relationship at B/C and C/D junctures but can exist as three types of relationship at A/B: (5α-H), cis (5β-H), and Δ^5.

a

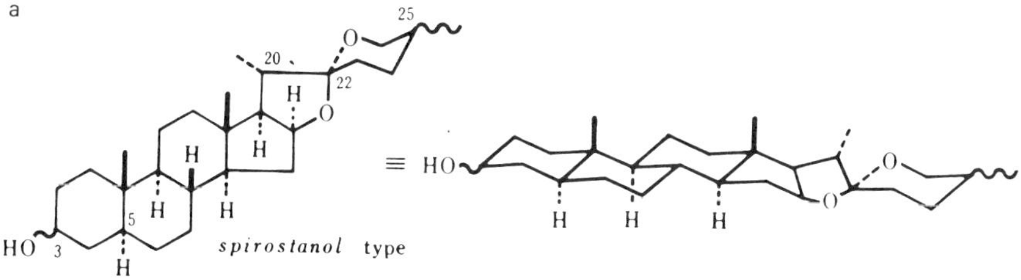

Structure I

Analysis of Sterols and Other Biologically Significant Steroids

The configuration at C-22 had been previously recognized to be only R; however, it has recently been found that 22S compounds occur in nature, accompanied by 22R and 25S compounds (Kudo *et al.*, 1984). With regard to the configuration at C-25, there are three types: a β-oriented methyl group (25S, neo, or 25L), an α-oriented methyl group (25R, iso, or 25D), and $\Delta^{25(27)}$. The 25R and 25S compounds usually coexist in approximately a 3:1 ratio. Furostanol derivatives are closely related to the previously mentioned spirostanol (Tschesche *et al.*, 1967) and are to be precursors of the spirostanols because they possess an opened F-ring of spirostane, almost all of which has a glycosidic linkage at C-26 OH and produces the corresponding spirostanol derivative upon treatment with β-glucosidase. Furostanol derivatives are predominantly found in the fresh plant (see Ib) (Kiyosawa *et al.*, 1968).

b

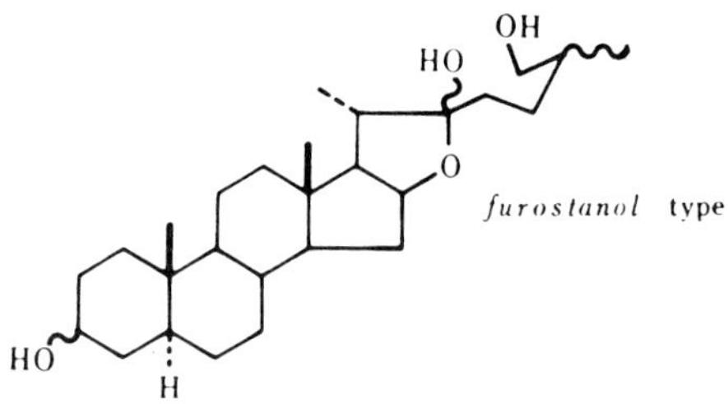

Structure I

B. Distribution in the Plant Kingdom

It is rare that spirostanols occur in free form in nature; most exist as glycosides. We shall refer here to the spirostanol and furostanol glycosides. These glycosides, distributed mainly in Monocotyledoneae (Liliaceae, Dioscoresceae, Amaryllidaceae, and Palmae), are also found in Scrophulariaceae, Solanaceae, Simarubaceae, Leguminosae, Zygophyllaceae, Primulaceae, and Gramineae.

C. Kinds of Spirostanols

More than about 130 kinds of spirostanols are so far known, among which tigogenin and sarsasapogenin are the most popular because they are typical and have been known a long time. Diosgenin is particularly important as the crude material for preparing various steroidal drugs (natural and artificial). The main spirostanols are listed in Table 1.

Atypical examples of spirostanols are nuatigenin [a spirostanol possessing a pentacyclic F-ring, *Avena sativa* (Gramineae)] (Tschesche and Richert, 1964), trillenogenin [an 18-norspirostanol, *Trillium kamtschaticum* (Liliaceae)] (Nohara *et al.*, 1975),

Table 1 Structures and distribution of spirostanols

Trivial Name	C-5-H	C-25	Substitution	Crude Drug or Plant
Sarsasapogenin	β	*S*	3β-OH	Sarsaparilla Radix, Anemarhenae Rhizoma
Smilagenin	β	*R*	3β-OH	Smilacis Rhizoma, Sarsaparilla Radix
Diosgenin	Δ^5	*R*	3β-OH	*Dioscorea tokoro* (Dioscoreaceae), Ophiopogosis Tuber, Smilacis Rhizoma
Tigogenin	α	*R*	3β-OH	*Digitalis lanata* (Scrophulariaceae)
Gitogenin	α	*R*	$2\alpha,3\beta$-OH	Digitalis (Scrophulariaceae)
Digitogenin	α	*R*	$2\alpha,3\beta,15\beta$-OH	Digitalis, *D. lanata*
Rhodeasapogenin	β	*S*	$1\beta,3\beta$-OH	*Rhodea japonica* (Liliaceae), *Convallaria majalis* var. *keiskei* (Liliaceae)
Convallamarogenin	β	$\Delta^{25(27)}$	$1\beta,3\beta$-OH	*C. majalis* var. *keiskei*
Ruscogenin	Δ^5	*R*	$1\beta,3\beta$-OH	*Ruscus aculeatus* (Liliaceae), Ophiopogonis Tuber
Pentologenin	β	*R*	$1\beta,2\beta,3\beta,4\beta,5\beta$-OH	*R. japonica*
Tokorogenin	β	*R*	$1\beta,2\beta,3\alpha$-OH	*D. tokoro*
Yonogenin	β	*R*	$2\beta,3\alpha$-OH	*D. tokoro*
Pennogenin	Δ^5	*R*	$3\beta,17\alpha$-OH	*Trillium smallii* (Liliaceae)
Metagenin	β	*R*	$2\beta,3\beta,11\alpha$-OH	*Metanarthecium luteo-viride* (Liliaceae)
Hecogenin	α	*R*	3β-OH, 12 C=O	*Agave americana* (Amaryllidaceae)

kryptogenin [a seco-furostanol carrying an opened F-ring, *T. kamtschaticum*], and others (see II).

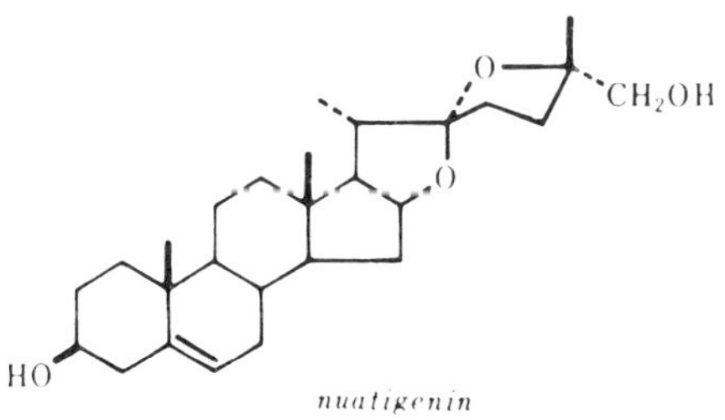

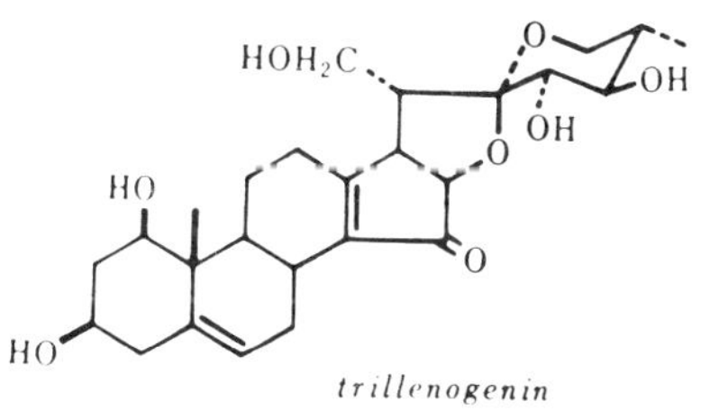

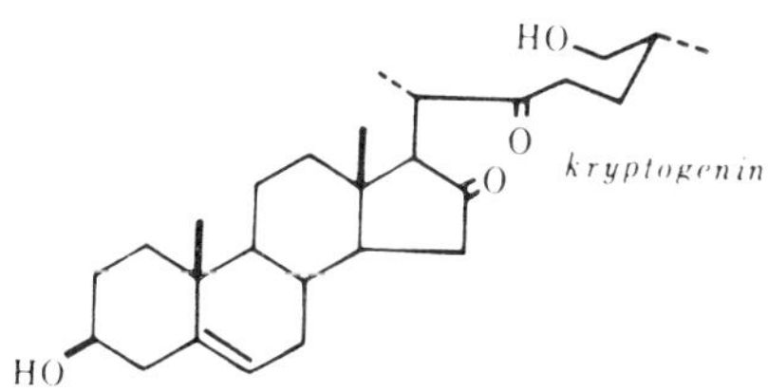

Structure II

D. Structural Types of Saponins

The glycosides of spirostanol are mainly saponins, a group of substances that upon shaking with water make soaplike suds. Since saponins are glycosides, they hydrolyze to give an aglycone (sapogenin) and sugar. Hemolytic and fish-poisoning reactions are characteristics of saponin that have been known for a long time; and steroidal saponin has the ability to form "molecular complexes" with steroids such as cholesterol that are only slightly soluble in water. Saponins are constituted mainly of the derivatives of spirostanol and furostanol and of transformed spirostane, cholestane, and ergostane. Although the sugar moiety is comprised chiefly of glucose, rhamnose, xylose, and arabinose, it is linked to the hydroxyl group at C-3 as an oligoglycoside, with a branched structure. With the increasing molecular weight of the sugar moiety in spirostanol glycosides, characteristics such as hemolysis, fish-poisoning, precipitation with cholesterol, and antimold activity tend to increase.

Since furostanol-type saponins are 26-*O*-glucosides, and the glucosidic moiety is easily released by reactions with enzymes, a ring closure to 26-OH takes place with dehydration with 22-OH, yielding a spirostanol. Thus, furostanol is recognized as the precursor in the biogenesis of spirostanol glycoside and is called its prototype (Kawasaki *et al.*, 1974). Furostanol glycosides show none of the characteristics of saponins and exhibit a clear red color with Ehrlich reagent (Kiyosawa *et al.*, 1968). It is generally known that the spirostanol glycosides show hemolysis, hemagglutination,

Table 2 Typical saponins

Saponin	Characteristics
Spirostanol-Type Saponins	
Dioscin	Widely distributed in Dioscoreae plants, e.g., *D. tokoro*; the first saponin of which structure was fully determined.
F-gitonin	Main saponin of digitalis.
Yononin	Contained in *D. tokoro*; the first example carrying sugar linkage except for C_3-OH.
Trillenoside	Contained in *Trillium tschonoskii* (Liliaceae); novel 18-norspirostanol oligoside.
Avenacoside	Contained in *Avena fatua* (Gramineae).
Furostanol-Type Saponins	
Sarsaparilloside	Contained in Sarsaparilla Radix. The C_{26}-*O*-glucoside is easily hydrolyzed to give a spirostanol-type glycoside, parillin. Used for treatment of rheumatism and syphilis in Europe and America in old times.
Protodioscin	Prototype saponin of dioscin; coexists with dioscin; abundant in the rhizomes of *T. tschonoskii*.
Others	
Osladin	Obtained as a sweetening material from the underground parts of *Polypodium vulgare* (Polypodiaceae); shows characteristics for saponin such as sudsing and hemolysis.
Thornasteroside A	Saponin of *Acanthaster planci*. Its aglycone is a cholestane-derivative; shows bioactivities of hemolysis, nervous poison, and antivirus.

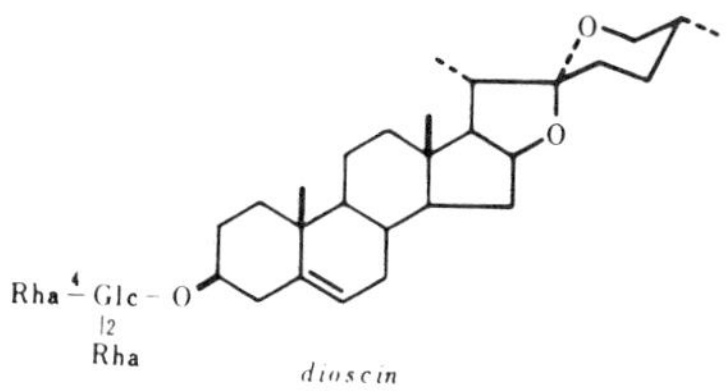

dioscin

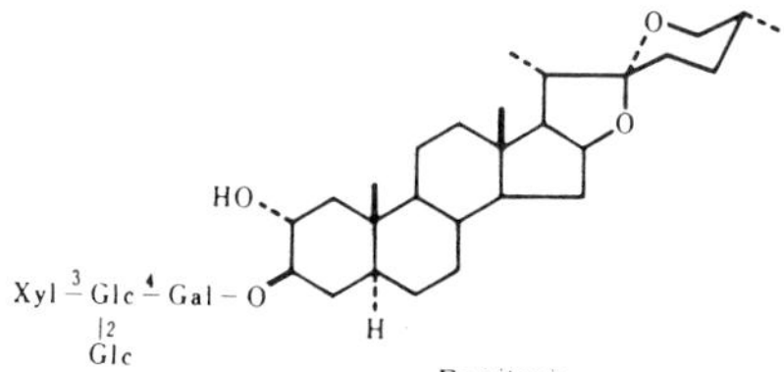

F-*gitonin*

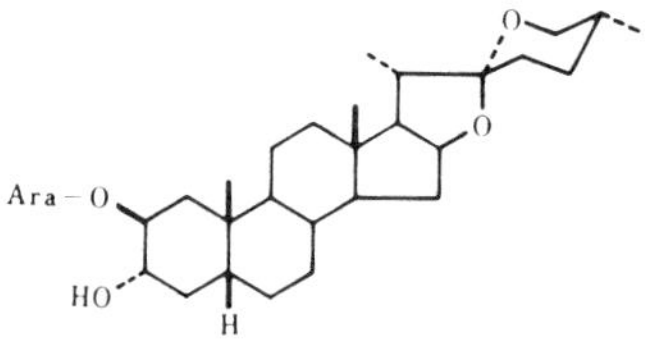

yononin

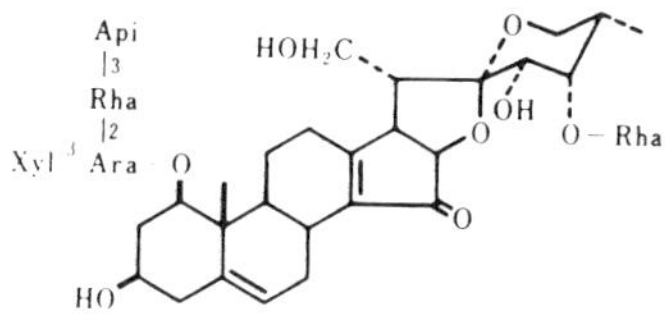

trillenoside

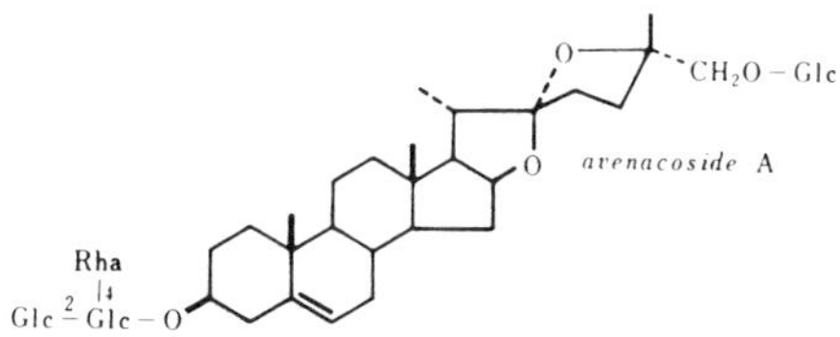

avenacoside A

Structure III

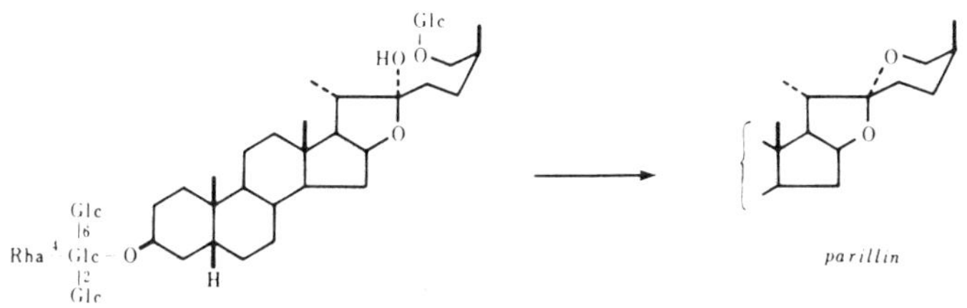

sarsaparilloside → *parillin*

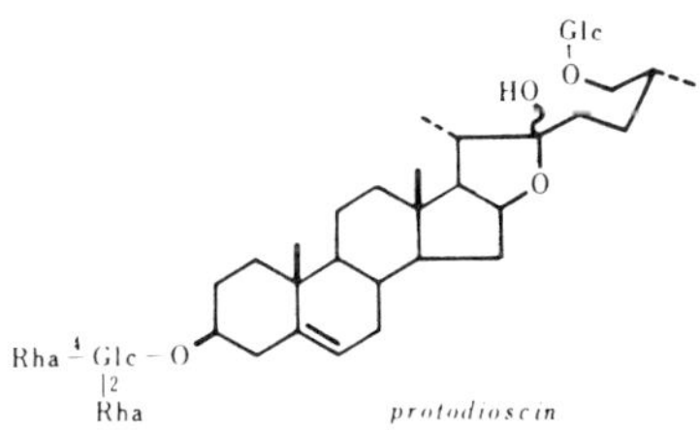

protodioscin

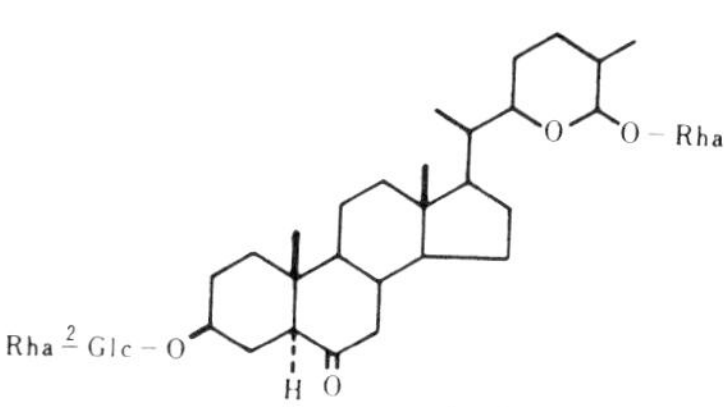

osladin

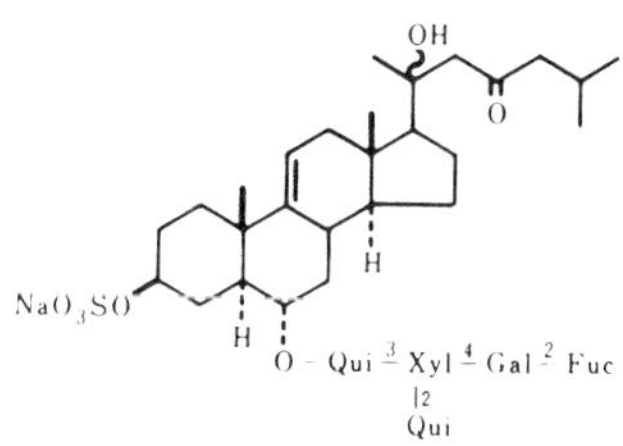

thornasteroside A

Structure IV

antibacterial action, antimold action, and poisonous reaction for molluscs, tadpoles, and fish, but these actions are weak or nonexistent in the furostanol glycosides. There is a hypothesis that the function of saponins in plants is as a defense against bacteria and plant viruses; that is, when a plant suffers injury, furostanol immediately changes into spirostanol, by the aid of an enzyme, to provide effective antibacterial action. With regard to the general chemistry of steroidal saponin, many reviews can be seen (Tschesche, 1973; Kawasaki, 1977a,b, 1982; Mahato *et al.*, 1982) (see Table 2 and structures III and IV).

II. QUALITATIVE ANALYSIS (COLORATION) AND DETECTION

There is no characteristic coloration for spirostanol, however, the Liebermann-Burchard reaction is usually applicable to the steroid with detection by thin-layer chromatography (TLC) using spraying reagents such as (1) chloroform solution (15%) of antimony chloride, (2) anisaldehyde/sulfuric acid reagent [0.5 ml anisaldehyde + g ml ethanol + 0.5 ml sulfuric acid (+0.1 ml acetic acid)], and (3) 10% sulfuric acid. In each case, spraying is followed by heating. Reagent (3) is the most conventional and convenient to use because the characteristics originating in aglycone can be observed by changes of color during heating and cooling. Tests for saponin are usually performed, such as for sudsing ability, fish poisoning, hemolysis, and formation of molecular complexes with cholesterol, as well as the Lieberman-Burchard reaction as color analysis. Moreover, the previously mentioned TLC color testing can also be applied to the spirostanols as can the color testing by chlorosulfonic acid/acetic acid (1:2), 30% sulfuric acid, 1% cerium sulfate in 10% sulfuric acid and cobalt chloride. Furthermore, it was found that furostanol glycoside shows a bright red color with Ehrlich reagent (1 g of *p*-dimethylaminobenzaldehyde + 50 ml of 36% hydrochloric acid + 50 ml of alcohol; spraying followed by heating). This color test is very useful (Kiyosawa *et al.*, 1968) for detecting furostanol glycoside because it can be distinguished from spirostanol glycoside, which is yellow.

III. EXTRACTION AND SEPARATION OF CRUDE SAPOGENOLS AND SAPONINS

Extraction is usually performed using water or alcohol (methanol and ethanol), repeatedly. However, because of the characteristics of saponin, water extraction foams strongly, and the solvent is very difficult to evaporate. Therefore, one should add antifoaming agents such as silicone oil and *n*-BuOH. The extract is defatted with petroleum ether, *n*-hexane, benzene, and ether. Excess chlorophyll can be eliminated with cyclohexane, chloroform, dichloromethane, and tetrachlorocarbon. Next, the residue is partitioned between water-saturated *n*-BuOH and water and separates comparatively easily into its components: sugar, water soluble contaminant (including strongly polar saponin), and regular saponin.

At this point, a recent typical separation method for saponin should be introduced. The BuOH layer is subjected to normal-phase silica-gel column chromatography. A good effect is obtained using various proportions of the solvent $CHCl_3/MeOH/H_2O$ (e.g., 7:3:0.5), which was developed by Kawasaki and Miyahara (1963). This solvent is considered to be the best one so far for separation. Moreover, chemical-bonding-type silica gel (octadodesyl silane, ODS), dextran derivative (Sephadex LH-20), and polystyrene high-porous resin column chromatographies are used effectively by slowly increasing the amount of MeOH in a dilute MeOH solvent system.

To check the separation of column chromatography, TLC is used with solvents such as $CHCl_3$/MeOH/water (65:35:10, 7:3:0.5, etc.), *n*-BuOH/AcOH/water (5:1:4), and *n*-BuOH-ethanol = 96% ammonia (3:6:5). The color test has already been mentioned.

The aqueous layer, after shaking *n*-BuOH and water, is passed through polystyrene high-porous resin (e.g. Amberlite XAD-2, Diaion CHP 20P). Major salts and sugar components pass through the column with water elution, and saponin remains in the resinous column. Subsequently, gradient elution using increasing amounts of MeOH (30% MeOH → 40% MeOH → MeOH) achieves separation of the saponins. Then the respective fractions are subjected to reversed silica-gel column chromatography to give a homogeneous saponin. In addition, droplet countercurrent chromatography (DCCC), designed by Tanimura *et al.* (1970), is sometimes effective for separating saponin. The solvent can be $CHCl_3$/MeOH/propanol/water (45:60:10:40), $CHCl_3$/MeOH/water (35:65:40), *n*-BuOH/AcOH/water (4:1:5), *n*-BuOH/propanol/water (2:1:3), $CHCl_3$/benzene/water (15:15:23:7) or AcOEt/propanol/water (4:2:7). Except for the above-mentioned recent methods, column chromatography has used dextran derivative (Sephadex LH-20, G-15), alumina, active charcoal, celite-florisil, or silicic acid-celite. Although separation of sapogenins that differ in the nature, number, and position of oxygen substituents is relatively easy, difficulties are encountered in the resolution of Δ^5- and 5α-sapogenins and are further compounded by isomerism at C-25. The 5β-sapogenins (smilagenin and sarsasapogenin) are less polar than their corresponding 5α-analogs (tigogenin and neotigogenin) in $CHCl_3$/toluene (9:1) on Kieselguhr G/silica gel G (1:1); however, the reverse order was observed when the sapogenin acetates were chromatographed in $CHCl_3$/toluene (9:1) on silica gel G. The 5α-compound, tigogenin acetate, moved faster than its Δ^5-analog, diosgenin acetate, in water-saturated dichloromethane/hexane (7:3) on silica gel G, developed continuously for 5 h. The 25R-sapogenins were consistently more mobile than their 25S-epimers in water-saturated dichloromethane/ether (199:1) on silica gel G, developed continuously for 6 h (Heftmann, 1967). It is dangerous to decide purity and to identify saponin only by physical constants such as melting point and $[\alpha]_D$. Besides the observations with TLC using various developers, HPLC and ^{13}C-NMR spectra have recently appeared as new and powerful methods. The ^{13}C-NMR measurement is assumed to be the most appropriate method for detecting purity because impurities appear as extra signals. Recently, Kawasaki *et al.* (1984) achieved separation of isomers at C-20 and C-25 of spirostanol by HPLC and substantiated their structures by the ^{13}C-NMR spectra.

IV. SPECTROSCOPIC ANALYSIS OF SAPOGENOLS AND SAPONINS

A. Infrared Spectra

It was found by Rothman *et al.* (1952) that several characteristic absorption bands due to spiroketal appeared between 850 and 990 cm^{-1}. Usually, four absorption bands (at 980, 918, 900, and 868 cm^{-1}) can be observed in the case of diosgenin, and by comparing their intensities at 900 and 920 one can decide whether the configuration at C-25 is R or S. That is, if the intensity of absorption at 900 is stronger than at 920, it is 25R; and the contrary case is 25S (Fig. 1). In the case of glycosides, their IR charts usually show a broad absorption band; however, spirostanol glycoside has the above-mentioned characteristic absorptions, which furostanol glycoside does not.

B. Electron-Impact, Field-Desorption, and Fast-Atom-Bombardment Mass Spectrometries

Electron-impact mass spectrometry (EI-MS) fragmentation of spirostanol was reported by Budzikiewicz *et al.* (1964), and the characteristic peak appears at *m/z* 139 (a) as a base peak originating from spiroketal (Fig. 2). Hydroxyl group(s) on the F-ring show a corresponding peak. In the case of the EI-MS of diosgenin, prominent peaks at *m/z* 414 (b, M^+), 396 (c), 282 (d), 267 (f), and 253 (g) originating from the steroidal main skeleton are observed (Fig. 3).

When the glycosidic sample is directly subjected to EI-MS without loading the appropriate derivative (methyl ether or acetate) (Nakano *et al.*, 1984), no fragment due to sugar moiety appears, but its spectrum shows a simplified fragmentation pattern ascribable to the aglycone residue. The diosgenin glycoside (e.g., dioscin) affords the above fragments (a–f). In the case of furostanol glycoside, a 26-glucosidic fragment at

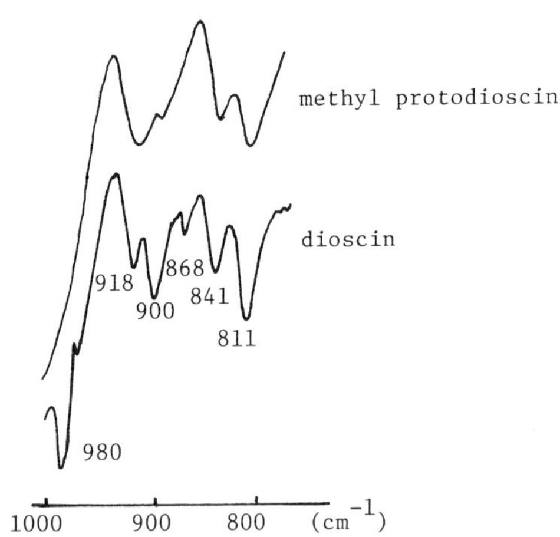

Figure 1 IR spectra of methyl protodioscin and dioscin.

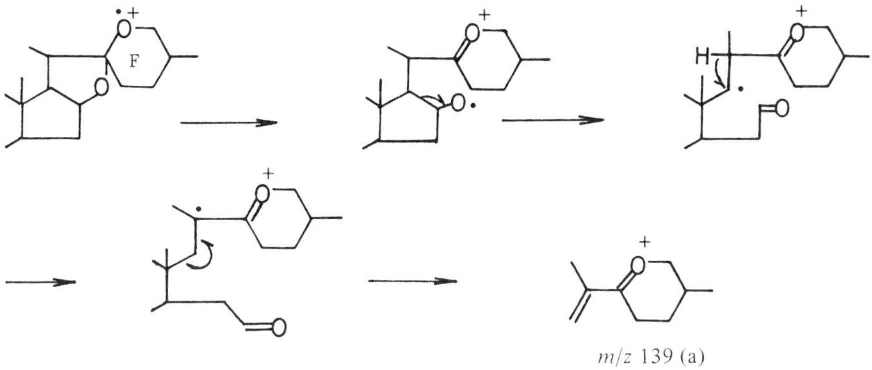

Figure 2 Fragmentation of spiroketal.

m/*z* 576 (g) is characteristic, though its intensity is not so strong. When the furostanol glycoside is subjected to electron impact, it changes partly into the spirostanol, and at the same time it gives the fragments (a–d and f) due to the spirostanol (Fig. 4). The EI-MS measurement of the appropriate derivatives (methyl ether or acetate) of saponins were reported (Komori *et al.*, 1975); however, the mass number of these molecular ions is larger. In the case of a compound, of which the molecular ion is over a thousand, it is difficult to detect the molecular ion because of the small intensities. But considerable information about the sugar sequence can be obtained. For example, the EI-MS of P-b permethyl ether afforded a M^+ at *m*/*z* 1154, though its intensity is weak, together with sugar fragments, terminal permethylated pentosyl cation at *m*/*z* 189, terminal permethylated methylpentosyl-methylpentosyl cation at *m*/*z* 363, and permethylated tetraosyl cation at *m*/*z* 741 (Komori *et al.*, 1975). Since the aglycone is

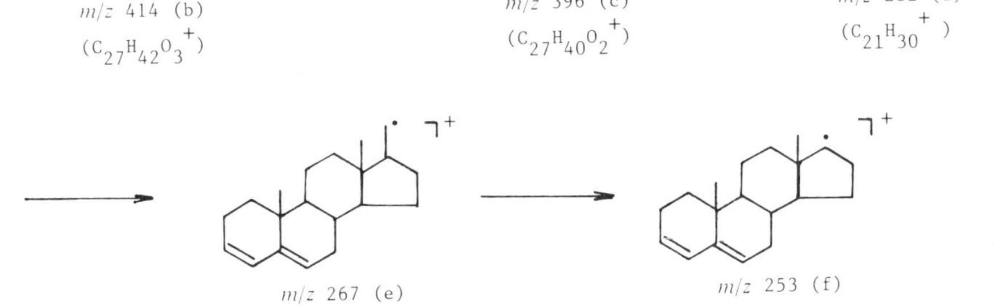

Figure 3 EI-MS spectrum of diosgenin.

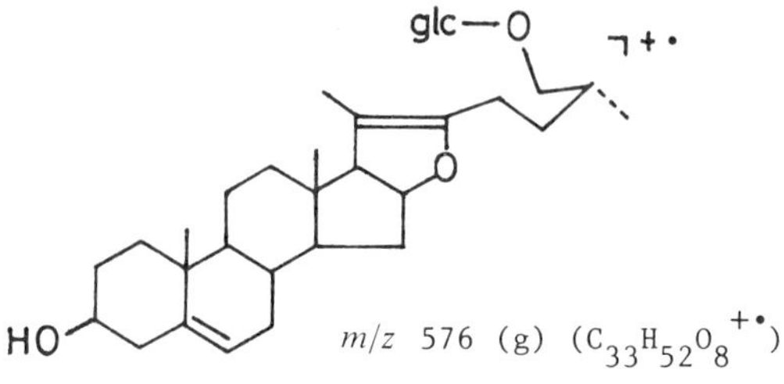

Figure 4 A fragment of furostanol.

diosgenin, the before-mentioned fragments a, c, d, and f appear. In the EI-MS of the acetate, for example, the EI-MS of gracillin acetate showed an M^+ at *m/z* 1262, peracetylated triosyl cation at *m/z* 849, peracetylated methylpentosyl cation at *m/z* 273, and peracetylated hexosyl cation at *m/z* 331 (Komori *et al.*, 1975).

Also, in the field of spirostanol glycoside (namely, saponin) chemistry, field-desorption mass spectrometry (FD-MS) has recently proven to be powerful. Until now, to measure a molecule of saponin, one had to measure the derivatives (acetate, silylate, methyl ether, etc.) of saponin. However, molecular ions could not sometimes be observed; and if they could be detected, they were of very small intensity and were difficult to discriminate. But the new methods of FD-MS and fast-atom bombardment mass spectrometry (FAB-MS) can solve the problem and determine the M^+ of the saponin. Schulten *et al.* (1978) rapidly adopted these methods in the saponin region, ascertained the complete occurrence of the M^+, and made clear that a large amount of information about the sugar sequence can be obtained. The FD-MS of methyl protodioscin showed peaks at *m/z* 1069 $[(M + K)\text{-MeOH}]^+$, 1053 $[(M + Na)\text{-MeOH}]^+$, 1030 $[M\text{-MeOH}]^+$, 923 $[1069\text{-rhamnose}]^+$, 907 $[1057\text{-rhamnose}]^+$, 891 $[1053\text{-glucose}]^+$, and 884 $[1030\text{-rhamnose}]^+$ (Komori *et al.*,1981). Moreover, they found that the ratio of the fragments in the FD-MS is nearly proportional to the yields of the prosapogenins obtained chemically by partial acid hydrolysis of saponin (Komori *et al.*, 1981). FAB-MS of methyl protodioscin showed peaks at *m/z* 1031 $[M + H\text{-}CH_3OH]^+$, 885 $[1031\text{-rhamnose}]^+$, 869 [1031-glucose], and 557 $[1031\text{-(glucose} + 2 \times \text{rhamnose)}]^+$. Both mass spectrometries can detect M^+ and are helpful methods for the determination of the purity and structures of saponins.

C. ^{1}H Nuclear Magnetic Resonance Spectra

First, it should be stated that a characteristic of the ^{1}H nuclear magnetic resonance (NMR) spectra of the ordinary spirostanols is that they show signals due to two angular methyl groups (10-Me and 13-Me) and two secondary methyl groups (20-Me and 25-Me). Diosgenin, as a typical example, shows signals ascribable to 3-H (m, δ 3.45), 16-H (m, δ 4.40), and 26-H_2 (m, δ 3.40). By the signal pattern due to 26-H_2 one can discriminate between 25R and 25S (Kutney, 1963). Since the chemical shifts of the α- and β-H at C-26 in the 25R compound are almost the same, they show a virtual

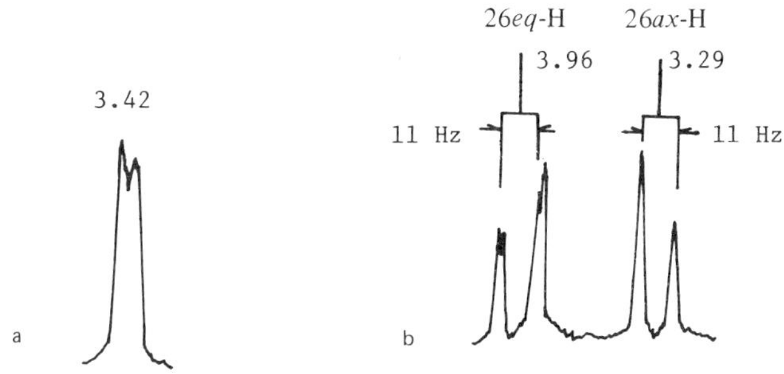

Figure 5 ^{1}H-NMR spectra showing C_{26} proton signals for (a) smilagenin (25R) and (b) neotigogenin (25S).

coupling, whereas signals due to 26-H_2 in the 25S compound can be observed as an AB quartet (Fig. 5). It is possible to estimate the ratio of a mixture of 25R and 25S by these signals. Whether a double bond, if present, is at C-5(6) or C-25(27) can easily be distinguished by the occurrence of its olefic proton. That is, C-5(6) shows signals due to 1H at around δ 5.32, and C-25(27) appears as a broad singlet signal due to 2H at around δ 4.79. When free saponin is measured in a solvent of $CDCl_3/CD_3OD/D_2O$ (7:3:0.5) and CF_3COOH (10%), signals due to anomeric protons that are hidden by the signals of many hydroxyl groups can be distinguished (Miyahara and Kawasaki, 1974). In measurement of dioscin by this method, signals ascribable to glucosyl and two rhamnosyl anomeric protons can be observed at about δ 4.5 (1H, d, J = 7 Hz), 4.9 (1H, br s), and 5.1 (1H, br s), respectively. By measurement of the ^{1}H-NMR spectrum of the methyl ether derived from saponin, in accordance with the Kuhn or Hakomori methods, these signals are also detectable at δ 4.2–5.4; and the mole number, juncture mode, and conformation of sugar can be discovered by the additional integration and J-value.

D. ^{13}C Nuclear Magnetic Resonance Spectra

1. Discrimination of Δ^5, 5α-H, 5β-H, 25R, 25S, and 25 Exomethylene-Spirostanols

Discrimination among 5β-H, 5α-H, and Δ^5 in the spirostanol derivatives can be made easily by the ^{13}C-NMR spectra. In the case of smilagenin (5β) and tigogenin (5α-H), significant differences at C-1–C-7, C-9, and C-19 can be observed in the chemical shift, as shown in Table 3. Moreover, in the case of the Δ^5 analog, the spectrum apparently differs from those of 5β-H and 5α-H because of sp^2 carbon intervention in the Δ^5 derivative. Furthermore, the 25R, 25S, and $\Delta^{25(27)}$ derivatives can be discriminated by the ^{13}C-NMR assignment of signals due to C-20–27 (Table 4).

2. Glycosidation Shift

With the formation of the glycosidic bond at the hydroxyl of sapogenol, the carbon adjacent to that hydroxyl group takes part in a significant change in the chemical shift (glycosidation shift; Kasai *et al.*, 1977; Tori *et al.*, 1977). This suggests that, in both

Table 3 ^{13}C-NMR spectra of smilagenin, tigogenin, and diosgenin

Carbon Site	Smilagenin (5β-H, 25R)	Tigogenin (5α-H, 25R)	Diosgenin (Δ^5, 25R)
C-1	30.6	37.5	37.8
C-2	28.6	32.5	32.5
C-3	66.0	70.6	71.2
C-4	34.4	39.3	43.4
C-5	37.0	45.2	142.0
C-6	27.2	29.1	121.0
C-7	26.9	32.5	32.3
C-8	35.6	35.4	31.8
C-9	40.4	54.6	50.4
C-10	35.6	35.9	37.0
C-11	21.2	21.4	21.2
C-12	40.2	40.3	40.0
C-13	41.0	40.8	40.5
C-14	56.6	56.6	56.8
C-15	32.2	32.1	32.3
C-16	81.2	81.1	81.1
C-17	63.2	63.1	62.9
C-18	16.6	16.7	19.1
C-19	24.2	12.5	19.6

sapogenol and its glycoside, the location of the glycosidic linkage can be determined by observing differences in the chemical shifts of the carbons that carry the hydroxyl group. Moreover, in the furostanol glycoside (22-OMe compound), which has an opened F-ring of spirostanol and a 26-*O*-glycosidic bond, the signals due to C-22–26 are shifted, respectively, by +3.5, −0.9, −1.1, +3.6, and +8.3 ppm compared with those of spirostanol (Fig. 6).

Table 4 ^{13}C-NMR spectra of diosgenin, yamogenin, and convallamarogenin

Carbon Site	Diosgenin (Δ^5, 25R)	Yamogenin (Δ^5, 25S)	Convallamarogenin (1β,3β-diacetoxy 5β-H, $\Delta^{25(27)}$)
C-20	42.0	42.5	42.0
C-21	15.0	14.9	15.0
C-22	109.2	109.7	109.4
C-23	31.9	26.4	29.0[a]
C-24	29.3	26.2	33.3[a]
C-25	30.6	27.5	144.5
C-26	66.9	65.1	65.1
C-27	17.3	16.3	108.1

[a] May be reversed.

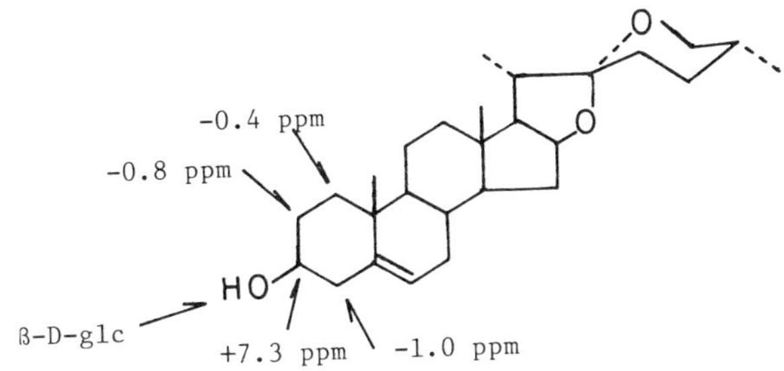

Figure 6 Shifts due to glucosidic linkage to C_3—OH of diosgenin.

3. Mole Number of Sugar and Linkage Mode

Anomeric carbons appear appropriately at around δ 95–110 ppm; thus, sugar mole numbers can be easily guessed by counting anomeric carbon peaks. Furthermore, by measuring $J_{C_1\text{-}H_1}$ of anomeric carbon (e.g., glucose: β-D-glc, 155 Hz and α-D-glc, 165 Hz; rhamnose: α-L-rha, 168 Hz and β-L-rha, 158 Hz), information can be obtained with regard to linkage modes.

REFERENCES

Budzikiewicz, H., Djerassi, C., and Williams, D. H. (1964). Steroidal sapogenins. *In* "Structure Elucidation of Natural Products by Mass Spectrometry," Vol 2, pp. 110–120. Holden-Day, San Francisco, California.

Heftmann, E., ed. (1967). "Chromatography," 2nd ed., pp. 550–553. Reinhold, New York.

Kasai, R., Suzuo, M., Asakawa, J., and Tanaka, O. (1977). Carbon-13 chemical shifts of isoprenoid-β-D-glucopyranosides and -β-D-mannopyranosides. Stereochemical influences of aglycone alcohols. *Tetrahedron Lett.* pp. 175–178.

Kawasaki, T. (1977a). Steroid saponin chemistry. *Proc. Symp. WAKAN-YAKU* **10**, 12–26.

Kawasaki, T. (1977b). Detection and isolation of steroidal saponin. *In* "Experimental of Natural Organic Compounds" (S. Natori, ed.), pp. 346–361. Kodansya Scientific Co., Tokyo.

Kawasaki, T. (1982). Spirostanol and furostanol type. *In* "Natural Products for Medicinal Use" (S. Shibata, ed.), pp. 430–436. Nanzando Co., Tokyo.

Kawasaki, T., and Miyahara, K. (1963). Thin layer chromatography of steroid saponins and their derivatives. *Chem. Pharm. Bull.* **11**, 1546–1550.

Kawasaki, T., Komori, T., Miyahara, K., Nohara, T., Hosokawa, I., and Mihashi, K. (1974). Furostanol bisglycosides corresponding to dioscin and gracillin. *Chem. Pharm. Bull.* **22**, 2164–2175.

Kiyosawa, S., Hutoh, M., Komori, T., Nohara, T., Hosokawa, I., and Kawasaki, T. (1968). Detection of proto-type compounds of diosgenin- and other spirostanol-glycoside. *Chem. Pharm. Bull.* **16**, 1162–1164.

Komori, T., Ida, Y., Mutou, Y., Miyahara, K., Nohara, T., and Kawasaki, T. (1975). Mass spectra of spirostanol and furostanol glycosides. *Biomed. Mass Spectrom.* pp. 65–77.

Komori, T., Maetani, I., Okamura, N., Kawasaki, T., Nohara, T., and Schulten, H.-R. (1981). Zur analogie der zuckerabspaltung aus oligoglykosidischen naturstoffen bei der säurehydrolyse und der felddesorptions-massenspektrometrie. *Liebigs Ann. Chem.* pp. 683–695.

Kudo, K., Miyahara, K., Marubayashi, N., and Kawasaki, T. (1984). Characterization of a minor compound, which accompanies the usual 22(R)-O,25β(S)-spirostanol glycoside, as a novel type of 22β(S)-O,25(S) analog. *Chem. Pharm. Bull.* **32**, 4229–4232.

Kutney, J. P. (1963). An nmr study in the steroidal sapogenin series. The sterochemistry of the spiroketal system. *Steroids* **1**, 225–235.

Mahato, S. B., Ganguly, A. N., and Sahu, N. P. (1982). Steroid saponins. *Phytochemistry* **21**, 959–978.

Miyahara, K., and Kawasaki, T. (1974). Anomeric proton signals of the component monosaccharides of free oligoglycosides in nuclear magnetic resonance spectroscopy. *Chem. Pharm. Bull.* **22**, 1407–1410.

Nakano, K., Miyamura, M., Ohe, M., Yoshioka, Y., Nohara, T., and Tomimatsu, T. (1984). Discrimination of the aglycones of diosgenin, pennogenin glycosides and their corresponding proto-type glycosides by the electron inpacting mass spectrometry. *Yakugaku Zasshi* **104**, 1140–1146.

Nohara, T., Nakano, A., Miyahara, K., Komori, T., and Kawasaki, T. (1975). Structure of a novel type steroid glycoside, 18-norspirostanol oligoglycoside. *Tetrahedron Lett.* pp. 4381–4384.

Rothman, E. S., Wall. M. E., and Eddy, C. R. (1952). Steroidal sapogenins. III. Structure of steroidal sapogenins. *J. Am. Chem. Soc.* **74**, 4013–4016.

Schulten, H. -R., Komori, T., Nohara, T., Higuchi, R., and Kawasaki, T. (1978). Field desorption mass spectrometry of natural products. II. Physiologically active pennogenin- and hederagenin-glycosides. *Tetrahedron* **34**, 1003–1010.

Tanimura, T., Pisano, J. J., Ito, Y., and Bowman, R. L. (1970). Droplet countercurrent chromatography. *Science* **169**, 54–56.

Tori, K., Seo, S., Yoshimura, Y., Arita, H., and Tomita, T. (1977). Glycosidation shifts in carbon-13 NMR spectroscopy: Carbon-13 signal shifts from aglycone and glucose to glucoside. *Tetrahedron Lett.* pp. 179–182.

Tschesche, R. (1973). Saponins. *Fortschr. Chem. Naturst.* **30**, 462.

Tschesche, R., and Richert, K. H. (1964). Über saponine der spirostanolrheihe. XI. Nuatigenin, ein cholegenin-analogon des pflanzenreiches. *Tetrahedron* **20**, 387–398.

Tschesche, R., Lüdke, G., and Wulff, G. (1967). Über sarsaparillosid, ein saponinderivat mit bisglykosidischer furostanolstruktur. *Tetrahedron Lett.* pp. 2785–2790.

8

Analysis of Oxysterols

Edward J. Parish
Department of Chemistry
Auburn University
Auburn, Alabama

I. INTRODUCTION

As a class of compounds, oxysterols can be defined as sterols bearing a second oxygen function, in addition to that at carbon-3, and having an iso-octyl or modified iso-octyl side chain. These compounds have demonstrated a variety of biological properties, including cytotoxicity, atherogenicity, carcinogenicity, mutagenicity, hypocholesterolemia, and effects on specific enzymes. Widely distributed in nature, they have been found in animal tissues and food stuffs (Smith, 1981) and have been isolated from drugs used in folk medicine for the treatment of cancer (Cheng *et al.*, 1977a,b, Nagano *et al.*, 1977a,b; Zandler *et al.*, 1977a,b). Other studies have shown that certain oxysterols have significant activity in the inhibition of DNA synthesis in cultured cells (De Fay *et al.*, 1982; Astruc *et al.*, 1978). A number of oxygenated derivatives of cholesterol and sterol intermediates in cholesterol biosynthesis have been found to be potent inhibitors of sterol biosynthesis in animal cells in culture (Schroepfer, 1981; Gibbons, 1983; Sinensky *et al.*, 1981). The specific inhibition of cholesterol biosynthesis in mammalian cells by oxygenated derivatives of cholesterol and lanosterol has been shown in many cases to decrease cellular levels of HMG-CoA reductase, a key regulatory enzyme in sterol biosynthesis (Sinesky *et al.*, 1981; Faust *et al.*, 1982; Tanaka *et al.*, 1983).

A large number of oxysterols have been evaluated for their abilities to repress HMG-CoA redustase activity in cultured mammalian cells (Schroepfer, 1981; Gibbons, 1983; Taylor *et al.*, 1984) and evidence for the existence of a specific cytrosolic receptor protein for oxysterols has been presented (Taylor *et al.*, 1984; Kandutsch *et al.*, 1984). After the activities of a number of sterols were evaluated, a good correlation was found between the actions of certain oxysterols on HMG-CoA reductase in L cells and their affinity for an oxysterol binding protein.

It has been shown that mammalian systems produce oxysterols. Derivatives of cholesterol hydroxylated in the 7α-, 25-, or 26-positions are produced in liver during bile acid biosynthesis (Vlahcevic *et al.*, 1980; Pederson *et al.*, 1979) and in side-chain hydroxylation in the 20α- and 22R- positions in the initial step in the conversion of cholesterol to steroid hormones in endocrine organs. Also, all cells produce 32-hydroxylanosterol and 32-oxolanosterol during the conversion of lanosterol to cholesterol (Gibbons *et al.*, 1980a; Tabacik *et al.*, 1981). Another mode of oxysterol biosynthesis has been described that uses the isopentenoid pathway to produce side-chain oxygenated derivatives of cholesterol and lanosterol (Nelson *et al.*, 1981; Panini *et al.*, 1984). Such compounds are derived from squalene 2,3-epoxide by the introduction of a second oxygen function to form squalene 2,3:22,23-dioxide prior to cyclization. Thus, this intermediate has been shown to form 24(S),25-epoxylanosterol, 24(S),25-epoxycholesterol, and 25-hydroxycholesterol in mammalian systems (Nelson *et al.*, 1981; Panini *et al.*, 1986). 24(S),25-Epoxycholesterol has been isolated from cultured mouse L cells, Chinese hamster lung fibroblasts, and human liver (Spencer *et al.*, 1985; Saucier *et al.*, 1985). These results add support to the hypothesis that oxysterols may be natural regulators of cholesterol biosynthesis in mammalian cells (Kandutsch *et al.*, 1978). Many oxygenated sterols are known to exist in and have been isolated from plants; these may be precursors to sterols required for growth and/or reproduction or may be secondary plant metabolites (Overton *et al.*, 1971–1976; Hanson *et al.*, 1977–1983). Another major source of oxysterols is the autoxidation of cholesterol, lanosterol, and other related sterols (Smith, 1981, 1987).

Due to the general interest in oxysterols and their wide distribution (both as naturally occurring and as synthetic substances), their analysis and structural characterization are topics of concern to both chemists and biochemists. During the isolation, chemical synthesis, and use of these compounds, specific methods have evolved for the analysis of this class of sterol. The purpose of the present work is to collect and categorize a number of these methods and techniques.

II. ISOLATION AND PURIFICATION

Many oxysterols contain functional groups (e.g., epoxides and ketones) that may be sensitive to high concentrations of acids or bases. Epoxides may undergo nucleophilic attack by strong bases (e.g., NaOH and KOH) and undergo ring opening. Moreover, treatment with strong acids can result in ring opening to form alcohols, alkenes, and ketones. The hydrolysis of cholesterol epoxides under mildly acidic conditions has been studied (Maerker and Bunick, 1986). Modified procedures are available for the isolation of steroidal epoxides from tissues and cultured cells by a saponification and/or extraction. (Saucier *et al.*, 1985; Spencer *et al.*, 1985; Panini *et al.*, 1986; Watabe and Sawahata, 1979; Watabe *et al.*, 1981). Ketones are known to form enolates under the influence of strong bases, which may then form condensation products of higher molecular weight (Maerker and Unruh, 1986). To circumvent these potential problems, procedures using direct extraction techniques are sometimes preferred to a saponification followed by extraction. Mild methods for the removal of the ester function without ketone enolization include the use of sodium or potassium carbonate in heated aqeuous solutions of methanol or ethanol. The addition of tetrahydrofuran to these mixtures has been found to significantly increase the solubility of more polar oxysterols (Parish and Schroepfer, 1980a; Parish *et al.*, 1984; E. J. Parish, M. Tsuda, and G. J. Schroepfer, Jr., unpublished results, 1988; Kumar *et al.*, 1987; Poyser and Ourisson, 1974; Burrows *et al.*, 1969).

Since most oxysterols, whether synthesized or obtained from a natural source, are seldom found in a pure state, a chromatographic purification is usually required. Conventional column chromatography using silica gel and eluting with solvent or a gradient of solvents of increasing polarity can produce excellent results if carefully conducted (Parish and Scott, 1983; Parish *et al.*, 1984). Other improvements include the use of medium-pressure liquid chromatography for difficult separations (Parish and Schroepfer, 1979, 1981a). In general, a steroidal mixture that can be resolved by thin-layer chromatography can be satisfactorily resolved by this procedure. High-performance liquid chromatography can also be used to isolate oxysterols in quantities large enough to permit characterization (Nelson *et al.*, 1981; Saucier *et al.*, 1985; Panini *et al.*, 1986).

Certain Δ^7-14-alkyl-15-hydroxy sterols cannot be separated by conventional chromatography. To facilitate isolation, their C-15 epimeric mixtures can be resolved by selective acetylation of the 15α-hydroxy epimer and chromatography of the resulting reaction products (Schroepfer *et al.*, 1977a; Parish *et al.*, 1979a,b).

Steroids (including oxysterols) are usually not highly crystalline substances. By using the benzoate (in preference to the acetate) ester, one can achieve a greater degree of crystallinity. This technique was used during the synthesis and isolation of 3β-benzoyloxy-14α,15α-epoxycholest-7-ene, a key intermediate in the synthesis of many 15 oxygenated sterols (Parish *et al.*, 1977, 1986). Benzoate esters are easily crystallized from systems and can be used to advantage during purification. A variety of solvent systems are reported for recrystallizing oxysterols. Ethanol/water, methanol/water, and particularly acetone/water have produced good results and are commonly used (Parish *et al.*, 1979a,b, 1984; Raulston *et al.*, 1976; Smith, 1981).

III. CHROMATOGRAPHIC ANALYSIS

A. Gas Chromatography

The sensitivity of the hydrogen flame-ionization detector, which is commonly found on most gas chromatographs, is sufficient to detect cholesterol at the nanogram level. Equal sensitivity for other sterols, including many oxysterols, should be expected. Unfortunately, the oxygenated functionality found in certain oxysterols may be labile to the thermal conditions used in gas chromatography (Smith, 1981).

A variety of oxysterols and oxysterol product mixtures, resulting from the oxidation of cholesterol, have been frequently analyzed by gas chromatography. Homberg and Bielefeld (1979) have reported the relative retention times of several A/B-ring oxysterols on nine different stationary phases of various polarities. Other work on the direct injection of underivatized and silylated cholesterol oxidation-product mixtures has led to the development of optimized procedures and conditions for analysis (Maerker and Unruh, 1986). Despite problems of incomplete derivatization and peak resolution, the application of gas chromatographic methods to this type of analysis has been somewhat more successful compared with the results obtained from high-performance liquid chromatography.

The use of capillary gas chromatography, particularly in combination with direct on-column injection, has increased the capability of gas chromatography as a useful and powerful tool in the analysis of cholesterol oxides. In this respect, the studies of Missler *et al.* (1985) and Krull *et al.* (1984) are especially noteworthy. Thin-layer chromatography has been used to enrich oxysterol fractions from complex mixtures prior to gas chromatographic analysis (Missler *et al.*, 1985; Maerker and Unruh, 1986; Maerker and Bunick, 1986).

A number of dioxygenated C_{27}-, C_{28}-, and C_{29}-sterols have been systematically separated on lipophilic Sephaxed gels followed by gas chromatographic analysis (Aringer and Nordstrom, 1981). Epimeric C-15 hydroxysterols have been analyzed by gas chromatography (Gibbons and Ramananda, 1975; Spike *et al.*, 1978). Preparative gas chromatography has been used to isolate oxysterols resulting from biological oxidations (Gibbons *et al.*, 1980b), and radio-gas chromatography was used to access the purity of radiolabeled oxysterols (Parish and Schroepfer, 1981b).

Due to their crystallinity, benzoate esters are commonly used during the chemical synthesis of oxysterols (Parish *et al.*, 1986). In contrast to acetates, the purity of benzoate esters is not routinely assessed by gas chromatographic methods because of the appearance of pyrolysis products. In one study that used capillary gas chromatography, the pyrolysis of benzoate esters was not observed (Parish *et al.*, 1987).

B. High-Performance Liquid Chromatography

High-performance liquid chromatography is increasingly used in oxysterol analysis. In many instances, oxysterols are quantitated using an ultraviolet detector operating at very short wavelengths. The relatively low molar absorbances, even at short wavelengths, for noncarbonyl and nondienoid oxysterols limits the sensitivity of detection, but sensitive measurements below 220 nm are routinely made. However, the 5,6-epoxides of cholesterol must be detected by the less sensitive differential refractive index detector. Ketosteroids can be detected with much greater sensitivity at wavelengths near their ultraviolet absorption maxima. Also, increased sensitivity can be attained by derivatization with reagents with a strong ultraviolet absorption. 3β-Benzoate and nitrobenzoate esters can be detected at nanogram levels. Thus, the 5,6-epoxides of cholesterol are readily detected as their 3β-benzoate esters (Smith, 1981; Ansari and Smith, 1979).

Cholesterol oxidation-product mixtures of varying complexities have been analyzed frequently by high-performance liquid chromatography. In spite of very significant recent advances, techniques have not yet reached the point of being useful in the separation and quantification of complex mixtures of cholesterol oxides (Maerker and Unruh, 1986). Tsai and Hudson (1981) have analyzed 24 oxygenated cholesterols and structurally related compounds with a silicic acid column and various mobile phases. The usual order of decreasing retention volumes were hydroxy on the ring, carbonyl on the ring, epoxy on the ring, hydroxy on the side chain, and carbonyl on the side chain. Synergistic effects of multiple hydroxyl substitutions on cholesterol were also observed.

High-performance liquid chromatography has recently been successfully used to quantify side-chain oxygenated derivatives of cholesterol and lanosterol isolated as products of cellular metabolism (Saucier *et al.*, 1985; Panini *et al.*, 1986, 1987). Also, similar techniques were used to discover the presence of 24(S),25-epoxycholesterol in human liver in an amount relative to cholesterol of approximately 10^{-3} (Spencer *et al.*, 1985). An earlier report describing the examination of human aorta, liver, and plasma for the presence of fatty acyl esters of oxidized cholesterol derivatives has also appeared (Smith, 1981). Recently, Chu and Schroepfer (1988) have developed conditions that permit the resolution of cholest-8(14)-en-3β-ol-15-one and cholesterol and fatty acyl esters of the two sterols.

C. Thin-Layer Chromatography

Thin-layer chromatography is a simple but effective method for the analysis of oxysterols. It has been described as possibly the best technique for resolving complex mixtures of cholesterol autoxidation products (Smith, 1981). Oxysterols have usually been detected by spraying with aqueous sulfuric acid and then warming to full color display using visible light or charring by more heat. Under these conditions, many oxysterols show different and distinctive color reactions. The phosphomolybdic acid or molybdic acid (Parish and Schroepfer, 1981a; Knapp and Schroepfer, 1975) reagents are also useful and give sensitive results, but in many instances they suffer from lack of color display for individual oxysterols. Using these methods one can detect as little as 5 μg of oxysterol. Other standard reagents and techniques have been used to detect cholesterol oxidation products (Smith, 1981).

Analysis of epimeric mixtures of steroidal alcohols by thin-layer chromatography can be useful for structural assignments; such mixtures are commonly the result of hydride reduction of the corresponding ketone. When mixtures of Δ^5-7-hydroxy sterols were examined on plates of silica gel G, the C-7β-epimer was less polar than the corresponding C-7α-epimer (Parish and Scott, 1983; Parish *et al.*, 1984; Kumar *et al.*, 1987). In the series of Δ^7-14α-alkyl-15-hydroxy sterols, similar results were found; the C-15β-epimeric alcohol was observed to be less polar than the C-15α-epimer (Martin *et al.*, 1970; Shcroepfer *et al.*, 1977c; Spike *et al.*, 1978; Parish *et al.*, 1979b). However, in the $\Delta^{8(14)}$-15-hydroxy series, the C-15β-epimeric alcohol was found to be more polar than the C-15α-epimer (Huntoon and Schroepfer, 1970 ; Phillips *et al.*, 1976). In another series, Δ^7-14β-15-hydroxy sterols (having an "unnatural" C/D-ring juncture) were resolved as an epimeric mixture, and the C-15β-epimer was found to be more polar than the C-15α-epimer (Parish *et al.*, 1976; Parish and Schroepfer, 1977a). Aringer and Nordstrom (1981) have described the analyses of a large number of oxygenated sterols, many of which were epimeric alcohols. Burrows *et al.* (1969) have reported the resolution of epimeric C-22 hydrosterols by both column and thin-layer chromatography.

A variety of solvent systems have been used to quantify natural and synthetic oxysterols. Some of the more common examples include various concentrations of benzene or toluene/ethyl ether, benzene or toluene/ethyl acetate, hexane/ethyl ether or ethyl acetate, and choloroform/ethyl ether or ethyl acetate, and chloroform/ethyl acetate (Parish and Schroepfer, 1981). Solvent systems have been discovered and developed for use with specific classes of oxysterols. Maerker and Bunick (1986) analyzed cholesterol autoxidation products using benzene/ethyl acetate/acetic acid (60:40:1) as the developing solvent. Oxysterols derived from the cellular cyclization of squalene 2,3:22,23-dioxide were resolved with a two-dimensional system using petroleum ether/acetone (90:10) as the first developing solvent. For the second dimension, a reverse-phase separation, the plate was impregnated with paraffin by dipping in a solution of 5% paraffin oil in petroleum ether and then developed in the second dimension with acetone/paraffin (saturated) water (85:15) as the developing solvent (Sexton *et al.*, 1987). Also, a solvent system of chloroform/ethyl ether/acetic acid (97:2.5:0.5) was used to successfully separate 32-oxygenated derivatives of 24,25-dihydrolanosterol (Parish and Schroepfer, 1981a).

IV. SPECTROSCOPIC METHODS

A. Nuclear Magnetic Resonance

Proton (^{1}H) nuclear magnetic resonance has been central to characterizing new oxysterols and confirming the structures of others. Without its use, structure determination would be difficult if not impossible in some cases. Examples of the application of proton nuclear magnetic resonance to the analysis of oxysterols are numerous indeed, and several notable examples are cited herein (Schroepfer, 1981; Parish *et al.*, 1986).

Shoolery and Rogers (1958) demonstrated that the frequency shifts of the C-18 and C-19 angular nmethyl protons of steroids were induced by several different functional groups and are approximately additive. This concept was further developed and extended by Zurcher (1963), who studied 260 steroids of known structure and derived many consistent chemical-shift values exhibited to specific functional groups at various nuclear locations. These results, and others, have been correlated into useful tables by Bhacca and Williams (1984); they are invaluable for the confirmation of oxygen functional groups on the sterol nucleus and have been extensively used in the identification of new oxysterol structures (Schroepfer, 1981; Parish *et al.*, 1986). Deviations from additivity, using these values, result from a deformed steroid frame, which is different from that of the basic ring conformations. The introduction of double bonds or epoxide rings at certain positions commonly cause this effect.

Because of their potent action as inhibitors of sterol biosynthesis, 15-oxygenated sterols have received a great deal of attention in recent years. During their chemical synthesis, it was noted that the C-7 vinyl proton of Δ^7-15-keto steroids was deshielded and shifted downfield to a lower resonance if the C/D-ring juncture was in the trans or "natural" configuration. This observation was useful in discerning the structure of the "unnatural" isomer with a C/D-cis ring juncture. Table 1 contains data derived from these and related compounds and exhibits the effects of an oxygen function at C-15 (15α-ol, 15β-ol, and 15-keto) on the resonance of the C-7 vinyl

Table 1 Effect of 15-oxygen function on the resonance of the C-7 proton in C-14α- and C-14β-Δ^7-sterols and their derivatives

	Oxygen Function at C-15			
		15-Hydroxy		
C-14-Substituent	None	15α-ol	15β-ol	15-Ketone
14α-Hydrogen				
3β-hydroxy	5.18	5.55	—	—
3β-acetate	5.18	—	—	—
3β-benzoate	5.18	—	—	—
14β-Hydrogen				
3β-hydroxy	—	5.50	5.49	—
3β-benzoate	—	—	—	5.44
3-ketone	—	5.45	5.45	—
14α-Hydroxyl				
3β-hydroxy	5.39	—	—	—
3 ketone	5.41	—	—	—
14α-Hydroxymethyl				
3β-hydroxy	5.30	—	—	—
3-ketone	5.32	—	—	—
14α-Acetoxymethyl				
3β-acetate	5.14	—	—	—
14α-Methyl				
3β-hydroxy	5.20	5.49	5.62	6.61
3β-acetate	5.20	—	—	—
3β-benzoate	—	—	—	6.54
3β-methoxy	—	5.49	5.58	6.60
14α-Ethyl				
3β-hydroxy	—	5.52	5.60	6.52
3β-acetate	—	—	5.63	—
3β-hydroxy	—	—	—	6.51
3β-benzoate	—	—	—	6.59
3β-ethoxy	—	—	—	6.58
14α-*n*-Propyl				
3β-hydroxy	—	5.48	5.68	6.53
3β-acetate	—	—	5.60	6.50
14α-Butyl				
3β-hydroxy	—	5.50	5.61	6.52
3β-acetoxy	—	—	5.62	6.52

Note: Resonances are given in ppm downfield from a tetramethylsilane internal standard.

Table 2 Effect of configuration of the 15-hydroxyl function on the resonance of the C-15 carbinol proton in C-14α- and C-14β-Δ^7-sterols

C-14-Substituent	15-Hydroxyl Function	
	15α-ol	15β-ol
14α-Hydrogen		
3β-hydroxy	4.25	—
14β-Hydrogen		
3β-hydroxy	3.75[a]	3.75[a]
3-ketone	4.02	3.81
14α-Methyl		
3β-hydroxy	4.33	4.12
3β-methoxy	4.25	4.05
14α-Ethyl		
3β-hydroxy	4.34	4.10
14α-*n*-Propyl		
3β-hydroxy	4.35	4.13
14α-*n*-Butyl		
3β-hydroxy	4.35	4.08

Note: Resonances are given in ppm downfield from a tetramethylsilane internal standard.

[a] These resonances overlap with those of the 3α-carbonyl proton.

proton in Δ^7-oxysterols (Parish *et al.*, 1979; Parish and Schroepfer, 1977b, 1979; Pascal and Schroepfer, 1980a,b; Schroepfer *et al.*, 1979a, 1980; Pascal *et al.*, 1979). Table 2 contains the effects of the configuration of the 15-hydroxyl function on the resonance observed from the C-15 carbinol proton in the same series of compounds. These results are useful in determining the configuration of the hydroxyl group at C-15.

In Δ^7-14α-alkyl sterols, the configuration of hydroxyl groups at C-15 can also be determined by observing the multiplet of the C-15 carbinol proton. The resonance due to the 15α-proton in these 15β-hydroxy sterols occurs as a doublet. Measurement from Dreiding models of the dihedral angles between the carbinol proton on C-15 and the protons on C-16 showed an angle of approximately 90° between the 16β-proton and the 15α-proton and an angle of approximately 30° between the 16α-proton and the 15α-proton. Using the methods of Karplus (1963) and Williamson and Johnson (1961), one finds that a dihedral angle of 90° should give a coupling constant *J* of approximately 0 whereas an angle of 30° should give a *J* value of approximately 6.2 cps. The resonance due to the 15β-proton in 15α-hydroxy sterols occurs as a doublet of doublets in the observed spectra of this class of sterol. Measurement from Drieding models of the dihedral angles between the carbinol proton at C-15 and the proton at C-16 show an angle of approximately 30° between the 15β-proton and 16β-proton and an angle of approximately 150° between the 15β-proton and the 16α-proton. A dihedral angle of 150° should result in a coupling constant of approximately 8.5 cps whereas, as noted previously, an angle of 30° should result in a coupling constant of approximately 6.2 cps. These calculated values are in close agreement with those observed with a number of Δ^{7}-14α-alkyl-15α- and β-hydroxy sterols (Schroepfer *et al.*, 1977b); Spike *et al.*, 1978; Parish *et al.*, 1979a). Another interesting phenomenon is the effect of a C-15-keto group on the C-7β-proton of $\Delta^{8(14)}$-15-keto sterols. The 15-keto function causes this proton (C-7β) to be deshielded to a lower frequency and easily observed in the spectrum. The C-7β-proton resonates at 4.18 ppm in cholest-8(14)-en-3β-ol-15-one, a compound with hypocholesterolemic activity (Raulston *et al.*, 1976; Schroepfer *et al.*, 1984). Since the C-7α-proton is not deshielded and observed downfield, the appearance or absence of the C-7α-proton can be used to determine the configuration of functional groups attached to C-7. Table 3 contains a variety of $\Delta^{8(14)}$-15-keto sterols and demonstrates the effects of structure on this diagnostic proton resonance (Parish and Schroepfer, 1976, 1977a, 1979, 1988; Schroepfer *et al.*,

Table 3 Effect of ring substitution on the resonance of the C-7β proton in $\Delta^{8(14)}$-15-keto sterols and their derivatives

$\Delta^{8(14)}$-15-Ketone	C-7β Proton
Cholest-8(14)-en-15-one	4.12
3β-hydroxyl	4.18
3α-hydroxyl	4.15
3β-acetate	4.13
3α-acetate	4.14
3β-benzoate	4.22
3α-benzoate	4.22
3β-hemisuccinate	4.20
3β-palmatate	4.15
3α-chloro	4.15
3α-pyridinium sulfate	4.25
3α-pyridinium sulfate	4.23
3β-potassium sulfate	4.25
3α-potassium sulfate	4.25
3-ketone	4.19
9α,3β-dihyroxyl	3.96
9α-hydroxyl-3β-acetate	3.95
9α-hydroxyl-3-ketone	3.96
9α-fluoro-3β-hydroxyl	3.90
9α-fluoro-3β-acetate	3.95
9α-fluoro-3β-benzoate	3.96
9α-fluoro-3-ketone	3.90
7α-^{2}H-3-ketone	4.21
7β-^{2}H-3β-benzoate	—
7α,3β-dihydroxyl	5.87
7α-hydroxyl-3-ketone	5.89
7α,3β-dibenzoate	6.95
7α-methyl-3β-hydroxyl	4.43
7α-methyl-3-ketone	4.43

Note: Resonances are given in ppm downfield from a tetramethylsilane internal standard.

1987; Kisic *et al.*, 1977; St. Pyrek and Schroepfer, 1987; St. Pyrek *et al.*, 1987; Parish *et al.*, 1979a).

The configuration of the epimeric Δ^5-C-7 alcohols can also be determined by analysis of the proton spectra resulting from each epimer (Parish *et al.*, 1984; Teng *et al.*, 1973). The vinyl proton at C-6 is shifted further downfield in the spectra of the C-7α-hydroxyl epimer, relative to the 7β-hydroxyl derivative. Gibbons and Ramanda (1975) have reported the use of the position of the C-18 methyl proton signal and the C-15 carbinol signal in assigning the correct configuration of the hydroxyl group at C-15 to lanost-7-en-3β,15α- and β-diols. Also, mixtures of the 5,6-epoxides of cholesterol and their esters are conveniently analyzed by proton spectra by observing the doublet resulting from the C-6-hydrogen (Smith, 1981). The C-6β-hydrogen of the 5α,6α-epoxide is a doublet (J = 3.3–4.1 cps) near 2.8 ppm and the C-6α-hydrogen of the isomeric 5β,6β-epoxide is also a doublet (J = 2.1–3.0 cps) near 3.0 ppm.

Carbon-13 (^{13}C) nuclear magnetic resonance studies can provide far more information concerning the structure of steroids than proton (^{1}H) nuclear magnetic resonance studies because most of the carbons exhibit separately resolved signals that can be assigned to specific carbon atoms with a high degree of confidence (Stothers, 1972). Since the first report by Reich *et al.* (1969), which clearly established the utility of the ^{13}C nuclear magnetic resonance studies of steroids, the field has expanded to include work on all classes of steroids.

The early work of Reich *et al.* (1969) and Blunt and Stothers (1977) included a few examples of oxysteroid spectral assignments. More recently, Tsuda *et al.* (1979) has undertaken the spectra analysis of cholest-8(14)-ene-3β,7α,15α-triol and in the process has examined the spectra of several C-7 and C-15 allylic hydroxysterols. Tsuda and Schroepfer (1981) have also analyzed the carbon spectra of 9α-fluorocholest-8(14)-en-3β-ol-15-one and some related compounds (steroid hypocholesterolemic agents). Parish *et al.* (1987) have reported the assignments for carbon atoms in 7-ketocholesteryl benzoate using a DEPT experiment and an additional C-H correlation experiment. With these techniques, assignments to individual carbons were conveniently made in a timely manner. Using similar techniques, St. Pyrek *et al.* (1987) have reported the analysis of the carbon, proton, and deuterium spectra of cholest-8(14)-en-3β-ol-15-one and its derivatives.

Djerassi *et al.* have reported both the ^{1}H and ^{13}C spectra of a number of oxysterols derived from marine sources or from intermediates in their chemical synthesis (Taylor and Djerassi, 1977; Cho and Djerassi, 1987; Jagodzinska *et al.*, 1985; Catalan *et al.*, 1983; Hirano and Djerassi, 1982). Anastasia *et al.* (1979a,b,c, 1983, 1986) have also published many examples of the carbon and proton spectra of a variety of oxysterols produced during the chemical synthesis of biologically significant steroids.

B. Mass Spectrometry

Mass spectrometry has had an important role in the identification and structural confirmation of oxysterols. In combination with gas chromatography, it is a powerful tool for identifying small amounts of oxysterols in complex mixtures. Since many oxysterols may be less than 100% pure, even after chromatography and recrystallization, the use of high-resolution mass spectrometry in exact mass measurements of molecular ions M^+ may be preferable to an elemental microanalysis in establishing structure (elemental composition).

Even though information obtained from the evaluation or analysis of a mass spectrum is included with the isolation and/or synthesis of almost all oxysterols, only a few significant systematic studies of the mass spectrometry of this class of sterol have appeared. Aringer and Nordstrom (1981) studied the fragmentation patterns of a number of dioxygenated C_{27}-, C_{28}-, and C_{29}-sterols and their trimethylsilyl (TMS) derivatives. Recently, an analysis of cholest-8(14)-en-3β-ol-15-one and a number of its fatty acid derivatives has appeared St. Pyrek and Schroepfer, 1987; St. Pyrek *et al.*, 1987). Djerassi *et al.* have published the analyzed spectra of a number of oxysterols derived from marine invertebrates (Jagodzinska *et al.*, 1985; Catalan *et al.*, 1983; Hirano and Djerassi, 1982; Roller *et al.*, 1970). In some instances, studies of ring fragmentations that would be relevant to oxysterol structure were facilitated by the removal of the 3-hydroxyl group, leaving the oxygen functionality on other ring positions (Midgley and Djerassi, 1973).

Wulfson *et al.* (1967) have proposed that the configuration of steroidal alcohols can be determined by study of the ratio of the abundances of the molecular ion M^+ to the ion due to loss of water ($M\text{-}H_2O$) with the axially substituted hydroxysteroid giving the lower ratio. This method was used to confirm the configuration of C-15 epimeric Δ^7-14-methyl hydroxysterols (Spike *et al.*, 1978; Schroepfer *et al.*, 1977a).

C. Infrared Spectrometry

Aside from the confirmation of certain functional groups, the use of infrared spectroscopy in oxysterol analysis is somewhat less diagnostic than other methods. One example of its utility is the use of the characteristic adsorption pattern of unsaturated ketones. Conjugation with a double bond results in delocalization of the electrons of both unsaturated groups (reduction of double-bond character) and causing absorption at a lower wavenumber (longer wavelengths). In this instance, the intensity of absorption of the olefinic bond in conjugation with the carbonyl is increased. The absorption of the carbonyl in sterolidal $\Delta^{8(14)}$-15-ketones is found at approximately 1700–1725 cm^{-1}, and an almost equally intense absorption for the olefinic group is observed at approximately 1612–1632 cm^{-1} (Raulston *et al.*, 1976; Parish *et al.*, 1977; Parish and Schroepfer, 1977a, 1979, 1980b; Schroepfer *et al.*, 1979b). Also, the spectral characterization of each of the isomeric 5,6-epoxides of cholesterol has been described (Chicoyte, 1968). The use of infrared spectrometry in the limited analysis of a number of cholesterol autoxidation products has been reviewed (Smith, 1981).

D. Optical Rotation

The measurement of the specific rotation $[\alpha]_D$ of steroids is usually conducted at 25°C in solutions of chloroform using a sodium-lamp light source. Steroid concentrations *c* of approximately 1% are common and are expressed as g/100 ml of solvent (Fieser and Fieser, 1949, 1959).

The usefulness of these measurements in oxysterol analysis results from the characteristic values exhibited by individual compounds as a means of identification. These values are particularly useful in the analysis of individual epimeric alcohols because, in many instances, these values differ greatly. The early work by Cook (1958) is especially noteworthy because he has recorded the specific rotations of a number of individual epimeric alcohols and other oxysterols. The recent use of these values, obtained from epimeric alcohols at C-7 and C-15, has been particularly significant in assigning configuration. At these carbons, a substantial levorotatory effect is observed for the 7β- or 15α-hydroxyl function whereas the values obtained from the 7α- or 15β-hydroxyl function are more dextrorotatory compared with the corresponding parent compounds containing no oxygen functionality at C-7 or C-15 (Fried *et al.*, 1964; Gibbons and Ramanada, 1975; Parish and Schroepfer, 1977b; Parish *et al.*, 1976, 1979b, 1984; Schroepfer *et al.*, 1977a, 1979b; Huntoon *et al.*, 1978). Table 4 contains some recently obtained values from C-7 and C-15 hydroxy sterols.

Table 4 Specific rotations $[\alpha]_D$ of C-15- and C-7-hydroxy sterols and their derivatives

Sterol	α-ol	β-ol
C-15-Hydroxyl function		
14α-methylcholest-7-ene-3β,15-diols	+33.0	−46.5
14α-methylcholest-7-ene-3β-methoxy-15-diols	+27.7	−27.9
14α-ethylcholest-7-ene-3β,15-diols	+9.8	−41.8
14α-ethylcholest-7-en-3β-acetate-15β-ol	—	−44.1
14α-ethylcholest-7-ene-3β-,15α-diacetate	+4.4	—
14α-ethylcholest-7-ene-3β-palmitate-15-diols	+11.5	−26.4
14α-ethylcholest-7-ene-3β,15α-dipalmitate	+7.0	—
14α-propylcholest-7-en-3β,15-diols	+21.8	−37.5
14α-propylcholest-7-en-3β-acetate-15β-ol	—	−32.9
14α-propylcholest-7-en-3β-15α-diacetate	+8.1	—
14α-butylcholest-7-ene-3β,15-diols	+17.1	−33.5
14α-butylcholest-7-ene-3β-acetate-15β-ol	—	−36.2
14α-butylcholest-7-ene-3β,15α-diacetate	+5.3	—
lanost-7-ene-3β,15-diols	+19.3	−23.8
lanost-8-ene-3β,15α-diol	+65.4	—
cholest-7-en-3β,15α-diol	+46.0	—
cholest-8-en-3β,15α-diol	+86.0	—
14β-cholest-7-ene-3β,15-diols	+20.6	−10.4
cholest-8(14)-ene-3β,15-diols	+17.6	−8.3[a]
7α-methylcholest-8(14)-ene-3β,15-diols	−16.5	−58.9
14β-cholestan-3β,15β-diol	—	+28.4
14β-cholestan-3β,15β-diacetate	—	−19.8
14β-cholestan-3β,15α-diol	+49.7	—
14β-cholestan-3β,15α-diacetate	+50.7	—
14β-cholestan-15α-ol-3-one	+68.8	—
C-7-Hydroxyl function		
4,4-dimethylcholest-5-ene-3β,7-diols	−80.6	−0.43

[a] This is a corrected value from that initially reported (Huntoon *et al.*, 1978).

E. X-Ray Crystallography

Difficult problems of oxysterol structural assignments have been very successfully resolved by X-ray crystallography. The successful use of X-ray methods is dependent on the availability of crystals of sufficient size and uniformity. In several studies, an available hydroxyl group(s) has been converted to the *p*-bromobenzoate ester function, which usually has sufficient crystallinity to produce viable crystals. In addition, the presence of the bromine atom simplifies the refinement of data required to solve a structural analysis.

Structural problems that have been resolved include the configuration of epimeric hydroxyl groups, the configuration of possible epimeric epoxides, and the configuration (cis or trans) of steroid ring junctures. To this end, analyses of the following molecules have been completed:

3β-*p*-bromobenzoyloxycholest-8(14)-en-15β-ol (Phillips *et al.*, 1976),

3β-*p*-bromobenzoyloxy-14α,15α-epoxycholest-7-ene (Conner *et al.*, 1977),

14β-cholest-7-ene-3β,15β-diol-*p*-bromobenzoate (Gilliland *et al.*, 1977),

3β-*p*-bromobenzoyloxy-14α-methylcholest-7-en-15β-ol (Spike *et al.*, 1978),

14α-ethylcholest-7-ene-3β,15α-diol di-*p*-bromobenzoate (Monger *et al.*, 1980),

and

3β-*p*-bromobenzoyloxy-15β-methyl-14β-cholest-7-ene-15α-ol (Schroepfer *et al.*, 1987; Bowen *et al.*, 1988).

V. SUMMARY

As a class of compounds, oxysterols have historically been found to exhibit a wide variety of biological activities. Due to the initial work by Kandutsch and Chen (1973, 1974, 1975), which demonstrated that oxysterols are significant regulators of mammalian sterol biosynthesis, further interest in these compounds was stimulated. As a result, a large number of new oxysterols have been prepared by chemical synthesis or have been isolated from biological systems. The amount of information from the analyses of these compounds has proliferated and is now an important facet of both chemical and biochemical studies. The use of many of these techniques for oxysterol analysis has been described in this brief overview. By the use of technology currently available, the unambigous structural characterization of any oxysterol is feasible.

REFERENCES

Anastasia, M., Fiecchi, A., and Scala, A. (1979a). *Chem. Commun.* p. 858.

Anastasia, M., Fiecchi, A., Gariboldi, P., and Scala, A. (1979b). *J. Org. Chem.* **44**, 4447.

Anastasia, M., Fiecchi, A., and Scala, A. (1979c). *J. Chem. Soc., Perkin Trans. I* p. 1821.

Anastasia, M., Alleri, P., Fiecchi, A., Galli, G., Gariboldi, P., and Scala, A. *J. Org. Chem.* **48**, 686.
Anastasia, M., Allevi, P., Ciuffreda, P., and Riccio, R. (1986). *Tetrahedron* **42**, 4843.
Ansari, G. A. S., and Smith, L. L. (1979). *J. Chromatogr.* **175**, 307.
Aringer, L., and Nordstrom, L. (1981). *Biomed. Mass Spectrom.* **8**, 183.
Astruc, M., Laporte, M., Takacik, C., and Crastes de Paulet, A. (1978). *Biochem. Biophys. Res. Commun.* **85**, 691.
Bhacca, N. S., Williams, D. H. (1984). "Applications of NMR Spectroscopy in Organic Chemistry." Holden-Day, San Francisco, California.
Blunt, J. W., and Stothers, J. B. (1977). *Org. Magn. Reson.* **9**, 439.
Bowen, S. T., Parish, E. J. Wilson, W. K., Schroepfer, G. J., Jr., and Quiocho, F. A. (1988). *Chem. Phys. Lipids* **46**, 245.
Burrows, E. P., Hornby, G. M., Caspi, E. (1969). *J. Org. Chem.* **34**, 193.
Catalan, C. A. H., Kokke, W. C. M. C., Duque, C., and Djerassi, C. *J. Org. Chem.* **48**, 5207.
Cheng, K.-P., Nagano, N., Bang, L., and Ourisson, G. (1977a). *J. Chem. Res., Synop.* p. 217.
Cheng, K.-P., Nagano, N., Bang, L., and Ourisson, G. (1977b). *J. Chem. Res., Minprint* p. 2501.
Chicoyte, E., Powrie, W. D., and Fennema, O. (1968). *Lipids* **3**, 335.
Cho, J. H., and Djerassi, C. (1987). *J. Org. Chem.* **52**, 4517.
Chu, A., and Schroepfer, G. J., Jr. (1988). *J. Lipid Res.* **29**, 235.
Cook, R. P. (1958). "Cholesterol." Academic Press, New York.
Conner, B. N., Parish, E. J., Schroepfer, G. J., Jr., and Quiocho, F. A. (1977). *Chem. Phys. Lipids.* **18**, 240.
De Fay, R., Astruc, M. E., Roussillon, S., Descomps, B., and Crastes de Paulet, A. (1982). *Biochem. Biophys. Res. Commun.* **106**, 362.
Faust, J. R., Kuskey, K. L., Chin, D. J., Goldstein, J. L., and Brown, M. S. (1982). *Proc. Natl. Acad. Sci. U.S.A.* **79**, 5205.
Fieser, L. F., and Fieser, M. (1949). "Natural Products Related to Phenanthrene." Reinhold, New York.
Fieser, L. F., and Fieser, M. (1959). "Steroids." Reinhold, New York.
Fried, J., Grabowich, P., Sabo, E. F., and Cohen, A. I. (1964). *Tetrahedron* **20**, 2279.
Gibbons, G. F. (1983). *Biochem. Soc. Trans.* **11**, 649, and references therein.
Gibbons, G. F., and Ramananda, K. (1975). *J. Chem. Soc. Chem. Commun.* p. 213.
Gibbons, G. F., Pullinger, C. R., Baillie, T. A., and Clare, R. A. (1980a). *Biochim. Biophys. Acta* **619**, 98.
Gibbons, G. F., Pullinger, C. R., Chen, H. W., Cavenee, W. K., and Kandutsch, A. A. *J. Biol. Chem.* **255**, 395.
Gilliland, G. L., Newcommer, M. E., Parish, E. J., and Schroepfer, G. J., Jr. (1977). *Acta Crystallogr., Sect. B* **B33**, 3117.
Hanson, J. R. *et al.* (1977–1983). "Terpenoids and Steroids," Vols. 7–12. Chemical Society, London.
Hirano, T., and Djerassi, C. (1982). *J. Org. Chem.* **47**, 2420.
Homberg, E., and Bielefeld, B. (1979). *J. Chromatogr.* **180**, 83.
Huntoon, S., and Schroepfer, G. J., Jr (1970). *Biochem. Biophys. Res. Commun.* **40**, 476.
Huntoon, S., Fourcans, B., Lutsky, B. H., Parish, E. J., Emery, H., Knapp, F. F., Jr., and Schroepfer, G. J., Jr. (1978). *J. Biol. Chem.* **253**, 775.
Jagodzinska, B. M., Trimmer, J. S., Fenical, W., and Djerassi, C. (1985). *J. Org. Chem.* **50**, 1435.
Jagodzinska, B. M., Trimmer, J. S., Fenical, W., and Djerassi, C. (1985). *J. Org. Chem.* **50**, 2988.
Kandutsch, A. A., and Chen, H. W. (1973). *J. Biol. Chem.* **248**, 8408.
Kandutsch, A. A., and Chen, H. W. (1974). *J. Biol. Chem.* **249**, 6057.

Kandutsch, A. A., and Chen, H. W. (1975). *J. Cell. Physiol.* **85**, 415.
Kandutsch, A. A., Chen, H. W., and Heiniger, J.-H. (1978). *Science* **201**, 498.
Kandutsch, A. A., Taylor, F. R., and Shown, E. P. (1984). *J. Biol. Chem.* **259**, 12388.
Karplus, M. (1963). *J. Am. Chem. Soc.* **85**, 2870.
Kisic, A., Monger, D., Parish, E. J., Satterfield, S., Raulston, D. L., and Schroepfer, G. J., Jr. (1977). *Artery* **3**, 421.
Knapp, F. F., Jr., and Schroepfer, G. J., Jr. (1975). *Steroids* **26**, 339.
Krull, V. J., Thompson, M., and Arya, A. (1984). *Talanta* **31**, 489.
Kumar, V., Amann, A., Ourisson, G., and Luu, B. (1987). *Synth. Commun.* **17**, 1279.
Maerker, G., and Bunick, F. J. (1986). *J. Am. Oil Chem. Soc.* **63**, 771.
Maerker, G., and Unruh, J., Jr. (1986). *J. Am. Oil. Chem. Soc.* **63**, 767.
Martin, J. A., Huntoon, S., and Schroepfer, G. J., Jr. (1970). *Biochem. Biophys. Res. Commun.* **39**, 1170.
Midggley, I., and Djerassi, C. (1973). *J. Chem. Soc., Perkin Trans I* p. 155.
Missler, S. R., Wasilchuk, B. A., and Meritt, C., Jr. (1985). *J. Food Sci.* **50**, 595.
Monger, D., Parish, E. J., Schroepfer, G. J., Jr., and Quiocho, F. A. (1980). *Acta Crystallogr., Sect. B* **B36**, 1460.
Nagano, M., Poyser, J. P., Bang, L., and Ourisson, G. (1977a). *J. Chem. Res. Synop.* p. 218. (M).
Nagano, M., Poyser, J. P., Bang, L., and Ourisson, G. (1977b). *J. Chem. Res., Miniprint* p. 2522.
Nelson, J. A., Steckbeck, S. R., and Spenser, T. A. (1981). *J. Biol. Chem.* **256**, 1067.
Overton, K. H., *et al.* (1971–1976). "Terpenoids and Steroids," Vols. 1–6. Chemical Society, London.
Panini, S. R., Sexto, R. C., and Rudney, H. (1984). *J. Biol. Chem.* **259**, 7767.
Panini, S. R., Sexton, R. C., Gupta, A. K., Parish, E. J., Chitrakorn, S., and Rudney, H. (1986). *J. Lipid Res.* **27**, 1190.
Panini, S. R., Gupta, A., Sexton, R. C., Parish, E. J., and Rudney, H. (1987). *J. Biol. Chem.* **262**, 14435.
Parish, E. J., and Schroepfer, G. J., Jr. (1976). *Tetrahedron Lett.* p. 3775.
Parish, E. J., and Schroepfer, G. J., Jr. (1977a). *Chem. Phys. Lipids* **18**, 258.
Parish, E. J., and Schroepfer, G. J., Jr. (1977b). *Chem. Phys. Lipids* **19**, 107.
Parish, E. J., and Schroepfer, G. J., Jr. (1979). *Chem. Phys. Lipids* **25**, 381.
Parish, E. J., and Schroepfer, G. J., Jr. (1980a). *J. Org. Chem.* **45**, 4034.
Parish, E. J., and Schroepfer, G. J., Jr. (1980b). *Chem. Phys. Lipids* **27**, 281.
Parish, E. J., and Schroepfer, G. J., Jr. (1981a). *J. Lipid Res.* **22**, 859.
Parish, E. J., and Schroepfer, G. J., Jr. (1981b). *J. Labelled Compd. Radioipharm.* **18**, 1429.
Parish, E. J., and Scott, A. D. (1983). *J. Org. Chem.* **48**, 4766.
Parish, E. J., Newcomer, M. E., Gilliland, G. L., Quiocho, F. A., and Schroepfer, G. J., Jr. (1976). *Tetrahedron Lett.* p. 4401.
Parish, E. J., Spike, T. E., and Schroepfer, G. J., Jr. (1977). *Chem. Phys. Lipids* **18**, 233.
Parish, E. J., Tsuda, M., and Schroepfer, G. J., Jr. (1979a). *Chem. Phys. Lipids.* **24**, 167.
Parish, E. J., Tsuda, M., and Schroepfer, G. J., Jr. (1979b). *Chem. Phys. Lipids.* **24**, 209.
Parish, E. J., Chitrakorn, S., Taylor, F. R., and Saucier, S. R. (1984). *Chem. Phys. Lipids.* **36**, 179.
Parish, E. J., Nanduri, V. B. B., Kohl, H. H., and Taylor, F. R. (1986). *Lipids* **21**, 27, and references therein.
Parish, E. J., Wei, T.-Y., and Livant, P. (1987). *Lipids* **22**, 760.
Pascal, R. A., Jr., Shaw, R., and Schroepfer, G. J., Jr. (1979). *J. Lipid Res.* **20**, 570.
Pascal, R. A., Jr., and Schroepfer, G. J., Jr. (1980a). *J. Lipid Res.* **21**, 118.

Pascal, R. A., Jr., and Schroepfer, G. J., Jr. (1980b). *J. Biol. Chem.* **255**, 3565.
Pederson, J. I., Bjorkhem, I., and Gustafsson, J. (1979). *J. Biol. Chem.* **254**, 6464.
Phillips, G. N., Jr., Quiocho, F. A., Sass, R. L., Werness, P., Emery, H., Knapp, F. F., Jr., and Schroepfer, G. J., Jr. (1976). *Bioorg. Chem.* **5**, 1.
Poyser, J. P., and Ourisson, G. (1974). *J. Chem. Soc., Perkin Trans. I* p. 2061.
Raulston, D. L., Mishaw, C. O., Parish, E. J., and Schroepfer, G. J., Jr. (1976). *Biochem. Biophys. Res. Commun.* **71**, 984.
Reich, H. J., Jautelat, M., Messe, M. T., Weigert, F. J., and Roberts, J. D. (1969). *J. Am. Chem. Soc.* **91**, 7445.
Roller, P., Tursch, B., and Djerassi, C. (1970). *J. Org. Chem.* **35**, 2585.
St. Pyrek, J., and Schroepfer, G. J., Jr. (1987). *J. Lipid Res.* **28**, 1308.
St. Pyrek, J., Wilson, W. K., and Schroepfer, G. J., Jr. (1987). *J. Lipid Res.* **28**, 1296.
Saucier, S. E., Kandutsch, A. A., Taylor, F. R., Spencer, T. A., Phirwa, S., and Gayen, A. K. (1985). *J. Biol. Chem.* **260**, 1457.
Schroepfer, G. J., Jr. (1981). *Annu. Rev. Biochem.* **51**, 585, and references therein.
Schroepfer, G. J., Jr., Parish, E. J., Chen, H. W., and Kandutsch, A. A. (1977a). *J. Biol. Chem.* **252**, 8975.
Schroepfer, G. J., Jr., Parish, E. J., and Kandutsch, A. A. (1977b). *J. Biol. Chem.* **252**, 8975.
Schroepfer, G. J., Jr., Parish, E. J., and Kandutsch, A. A. (1977c). *J. Am. Chem. Soc.* **99**, 5494.
Schroepfer, G. J., Jr., Parish, E. J., and Kandutsch, A. A. (1979a). *Chem. Phys. Lipids* **25**, 265.
Schroepfer, G. J., Jr., Pascal, R. A., Jr., and Kandutsch, A. A. (1979 b). *Biochem. Pharmacol.* **28**, 249.
Schroepfer, G. J., Jr., Pascal, R. A., Jr., and Kandutsch, A. A. (1980). *Experientia* **36**, 518.
Schroepfer G. J., Jr., Parish, E. J., Kisic, A., Frome, D. M., and Kandutsch, A. A. (1981). *Chem. Phys. Lipids* **29**, 201.
Schroepfer, G. J., Jr., Sherrill, B. C., Wang, K.-S., Wilson, W. K., Kisic, A., and Clarkson, T. B. (1984). *Proc. Natl. Acad. Sci., U.S.A.* **81**, 6861.
Schroepfer, G. J., Jr., Parish, E. J., Kandutsch, A. A., Bowen, S. T., and Quiocho, F. A. (1987). *Biochem. Int.* **15**, 403.
Sexton, R. C., Panini, S. R., Azran, F., and Rudney, H. (1987). *Biochemistry* **22**, 5687.
Shoolery, J. N., and Rogers, M. T. (1958). *J. Am . Chem. Soc.* **80**, 5121.
Sinensky, M., Target, R., and Edwards, P. A. (1981). *J. Biol. Chem.* **256**, 11774.
Smith, L. L. (1981). "Cholesterol Autoxidation," and references therein. Plenum, New York.
Smith, L. L. (1987). *Chem. Phys. Lipids* **44**, 87.
Spencer, T. A., Gayen, A. K., Phirwa, S., Nelson, J. A., Taylor, F. R., Kandutsch, A. A., and Erickson, S. (1985). *J. Biol. Chem.* **260**, 13391.
Spike, T. E., Martin, J. A., Huntoon, S., Wang, A. H.-J., Knapp, F. F., Jr., and Schroepfer, G. J., Jr (1978). *Chem. Phys. Lipids* **21**, 31.
Stothers, J. B. (1972). "Carbon-13 NMR Spectroscopy." Academic Press, New York.
Tabacik, C., Aliau, S., Serrou, B., and Crastes de Paulet, A. (1981). *Biochem. Biophys. Res. Commun.* **101**, 1087.
Tanaka, R. D., Edwards, P. A., Lan, S.-F., and Fogelman, A. M. (1983). *J. Biol. Chem.* **258**, 13331.
Taylor, E. J., and Djessari, C. (1977). *J. Org. Chem.* **43**, 3571.
Taylor, F. R., Saucier, S. E., Shown, E. P., Parish, E. J., and Kandutsch, A. A. (1984). *J. Biol. Chem.* **259**, 12382.
Teng, J. I., Kulig, M. J., Smith, L. L., Kam, G., and van lier, J. E. (1973). *J. Org. Chem.* **38**, 119.
Tsai, L.-S., and Hudson, C. A. (1981). *J. Am. Oil. Chem. Soc.* **58**, 931.
Tsuda, M., Parish, E. J., and Schroepfer, G. J., Jr. (1979). *J. Org. Chem.* **44**, 1282.

Tsuda, M., and Schroepfer, G. J., Jr., (1981). *J. Lipid Res.* **22**, 1188.

Vlahcevic, Z. R., Schwartz, C. C., Gustafsson, J., Halloran, L. G., Danielson, H., and Swell, L. (1980). *J. Biol. Chem.* **255**, 2925.

Watabe, T., and Sawahata, T. (1979). *J. Biol. Chem.* **254**, 3854.

Watabe, T., Kanai, M., Isobe, M., and Ozawa, N. (1981). *J. Biol. Chem.* **256**, 2900.

Williamson, K. L., and Johnson, W. S. (1961). *J. Am. Chem. Soc.* **83**, 4623.

Wulfson, N. S., Zaretskii, V. I., and Zaikin, V. G. (1967). *Khim. Prir. Soedin.* **3**, 369.

Zandler, M., Patrick, K., Bang, L., and Ourisson, G. (1977a). *J. Chem. Res. Synop.* p. 219.

Zandler, M., Patrick, K., Bang, L., and Ourisson, G. (1977b). *J. Chem. Res., Miniprint* p. 2572.

Zurcher, R. F. (1963). *Helv. Chim. Acta* **46**, 2054.

9

Lipoprotein Analysis

Arnis Kuksis
Banting and Best Department of Medical Research
University of Toronto
Toronto, Canada

I. INTRODUCTION

An essential part of lipoprotein analysis is a determination of cholesterol (Skipski, 1969; Scanu, 1972; Gotto *et al.*, 1986). An estimate of total cholesterol provides a simple method for quantitating plasma lipoproteins in various density fractions obtained by ultracentrifugation, polyanionic precipitation, or other means of separation (Lipid Research Clinics Program, 1974). Indeed, abnormalities in plasma lipoproteins and specific disease conditions are commonly described in terms of total and specific lipoprotein cholesterol levels (Fredrickson *et al.*, 1978; Gotto *et al.*, 1986). Further insight into lipoprotein structure and metabolism is provided by separate estimation of the ratios of free to esterified cholesterol and of free cholesterol to phospholipid, as well as determination of the fatty acid composition of the cholesteryl esters (Kuksis *et al.*, 1981, 1982a). Lecithin-cholesterol acyltransferase (LCAT) deficiency (Glomset *et al.*, 1983), phytosterolemia (Bhattacharya and Connor, 1978), and cerebrotendinous xanthomatosis (CTX) (Salen *et al.*, 1983) provide special instances of plasma sterol and steryl ester abnormalities. The popularity of cholesterol measurements is based on the characteristic quantitative presence of cholesterol in the lipoprotein fractions (Scanu, 1972, 1981) and the relative ease of its measurement by colorimetric methods (Abell *et al.*, 1952; Cooper *et al.*, 1986), which can be automated (Bachorik *et al.*, 1979; MacAulay *et al.*, 1980; Naito and David, 1984).

Chromatographic methods of sterol analyses permit the estimation of lipoprotein cholesterol and other sterols, such as the biosynthetic precursors of cholesterol (Miettinen, 1971; Hansbury and Scallen, 1980), the products of its metabolic transformation (Ishikawa *et al.*, 1976; Javitt *et al.*, 1981, 1982; Salen *et al.*, 1985a,b), and the related plant sterols (Kuksis and Huang, 1962; Rao *et al.*, 1975; Kuksis *et al.*, 1976; 1986a; Miettinen, 1980). These compounds occur as major components in the surface coating of the lipoprotein particle and as minor solutes in its hydrophobic interior, as demonstrated for cholesterol (Zilversmit, 1965, 1969; Huang and Kuksis, 1967a; Miller and Small, 1983a,b), of the very low and low density lipoproteins. Identification and quantitiation of these sterol derivatives is of interst in the diagnosis of CTX and phytosterolemia (Bhattacharyya and Connor, 1978; Salen *et al.*, 1983).

Cholesterol, its metabolites, and the plant sterols also occur as part of the lymph lipoproteins (Zilversmit, 1965, 1969; Huang and Kuksis, 1967a; Yang and Kuksis, 1987) and milk lipoproteins (Huang and Kuksis, 1967b; Mellies *et al.*, 1978; Huang and Harzer, 1984; Steiner *et al.*, 1985).

Estimation of the quantitatively minor steroid hormones in plasma (Patterson *et al.*, 1984) and in milk (Gyawu and Pope, 1983) is also of great clinical and biochemical interest but is difficult because of the greater polarity of these compounds and their occurrence as complexes with special protein carriers (Dunn *et al.*, 1981). Although these steroids are not usually considered to be components of the common lipoproteins, they are mentioned here to complete the coverage of plasma neutral sterols and steroids.

This chapter, after opening with a brief discussion of the structure of lipoproteins and their content of sterols and describing quantitative colorimetric, chromatographic, and mass spectrometric analyses of sterols and steroids; is devoted to applications of sterol and steryl ester analyses in clinical studies and in studies with synthetic and animal models of clinical disease. Gas-liquid chromatography (GLC) of cholesterol and cholesteryl esters of human plasma has been reviewed recently by Kuksis and Myher (1986) and Mares (1987).

II. LIPOPROTEIN STRUCTURE AND STEROL CONTENT

Lipoproteins are made up of polar and nonpolar lipids and apoproteins in variable proportions that are related to particle size and density. The exact arrangement of the lipid and protein in the lipoproteins is unknown, but there is evidence that the phospholipids, free sterols, and protein are in an outer hydrophilic shell, whereas the triacylglycerols and cholesteryl esters are in a hydrophobic core (Edelstein *et al.*, 1979; Scanu, 1981). This spherical model is supported by various calculations of the size, volume, and surface area of the lipoproteins and by the data from some reconstitution studies (Scanu, 1972, 1981; Jonas, 1986). Miller and Small (1983a,b) have separated chylomicrons and very low density lipoprotein (VLDL) into pure surface and oil (core) phases by centrifugation and have shown that minor amounts of triacylglycerols (2–5%) and cholesteryl esters (less than 1%) are soluble in the surface, where they assume a horse-shoe shape (Chana *et al.*, 1985). Minor amounts of free cholesterol (less than 2%) dissolve in the oil at 22° to 24°C, but none of the phospholipid is partitioned into the oil phase. Although somewhat more free cholesterol would be expected to dissolve into the largely cholesteryl ester cores of low density lipoprotein (LDL) and high density lipoprotein (HDL), these minor alterations in the distribution of free cholesterol do not invalidate the spherical lipid emulsion model of lipoprotein structure. Newly synthesized HDL, however, appears as disks that tend to form roleaux in negatively stained preparations (Hamilton *et al.*, 1976). When a critical amount of the free sterol in these nascent particles is converted to cholesteryl ester through the action of LCAT, the particle assumes a spherical shape. The free cholesterol in the surface phase of the chylomicrons, VLDL, and LDL approaches saturating levels, that is, a phosphatidyl choline/free cholesterol (PC/FC) molar ratio of 1 (Kuksis *et al.*, 1981). The surface monolayers of normal HDL contain much less free cholesterol (PC/FC ratio of 4–5) (Kuksis *et al.*, 1981, 1982a,b). There is evidence that the PC/FC ratios in plasma lipoproteins vary with metabolism (Miller and Small, 1983b) and disease (Kuksis *et al.*, 1982a,b; Fielding, 1984; Fielding *et al.*, 1984). Lymph chylomicrons possess a composition and structure comparable to that of the plasma chylomicrons (Zilversmit, 1965, 1969; Huang and Kuksis, 1967a). The distribution of cholesterol in plasma lipoproteins is closely paralleled by the distribution of plant sterols, campesterol and sitosterol, as well as other minor sterols (Sugano *et al.*, 1978; Kakis and Kuksis, 1984; Kakis *et al.*, 1988). Other steroids, however, can be carried by special carrier proteins in the aqueous phase (Dunn *et al.*, 1981) or be associated with albumin. Usually, the subparticle distribution of cholesterol and other sterols in lipoproteins is not determined, but it may provide a valid subject of inquiry (Miller and Small, 1983a,b; Lippi *et al.*, 1986), as may the existence of free cholesterol not carried by lipoprotein (Deliconstantinos, 1983). In addition, cholesterol may be carried in plasma or serum as xenobiotic conjugates (Fears, 1985) and sulfate (Van Doormaal *et al.*, 1986).

III. ISOLATION OF LIPOPROTEINS

Provided the samples are properly prepared, either plasma or serum is suitable for lipoprotein isolation and sterol analysis (Naito and David, 1984; Ferreri, 1984). When left at room temperature too long, serum or plasma can have increased LCAT activity, which causes altered lipoprotein composition with respect to the free and esterified cholesterol ratio. Plasma is usually preferred when lipoproteins are analyzed and ethylenediamine tetraacetate (EDTA) (1 mg/ml blood) is used as the anticoagulant. EDTA retards autoxidation, which leads to alterations in physical properties and degradation of the lipoproteins (Hatch and Lees, 1968; Schuh *et al.*, 1978). The lipoproteins can be isolated by a variety of techniques in amounts sufficiently large for determination of the component sterols and steryl esters. None of the methods are perfect, and caution must be exercised in their adoption for untried purposes.

A. Sequential Ultracentrifugation

This classical method of lipoprotein separation provides the VLDL, LDL, and HDL classes and is well defined for human lipoproteins (Hatch and Lees, 1968; Lipid Research Clinics Program, 1974; Ferreri, 1984). Postprandial plasma or certain pathological states provide also a chylomicron fraction. In many instances the LDL and HDL are resolved into two or more subfractions. Kupke and Worz–Zeugner (1986) have demonstrated the feasibility of sequential separation by microultracentrifugation of VLDL, LDL, and HDL from 100 μl of serum. The lipoprotein sterol and lipid recoveries were 98–101% as determined by high-performance thin-layer chromatography (HPTLC). The procedure was standardized by comparison with an electrophoresis-enzymatic procedure. It was adequate for analysis of capillary serum from children, including premature neonates. A serious disadvantage of classical ultracentrifugation is the lengthy time (3–5 days) required for completion of the separation. A significant time saving results from using gradient ultracentrifugation in a swing-out rotor (Foreman *et al.*, 1977). After 24 h of centrifugation in a salt gradient, the lipoproteins are resolved as discrete bands. Chung *et al.* (1986) have developed methods that separate plasma lipoproteins using density-gradient ultracentrifugation in vertical rotors. These separations are comparable to those obtained in swing-out rotors, but the separation is completed in less than a tenth of the time. Of special interest to cholesterol determinations are the lipoprotein subfractions, which are readily obtained on zonal centrifugation (Patsch and Patsch, 1986).

The lipoprotein density ranges established for humans are not directly applicable to animal species, which show considerable overlapping of ranges (Chapman, 1980). Thus, the large HDL in dog, cow, and pig extends into the LDL range (Weisgraber and Mahley, 1986). Traditional ultracentrifugation also has failed to provide complete separation of individual lipoproteins in the rhesus monkey (Rudel *et al.*, 1986), rat (Breckenridge *et al.*, 1979), and mouse (Breckenridge *et al.*, 1985); so other methods of separation have been sought.

B. Gel Filtration

This method separates lipoprotein molecules according to size, the smaller molecules emerging last. When the separations are performed in 4% agarose gel, human serum yields separate fractions for chylomicrons, VLDL, LDL, and HDL (Rudel *et al.*, 1986). In addition, the chylomicrons and VLDL yield subfractions (Ferreri, 1984). The technique has also been shown to give subfractions of LDL and HDL when monkey

(Rudel *et al.*, 1986) or bovine (Ferreri, 1984) serum is used. For the purpose of sterol measurement, it is possible to apply the serum directly to the column. The total running time is 20–30 h.

More recently high performance liquid chromatography (HPLC) methods have been applied to gel filtration of serum lipoproteins (Hara and Okazaki, 1986), which allows the separation of chylomicrons, VLDL, LDL, HDL_2, and HDL_3. The lipoprotein fractions are eluted from a series of columns using 0.15-M sodium chloride as eluant. These separations are performed over a period of 69–90 min with as little as 10–50 μl of serum, which is sufficient for a sensitive colorimetric assay for total cholesterol and choline-containing phospholipids and an ultraviolet (UV) assay of protein during fractionation of human whole serum. Clifton *et al.* (1987) have described a simple technique for isolating subfractions of HDL in quantities sufficient for chemical characterization using a fast protein liquid chromatography on a column of Sepharose 6B (250 minutes).

A variation of the gel filtration method is provided by affinity chromatography. Thus, chromatography on heparin-Sepharose (Shelburne and Quarfordt, 1977) or heparin-agarose (Fielding *et al.*, 1984) brings about a specific retention of the apoprotein B-containing lipoproteins, whereas the other lipoproteins pass through the column unabsorbed in 0.15-M NaCl/1-mM EDTA. The adsorbed fractions are recovered with 3-M NaCl/1-mM EDTA (Fielding *et al.*, 1984). Both adsorbed and unabsorbed fractions can be subjected to subsequent ultracentrifugation to effect further separation and purification of the fractions.

C. Electrophoresis

This technique is used mainly for analytical purposes. Human VLDL, LDL, and HDL exhibit pre-β-, β- and α-migration, respectively, on paper, agarose, and cellulose acetate electrophoresis. However, preparative systems for fractionation of larger quantities of lipoproteins exist. Weisgraber and Mahley (1986) have used such a system to isolate pure HDL_c, which overlaps the LDL prepared by sequential ultracentrifugation, and to determine its cholesterol content. Commercial systems are now available for quantitative electrophoresis of lipoproteins, which can be resolved in sufficiently large quantities for effective cholesterol analysis (Marz and Gross, 1986).

D. Polyanionic Precipitation

Plasma lipoproteins can be separated to a considerable extent by precipitation with polyanionic reagents, such as dextran sulfate-Mn^{2+} (Warnick, 1986), heparin-Mn^{2+} (Gidez *et al.*, 1982; Bachorik and Albers, 1986), and Mg^{2+}-phosphotungstic acid (Burnstein and Legmann, 1982; Assmann *et al.*, 1983; Tong and Kuksis, 1988). These methods have been extensively used for rapid determination of cholesterol in HDL (Bachorik and Albers, 1986), which remains in solution while the VLDL and LDL are precipitated. The obtained HDL fraction, however, is not completely free of VLDL and

LDL as shown by electrophoresis, which frequently indicates residual apoprotein B. In some instances the lipoprotein classes have been recovered from both the precipitate and the supernatant and, after a suitable adjustment of densities, have been subjected to conventional ultracentrifugation to yield better-defined fractions (Burnstein and Legmann, 1982; Gidez *et al.*, 1982; Tong and Kuksis, 1988). Improved phosphotungstic acid-$MgCl_2$ reagents (Drager *et al.*, 1982; Assmann *et al.*, 1983) are now commercially available along with kits for cholesterol determination. Recently. polyethyleneglycol (PEG 6000) has been used for the isolation of HDL (Lippi *et al.*, 1982; Lundberg *et al.*, 1984; Kostner *et al.*, 1985). Also, polyvinyl sulfate has been used to isolate LDL (Assmann *et al.*, 1984). All of these fractions are suitable for the determination of free and esterified cholesterol and other steroids by most of the quantitative methods discussed in the following sections.

IV. METHODS OF STEROL ANALYSIS

The sterols are usually extracted from plasma using chloroform-methanol mixtures, but isopropanol extraction has been found to be more selective (Gartzke, 1979). More recently, silica Sep-Pak cartridges (Wang and Peter, 1983) and aminopropyl bonded-phase (Bond Elut) cartridges (Kaluzny *et al.*, 1985) have been proposed for this purpose. For total sterol determination, the total lipid extract is saponified and the sterol content established by appropriate colorimetric, fluorometric, chromatographic, or mass spectrometric methods, or by a combination of these methods. When more than one sterol type is present, the colorimetric or fluorimetric assays can be preceded by a chromatographic resolution of the unsaponifiables. Chromatographic separation of the total lipid extract also is necessary for a separate estimation of the free and esterified sterol content and for identification of the steryl esters. Radioactive steroids are determined by such general methods as liquid scintillation counting, thin-layer chromatography scanning and flow-through monitoring (e.g., Child and Kuksis, 1980, 1986; Lin *et al.*, 1983).

A. Colorimetry and Fluorimetry

Simple colorimetric methods which are extensively used for serum cholesterol determination in clincial laboratories, are fast, relatively easy to perform and readily automated (Naito and David, 1984). However, their precision and especially their accuracy must be ascertained and closely monitored. Most of the colorimetric methods use the Liebermann–Burchard reaction (Abell *et al.*, 1952), but other reactions based on iron-acid (Burke *et al.*, 1974) and *o*-phthalaldehyde (Rudel and Morris, 1973) reagents have also been used.

Fluorometric assays for cholesterol and cholesteryl esters have been described (Bondjers and Bjorkerud, 1971; Huang *et al.*, 1975; Heider and Boyett, 1978; Daniels *et al.*, 1981). They provide increased sensitivity of detection (0.1–10 μg). According to Bondjers and Bjorkerud (1971), the sterols and steryl esters are first resolved by thin-layer chromatography (TLC) and the fractions recovered with chloroform. The solvent is evaporated, and the dry residue treated with a freshly prepared zinc chloride-glacial acetic acid reagent at 60°C for 30 min. The sample is measured at room temperature in a fluorimeter at an excitation wavelength of 528 nm and a fluorescence wavelength of 565 nm, between 40 and 80 min after heating.

In recent years, enzymatic (Warnick, 1986) cholesterol assays have largely replaced the more laborious, interference-susceptible, and less specific routine nonenzymatic methods. The enzymatic procedure usually involves cleavage of the cholesterol esters with cholesterol esterase and oxidation of the free cholesterol by cholesterol oxidase (Warnick, 1986). The reactions are quantitated photometrically or fluorometrically by use of H_2O_2-dependent color-forming reactions. The chromogenic indicator system of Trinder and Webster (1984) has given the greatest sensitivity.

B. Chromatography

In addition to sample purification prior to colorimetric analyses (Gartzke, 1979; Siedel *et al.*, 1983), chromatographic methods are extensively used to identify free sterols (Nes, 1985; Rodriguez and Parks, 1985) and to separate free and esterified sterols. Cholesteryl esters can be quantitated by chromatographic methods either directly or as the fatty acid methyl esters derived by transmethylation. Bianchini *et al.* (1985) recommend a combination of HPLC for the isolation, GLC for quantitation, and gas chromatography/mass spectrometry (GC/MS) for identifying natural sterol mixtures as the acetates. In combination with stable isotope internal standards and mass spectrometry, chromatographic methods offer the ultimate routines for the absolute identification and quantitation of cholesterol and other steroids in whole plasma or serum and in isolated lipoproteins.

1. Thin-Layer Chromatography

Thin-layer chromatography (TLC) is the most frequently used method for the separation of sterols and sterol esters prior to estimation by GLC or colorimetric methods. TLC also is suitable for the separation and isolation of sterols and steryl esters for determination of radioactivity (Perret *et al.*, 1987). A disadvantage of commonly used conventional plates is that they take a long time to develop, especially if a two-dimensional separation of a total lipid extract is attempted. Much more rapid development and more complete resolution of components can be obtained by means of smaller plates (Bowyer and King, 1977). Gartzke (1979) has described a two-solvent system for an improved resolution of the free and esterified cholesterol from other serum lipids.

More recently, rapid TLC separations have been obtained by high-performance thin-layer chromatography (HPTLC) (Siedel *et al.*, 1983), which uses much thinner layers made up of finer gel powders. The resolved components can be reliably quantitated by charring (Siedel *et al.*, 1983). In other instances the products of TLC purification and separation are quantitated by GLC (Gambert *et al.*, 1979; Jensen *et al.*, 1979; Kuksis *et al.*, 1986a) or are assayed by enzymatic methods (Siedel *et al.*, 1983). In special cases the products of chromatographic purification are quantitated by measuring optical activity (Kuo and Yeung, 1982) or by recording mass spectra using stable isotope-labeled internal standards (Bjorkhem *et al.*, 1974; Cohen *et al.*, 1980; Patterson *et al.*, 1984).

The use of quartz rods, to which silica gel is fused at high temperature, for separation and quantitation of neutral lipids including free and esterified cholesterol has been described by several workers (Vandamme *et al.*, 1978; Christie and Hunter, 1979; Farnworth *et al.*, 1982). For quantitation of lipids, the rods are passed through a hydrogen flame ionization detector. These methods also allow clean separation of cholesteryl esters from fatty acid methyl esters and hydrocarbons, and of free cholesterol from 1,2- and 1,3-diacylglycerols. When impregnated with silver nitrate, both adsorption plates and rods can be used for resolution of sterols (Gray *et al.*, 1971; Nes, 1985) and of steryl esters (Morris, 1963) on the basis of unsaturation.

2. Gas-Liquid Chromatography

Cholesterol, the related plant sterols, and their saturated analogs are readily separated on both packed gas-liquid chromatography (GLC) columns (Ishikawa *et al.*, 1976) and capillary GLC columns (Kuksis *et al.*, 1986a). Electron capture provides a sensitive method of detection and quantitation of sterols (desmosterol) as the pentafluorobenzoates (Pullinger and Gibbons, 1983). High-resolution GLC has been extensively studied as a reference method for cholesterol determination (Ambert *et al.*, 1976; Lillienberg and Svanborg, 1976; Hindricks *et al.*, 1977; Derks *et al.*, 1985). Quantitation is obtained by use of various internal standards. With high-temperature GLC and nonpolar columns, a carbon number separation can also be obtained for various fatty acid esters of cholesterol (Kuksis, 1964; Kuksis *et al.*, 1975), which can be quantitated (Kuksis *et al.*, 1978b; Mares *et al.*, 1979), and for various fatty acid esters of cholesterol and plant sterols (Kuksis *et al.*, 1986b).

High-temperature GLC on polar liquid phases enables separation of the cholesteryl esters, based on both molecular weight and degree of unsaturation (Smith, 1982, 1983; Kuksis and Myher, 1986; Kuksis *et al.*, 1986a). The separation of the steryl esters on polar capillary columns is comparable to that realized by a GLC analysis of the component fatty acids following transmethylation of the cholesteryl esters (Mookerjea *et al.*, 1975; Petty *et al.*, 1975; Jensen *et al.*, 1979; Wang and Peter, 1983; Mattson *et al.*, 1985). However, contamination of the sample and incomplete transmethylation or destruction of the steryl esters during the transesterification process is no longer a problem. The GLC systems are confined mainly to research laboratories because they are more difficult to execute and automate (Kuksis *et al.*, 1975; Myher and Kuksis, 1984).

3. High-Performance Liquid Chromatography

Free sterols have been chromatographed on high-performance liquid chromatography (HPLC) using packed reverse-phase, normal-phase, or silver nitrate-impregnated normal-phase columns, or a combination of column types. The advantages and disadvantages of the various combinations for resolving cholesterol precursors (Hansbury and Scallen, 1980) and cholesterol analogs (Rodriguez and Parks, 1985) have been discussed in the literature. The reversed-phase HPLC separation of the 7-dehydro derivatives of cholesterol and plant sterols (Child and Kuksis, 1983a) and of the ring-structure derivatives of cholesterol and plant sterols (Child and Kuksis, 1983b) has also been described. Reversed-phase HPLC is well suited for the resolution of intact cholesteryl esters (Smith *et al.*, 1980; Carroll and Rudel, 1981; Perkins *et al.*, 1981; Bernert *et al.*, 1982; Kuksis *et al.*, 1983a), as well as for the resolution of steryl esters differing in both sterol and fatty acid moiety (Bilheimer *et al.*, 1983; Kuksis *et al.*, 1986a; Poll *et al.*, 1985). Since only a few sterols absorb strongly in the ultraviolet, sensitive detection and quantitation of eluted components is a problem in HPLC of sterols and steryl esters. The use of a mass spectrometer as a detector for the HPLC greatly improves the quantitation of sterol and steryl ester peaks and insures their accurate identification (Kuksis *et al.*, 1983a, 1986a). Lagana *et al.* (1986) have proposed an HPLC separation and spectrophotometric detection of progesterone in serum.

C. Mass Spectrometry

Mass spectrometry also has been employed for identifying and quantitating sterols and steroids in plasma and plasma lipoproteins. In addition to direct probe analysis, mass spectrometry has been used in combination with GLC, HPLC, and even TLC. Of special interest is the method of mass fragmentography, in which losses in extraction or chromatography can be allowed for by the use of a stable isotope (deuterium)-labeled internal standard.

1. Direct-Probe Mass Spectrometry

Direct-probe mass spectrometry (DP-MS) is seldom employed for mass spectrometric quantitation of cholesterol and other relatively nonpolar steroids, though occasionally this method is still used for sterol and steroid identification. Most often. DP-MS is employed for identifying and quantitating polar steroids and steroid conjugates (Budzikiewicz, 1980). Although the invention of mass-spectrometry/mass-spectrometry (MS/MS) has raised hopes for a modern DP-MS, practical analyses of steroids have shown that chromatographic prefractionation is necessary (Gaskell *et al.*, 1985) prior to MS/MS analysis.

2. Gas Chromatography/Mass Spectrometry

One of the most widely used techniques in the investigation of sterols is gas chromatography/mass spectrometry (GC/MS) of the TMS ether derivatives. These derivatives greatly increase the sterol volatility, which facilitates their GLC separation and mass spectrometric structure identification (Budzikiewicz, 1980). Similarly, the TMS ethers of the plant sterols and the precursors of cholesterol can be identified by their molecular weight and characteristic fragment ions. Since many sterols have common molecular weights and give common fragment ions, an effective GLC resolution of the TMS ethers of the sterols is crucial for reliable identification. Quantitation is best obtained by stable isotope dilution (Bjorkhem *et al.*, 1974; Freudenthal *et al.*, 1981).

In the area of plasma cholesterol, most of the published isotope dilution GC/MS methods are now referred to as reference methodologies (Bjorkhem *et al.*, 1974; Siekmann *et al.*, 1976; Cohen *et al.*, 1980). Knowledge of the error propagation in the measurement process and the direct linking of definitive methodologies with the evaluation of candidate reference sera, have changed the requirements for a method to be definitive. Stable isotope dilution methods have also been proposed for plasma testosterone (Chapman and Bailey, 1974) cortisol (Siekmann and Breuer, 1982; Jonckheere and De Leenheer, 1983; Patterson *et al.*, 1984; Gaskell and Siekmann, 1986), progesterone (Gaskell *et al.*, 1984), and the androstanediols (Jacolot *et al.*, 1986).

Electron-impact mass spectrometry (EI-MS) analyses of steryl esters via direct probe or GC/MS have not provided ions directly indicative of the molecular weight (Murata *et al.*, 1975). Wakeham and Frew (1982) have used methane chemical-ionization mass spectrometry (CI-MS) of steryl esters and have produced fragment ions that indicate both the acid and sterol moieties but do not yield a molecular ion of the intact ester. Lusby *et al.* (1984), however, have reported the development of electron-impact (EI) and chemical-ionization (CI) techniques for GC/MS analyses of intact steryl esters, by which the latter produced ions indicative of the molecular weight as well as the sterol and fatty acid fractions of the molecule. Recently, Evershed and Goad (1987) have employed ammonia as a reagent gas, with negative-ion scanning, to obtain spectra from which the structure of the steryl and fatty acyl moieties could be readily deduced.

3. Liquid Chromatography/Mass Spectrometry

Since HPLC is capable of resolving thermally unstable, polar and high-molecular-weight solutes, it has an advantage over GC/MS when dealing with free sterols and polyunsaturated steryl esters. Of special interest is the reversed-phase liquid chromatography/mass spectrometry (LC/MS) method, which allows a resolution of cholesterol and related sterols and of their fatty acid esters on the basis of unsaturation within a carbon number (Kuksis *et al.*, 1983a, 1986a). LC/MS should also be well suited for work with isotope-labeled internal standards. The recent demonstration of the suitability of the thermospray interface for work with neutral steroid molecules (Watson *et al.*, 1987) promises to facilitate the analysis of the small amounts of sterols and related steroids in plasma and plasma lipoprotein extracts by combined LC/MS systems.

D. Radioimmunoassay and Chemiluminescence Immunoassay

In constrast to cholesterol and its esters, which are estimated by chemical and enzymatic methods, the steroid hormones of plasma are assayed almost exclusively by radioimmunological methods (Lantto *et al.*, 1980; Lantto, 1982; Hofman *et al.*, 1985; Dhar *et al.*, 1985, 1986). De Boever *et al.* (1984) have described a solid-phase chemiluminescence immunoassay for progesterone in unextracted serum.

V. ANALYSIS OF WHOLE PLASMA OR SERUM

Due to the clinical significance attached to the total cholesterol levels of plasma or serum, an enormous effort has been expended in arriving at accurate, precise, and rapid methods of cholesterol analysis. In specific instances, cholesterol content has been related to the content in serum of other lipid classes or molecular species.

A. Total Sterol Content

The Liebermann–Burchard method described by Duncan *et al.* (1982) is the most widely accepted reference method for cholesterol in serum. This colorimetric technique shows good precision and is claimed to compare favorably with the Definitive Method of the U.S. National Bureau of Standards (Cohen *et al.*, 1980). Recently, the transferability of the method from one laboratory to another by written specifications was tested in 14 laboratories, and a coefficient of variation (CV) ranging from 1.5% to less than 3% was obtained among them (Cooper *et al.*, 1986).

The Liebermann–Burchard reaction and its variants do not distinguish between cholesterol and related sterols that may be present in a plasma, though minor discrepancies in the rate of reaction and the yield of the color have been reported (Haust and Bedveridge, 1964). To limit the variety of sterols that react in the Liebermann–Burchard reaction, a preliminary isolation of cholesterol and other 3β-hydroxy sterols by digitonin precipitation has been used (Haust *et al.*, 1966). The sterols are determined colorimetrically after regeneration from the digitonides and after removal of the digitonin. Steroids with a structure similar to cholesterol, which are potential interferences, include cholestanol (5-cholestan-3β-ol), Δ-7-cholestenol (5-cholest-7-en-3β-ol), and 7-dehydrocholesterol (cholesta-5,7-dien-3β-ol). Similarly, the 24-alkyl derivatives of cholesterol (the plant sterols: campesterol, stigmasterol, and sitosterol) are determined as cholesterol, along with their saturated and unsaturated derivatives. Other methods for the segregation of different sterols and steroids, among themselves and from other extraneous material recovered during solvent extraction, are based on chromatography (Hansbury and Scallen, 1980). Thus, the fast-reacting methyl sterols can be removed by adsorption chromatography, whereas reversed-phase HPLC allows the segregation of the sterols on the basis of both polarity and molecular weight (Duncan *et al.*, 1979; Hansbury and Scallen, 1980; Child and Kuksis, 1983a,b).

An adaptation of the colorimetric method, which has been automated and widely used, relies on enzymatic hydrolysis and oxidation of the sterols and steryl esters (Warnick, 1986). The enzymatic methods are limited to the determination of the 3β-hydroxy sterol derivatives and cannot distinguish between cholesterol and other 3β-hydroxy sterols in the sample. Since 70–80% of serum total cholesterol is esterified with fatty acids of various chain lengths and degrees of unsaturation, the efficiency of the esterase reaction is a major factor governing the analytical performance of the enzymatic assays (Tel and Behrends, 1980; Noel *et al.*, 1983; Wiebe and Bernert, 1984). It has been shown that chemical hydrolysis of the esters yields 4–6% higher values for total cholesterol than enzymatic hydrolysis (Cooper *et al.*, 1982). Although the incompleteness of hydrolysis may be generally true of all cholesteryl esters, there is evidence (Tel and Behrends, 1980) that cholesteryl arachidonate and acetate may be less susceptible than the other cholesteryl esters to the esterase hydrolysis. Use of reagents with an improved lipolytic efficiency (95.5%) yields results for serum total cholesterol that are identical to those measured with a candidate reference procedure involving saponification of the cholesteryl esters (Siedel *et al.*, 1983; Wiebe and Bernert, 1984).

Transferability studies of enzymatic methods have confirmed the great utility of such routines in clinical laboratories and their potential as reference or reference equivalent methods (Svensson *et al.*, 1982; Katterman *et al.*, 1983). The combination of chemical hydrolysis and extraction, as used in the Centers for Disease Control (CDC) proposed reference method (Duncan *et al.*, 1982) with enzymatic measurement of the extracted cholesterol, has been examined and found to give suitable accuracy and precision (Franzini and Bessozzi, 1985; Cooper *et al.*, 1986).

Lillienberg and Svanborg (1976) proposed GLC with internal standards for plasma cholesterol estimation and noted that such methodology was easy to standardize and that results of GLC and enzymatic methods agreed on samples of free cholesterol. Hindricks *et al.* (1977) compared GLC with enzymatic and direct colorimetric methods for total cholesterol and considered GLC to be viable potential reference method. Brunnekreeft *et al.* (1983) investigated the suitability of GLC analysis without derivatization with the internal standard cholestanol and observed advantages in increased speed of analysis and in specificity. Derks *et al.* (1985) have reported a high-resolution capillary GLC method for plasma cholesterol analysis. The use of special precautions in weighing, novel calibration with bracketing standards, and a well-described chromatographic peak integration procedure that defines rigorously the integration boundaries so that they can be precisely calibrated with an internal standard, resulted in a remarkably low overall CV, in the range of 0.35 to 0.50%. The analyses were performed using the TMS derivatives prepared with *N,O*-bis(trimethylsilyl) trifluorocetamide in pyridine after an overnight reaction at room temperature. The internal standard was epicoprostanol in ethanol, such that the aliquots to be added to the standards and serum aliquots contained an amount of epicoprostanol equal to the amount of cholesterol expected in the serum sample. In special instances the serum can contain coprostanol (Gambert *et al.*, 1979) and cholestanol (Ishikawa *et al.*, 1976), which may be resolved from the other plasma sterols by GLC on appropriate chromatography columns. Figure 1 shows a capillary GLC separation of a mixture of cholesterol and plant sterols and their saturated analogs that was obtained from a patient with phytosterolemia (Kuksis *et al.*, 1986a). The presence of stanols was further visualized by an oxidative destruction of the unsaturated sterols, as reported by Serizawa *et al.* (1981). This complement of sterols is similar to that reported by Rao *et al.* (1975) and Miettinen (1980), who also noted the presence of avena sterol. Earlier, Miettinen (1968) had identified traces of lanosterol and methyl sterol precursors in normal serum by TLC, GLC, and GC/MS. Table 1 gives quantitative values for cholesterol and methyl sterols in fed and fasted obese human subjects (Miettinen, 1968). Thompson *et al.* (1981) have obtained separation of C_{24}-epimeric sterols by GLC on SP-2340. The 24β-epimer with saturated side chain eluted before the corresponding 24α-epimer. The order was reversed for the C_{24}-epimer sterol TMS ethers with a double bond in the side chain at C_{22}. This is of interest because one of the dietary plant sterols, campersterol, is a mixture of C_{24}-epimers.

More specifically, isotope-dilution mass spectrometry has been proposed as a Definitive Method for measurement of cholesterol and other steroids in plasma or

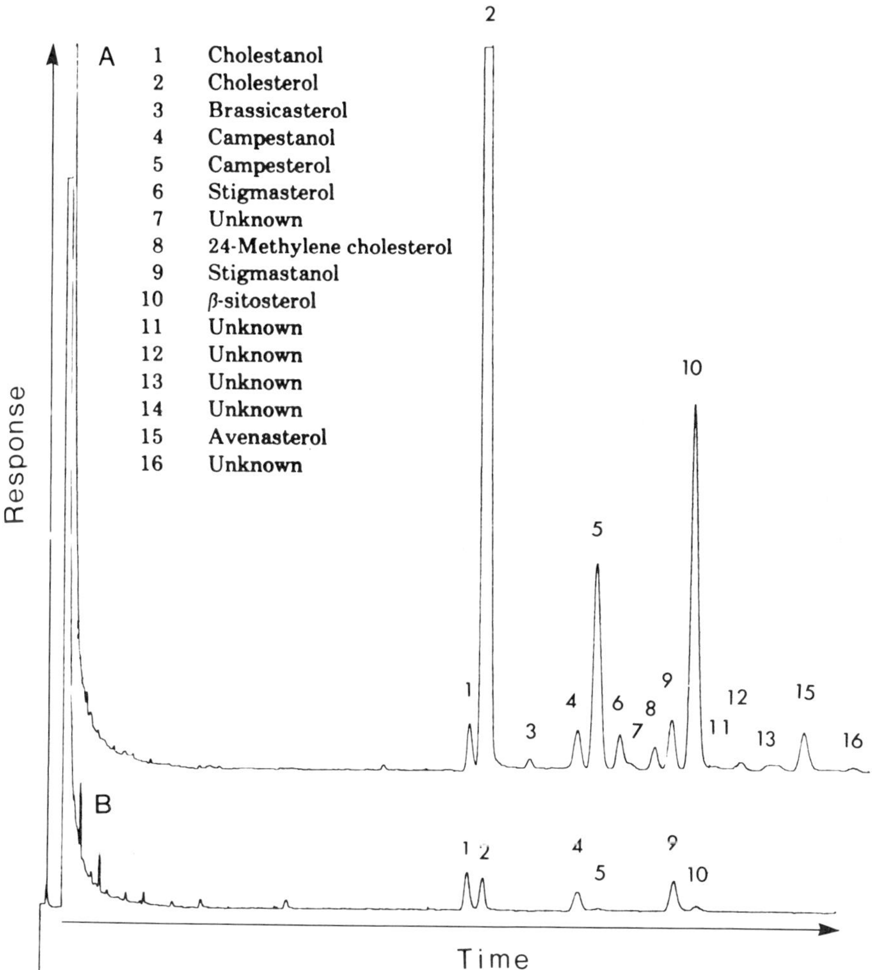

Figure 1 Capillary GLC separation of mixture of cholesterol and plant sterols and their saturated analogs as isolated from a patient with phytosterolemia. Profile A, Sterols from plasma total steryl ester fraction; profile B, oxidation products of A. Peak identification: as given in figure. Column: Supelcowax 10 on flexible quartz capillary column (15 m × 0.3 mm i.d.). Temperature: 250°C, isothermal. Carrier gas: H_2, 5 psi inlet pressure. Sample: steryl acetates. Instrument and other operating conditions as given elsewhere (Myher and Kuksis, 1987).

serum. Bjorkhem *et al.* (1974) have added a fixed amount of [2,2,3,4-$^2H_4$]cholesterol to a fixed amount of serum and have determined the amount of the unlabeled cholesterol from the ratio between the recordings of *m/z* 386 and *m/z* 389 obtained after analysis by GC/MS equipped with a multiple-ion detector. The sterols were analyzed in the free form on a nonpolar GLC column. The relative standard deviation was about 1.3%. A comparison of the GC/MS and the Liebermann–Burchard Autolab system gave a

Table 1 Serum cholesterol and methyl sterols in fed and fasted obese human subjects

Subject	Fasting (days)	Cholesterol (mg/100 ml)	Methyl Sterols[a] (μg/100 ml)				
			I	II	III	IV	V
1	0	159	10.5	8.4	7.4	12.2	5.4
	4	146	3.5	3.4	3.4	2.7	1.2
2	0	299	94.4	123.8	197.0	34.4	31.0
	5	259	76.0	106.4	270.4	25.4	19.1
3	0	160	21.6	27.1	17.7	48.3	6.5
	6	171	9.2	24.2	8.5	20.4	5.7
4	0	233	12.0	31.2	13.1	29.8	13.0
	10	165	18.0	16.6	10.2	4.2	2.7
5	0	262	38.1	56.5	48.3	38.6	22.3
	2	272	32.0	35.6	32.8	35.1	20.2
6	0	192	141.0	106.0	134.8	33.8	33.4
	6	218	30.8	38.6	46.9	13.1	11.6
7	0	260	14.1	37.30	24.7	59.6	27.0
	2	247	10.9	29.2	11.1	31.1	15.4
8	0	208	13.9	30.0	13.6	30.0	14.2
	4	188	4.8	27.3	9.4	4.3	3.2
9	0	116	8.6	22.1	11.9	15.9	6.0
	4	119	7.4	20.9	4.8	7.6	7.1

Source: Miettinen, 1968.

[a] I, Δ^8-methostenol + Δ^8-lanostenol; II, methostenol + dimethyl cholestenol (one double bond); III, lanostenol derivative; IV, lanosterol; V, dimethyl cholestenol (two double bonds).

regression coefficient of 1.01 with the two methods. The extraction step seemed to limit the sensitivity of the method. The accuracy and reliability of the method has been confirmed in several other laboratories (Cohen *et al.*, 1980; Wolthers *et al.*, 1980; Freudenthal *et al.*, 1981; Schafer *et al.*, 1982).

Kuo and Yeung (1982) have used reversed-phase HPLC to identify 7-dehydrocholesterol in human serum, which apparently is present in concentrations ranging from 5 to 40 mg/dl, with 20 mg/dl as the median. This optically active compound is a potential interference for cholesterol. About 80% of it is esterified. Individual concentrations for cholesterol and 7-dehydrocholesterol are readily obtained, since the two have distinct retention times. Δ-7-Cholesterol comprises about 1% of total cholesterol; therefore its interference on free cholesterol is within the possible error estimated for the present method. Cholestanol and cholesterol were not resolved by this reverse-phase system. Although the free plant sterols are readily resolved from each other and from free cholesterol on reversed-phase HPLC, the corresponding fatty acid esters overlap according to their partition numbers (Kuksis *et al.*, 1983a, 1986b). Child and Kuksis (1983a,b) have shown that higher-efficiency columns and gradient-elution yields improved separation between cholesterol and 7-dehydrocholesterol and their corresponding plant sterol derivatives.

GC/MS has been used to assess the performance of routine methods for the determination of steroids other than cholesterol in plasma or serum. The method has been especially important for the less-abundant steroids, which are difficult to analyze. Thus, GC/MS analysis of serum cortisol (Bjorkhem *et al.*, 1981) has been used to assess the performance of such routine methods as fluorometry, competitive protein binding, and radioimmunoassay (Lantto *et al.*, 1980). Special advantages have been demonstrated for radioimmunoassays incorporating plasma standards for which the cortisol concentrations have been determined by GC/MS (Lantto, 1982). Fluorometric assays for cortisol have been positively biased with respect to GC/MS targets, whereras the radioimmunoassay varies with the method or commercial kit employed. Jonckheere and De Leenheer (1983) have proposed a candidate definitive method for cortisol, which is a minor steroid in serum, based on addition of 4-[^{14}C]cortisol in approximately 1:1 peak-height ratio in the GLC. Following equilibration, solvent extraction of cortisol, and its internal standard from the serum matrix, the steroids are converted into the methoxine-TMS derivatives and the extract is purified by gel chromatography. Capillary GC/MS measurements are then made of the peak heights at *m/z* 605 and 607 for each sample and calibration mixtures. Suboptimal conditions of separation were deliberately chosen to provide no separation between syn-anti isomers of cortisol and labeled cortisol methoxylamine-TMS derivatives. Analysis of variance gave a coefficient of variation of 0.38% for a serum pool containing 90.79 ng cortisol per ml of serum.

B. Ratio of Free and Esterified Sterols

The early methods of chromatographic resolution of free and esterified plasma cholesterol have been described by Skipski (1969). A two-step determination of plasma total and free cholesterol based on liquid-solid chromatography and GLC measurement of free and esterified plasma cholesterol was suggested as a reference method by Ambert *et al.* (1976). Bowyer and King (1977) have proposed a "three-dimensional" separation of neutral lipids to improve the resolution of cholesteryl esters from methyl esters and hydrocarbons. The cholesterol and cholesteryl esters are assayed fluorometrically (Bondjers and Bjorkerud, 1971). Gartzke (1979) has described an effective TLC separation of free and esterified cholesterol, along with other plasma neutral lipids, using two developments in the same direction. The resolved components were quantitated by densitometry and the results compared with those obtained with colorimetric and enzymatic methods.

Vandamme *et al.* (1978) have reported on the resolution of free and esterified plasma cholesterol using the Chromarod method of TLC. Comparisons of the estimates of the free and esterified cholesterol by the Chromarod and classical chemical analysis showed that correction factors were necessary. Christie and Hunter (1979) have shown that better separations are obtained with the Chromarod system using a double-solvent development. Other workers (Farnworth *et al.*, 1982) have suggested the inclusion of an internal standard in the test solution, which improves the precision of the method.

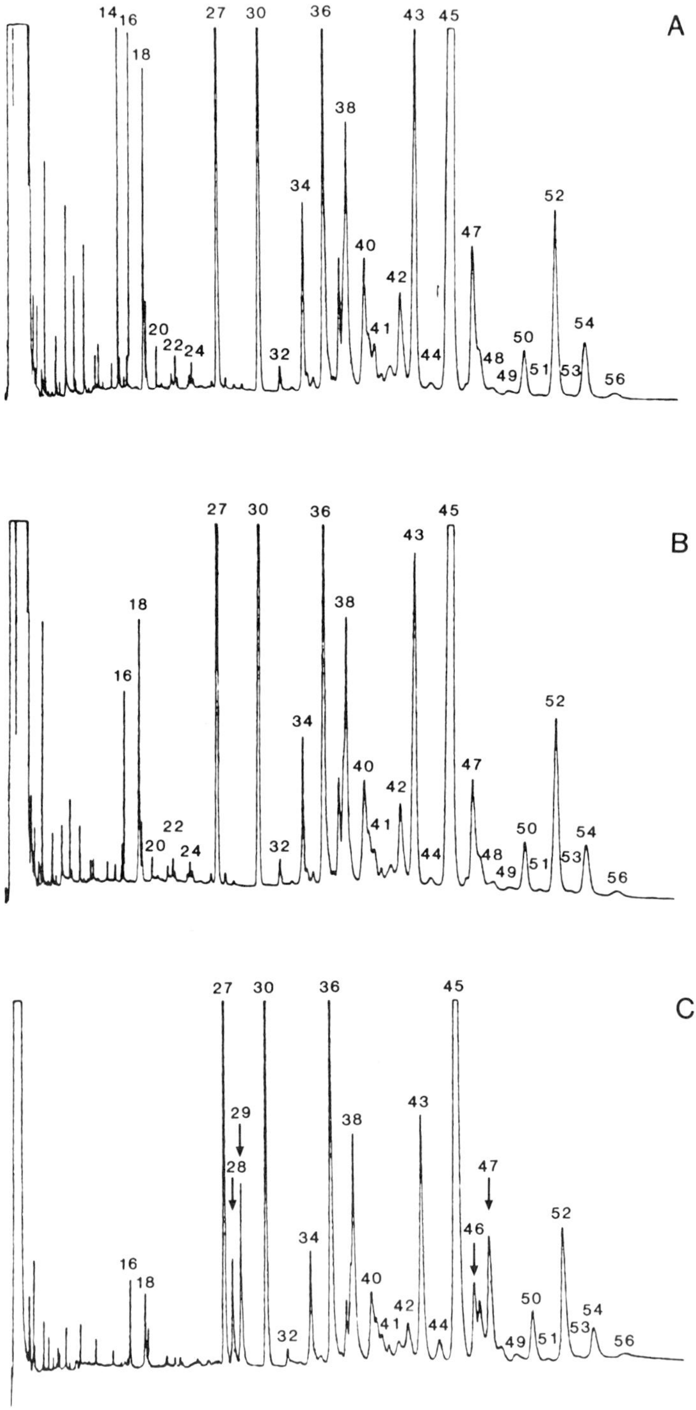
A
14 16 18 20 22 24 27 30 32 34 36 38 40 41 42 43 44 45 47 48 49 50 51 52 53 54 56
B
16 18 20 22 24 27 30 32 34 36 38 40 41 42 43 44 45 47 48 49 50 51 52 53 54 56
C
16 18 27 28 29 30 32 34 36 38 40 41 42 43 44 45 46 47 49 50 51 52 53 54 56

Separations of free and esterified sterols are readily accomplished by means of high-temperature GLC. Kuksis (1964), Kuksis *et al.* (1967, 1969), and, more recently, Mares *et al.* (1978, 1979, 1983) and Mares (1987) have reported applications to the quantitation of plasma neutral lipids, and Kuksis *et al.* (1975, 1978b) have reported similar success with total lipid extracts of plasma dephosphorylated with phospholipase C (*Bacillus cereus*). Both methods resolve free cholesterol from any plant sterols and provide a carbon number distribution for the mixed steryl esters. These techniques have been extensively applied in studies of plasma lipid composition in normal subjects (Kuksis *et al.*, 1978b, 1981, 1982c; Mares *et al.*, 1978, 1979, 1983) and in patients with hyperlipoproteinemia (Kuksis *et al.*, 1982a,b; Mares *et al.*, 1978, 1983; Skorepa *et al.*, 1976, 1979, 1983; Steiner *et al.*, 1985; Mares, 1987), phytosterolemia (Kuksis *et al.*, 1986a,b), hepatic lipase deficiency (Breckenridge *et al.*, 1982), and rheumatoid arthritis (Sonnenberg *et al.*, 1987). Figure 2 shows capillary GLC profiles of total plasma lipids from normal subjects and from a patient with phytosterolemia. Other applications of GLC estimations of free and esterified cholesterol have been made in studies of plasma lipid response to birth control pills (Hedlin *et al.*, 1978), dietary manipulations (Mercer and Holub, 1979; Kuksis *et al.*, 1982c), and intralipid infusion in infants (Griffin *et al.*, 1979). These techniques have also been applied to plasma lipid analyses of rats (Mookerjea *et al.*, 1975; Kuksis *et al.*, 1978a; Breckenridge *et al.*, 1979; Kakis and Kuksis, 1984) and mice (Kuksis *et al.*, 1983b; Breckenridge *et al.*, 1985). In addition to providing the free and esterified cholesterol ratio, the GLC profiles of total plasma lipids provide characteristic ratios of free and esterified sterols to other lipid classes, which are of interest in studies of lipoprotein structure and metabolism. Table 2 gives various lipid class ratios in VLDL, LDL_1, LDL_2, and HDL particles of fasting normolipemic and hyperlipemic subjects, as obtained by high-temperature GLC (Kuksis *et al.*, 1981, 1982a).

Figure 2 Capillary GCL profiles of plasma total lipids. Profile C, a patient with phytosterolemia; profiles A and B, two healthy family members (controls). Peak identification: 16 and 18, TMS esters of free fatty acids with 16 and 18 carbon atoms; 20, 22, 24, di-TMS ethers of monoacylglycerols with 16, 18, and 20 acyl carbons, respectively; 27, TMS ether of free cholesterol; 28, TMS ether of free campesterol (arrow); 29, TMS ether of free sitosterol (arrow); 30, tridecanoylglycerol, internal standard; 32–42, TMS ethers of diacylglycerol and ceramide moieties with 30–40 fatty chain carbons; 43–49, steryl esters with 43–49 total carbon atoms (46 is C_{18} fatty acid ester of campesterol and 47 is C_{18} fatty acid ester of β-sitosterol); 50–56, triacylglycerols with 50–56 acyl carbons. The *x*-axis is linear with respect to retention time. Peak 54 was eluted in 23 min GLC conditions: instrument, Hewlett-Packard Model 5880A gas chromatograph equipped with on-column capillary injector and a flame ionization detector; column, flexible quartz capillary (8 m × 0.30 mm i.d.) coated with permanently bonded nonpolar SE-54 liquid phase (Hewlett-Packard); temperature, programmed from 40° to 150°C at 30°C/min, then to 230°C at 20°C/min, to 280°C at 10°C/min, and to 340°C at 5°C/min; carrier gas, H_2 at a head pressure of 55.1 kPA. Sample: dephosphorylated and silylated total lipid extracts of plasma (Kuksis *et al.*, 1986a).

Table 2 Lipid class ratios in VLDL, LDL_1, LDL_2, and HDL particles of fasting normolipemic and hyperlipemic subjects

Chemical Components[a]	Normolipemics[b]		Hyperlipemics[b]	
	Males (7)	Females (4)	Type III (6)	Type IV (4)
VLDL				
FC/TC	0.44 ± 0.02	0.37 ± 0.01	0.20 ± 0.01	0.36 ± 0.02
FC/PL	0.62 ± 0.02	0.54 ± 0.01	0.73 ± 0.05	0.62 ± 0.04
EC/TG	0.29 ± 0.02	0.33 ± 0.01	0.58 ± 0.2	0.34 ± 0.08
FC/SPH	5.5 ± 0.08	5.3 ± 1.0	4.2 ± 1.0	3.5 ± 0.3
FC/PC	0.70 ± 0.05	0.60 ± 0.01	0.91 ± 0.05	0.78 ± 0.04
LDL_1				
FC/TC			0.28 ± 0.01	0.29 ± 0.02
FC/PL			0.73 ± 0.05	0.68 ± 0.05
EC/TG			1.9 ± 0.5	1.3 ± 0.5
EC/SPH			2.5 ± 0.1	2.7 ± 0.2
FC/PC			1.0 ± 0.1	0.9 ± 0.1
LDL_2				
FC/TC	0.27 ± 0.01	0.29 ± 0.01	0.23 ± 0.03	0.23 ± 0.02
FC/PL	0.72 ± 0.05	0.70 ± 0.01	0.60 ± 0.04	0.69 ± 0.02
EC/TG	7.9 ± 1.0	9.6 ± 0.2	3.2 ± 1.0	4.4 ± 1.0
FC/SPH	2.9 ± 0.3	2.7 ± 0.1	2.8 ± 0.5	2.8 ± 0.3
FC/PC	0.95 ± 0.05	0.95 ± 0.02	0.76 ± 0.1	0.90 ± 0.1
HDL				
FC/TL	0.20 ± 0.01	0.19 ± 0.01	0.20 ± 0.02	0.24 ± 0.01
FC/PL	0.26 ± 0.02	0.23 ± 0.01	0.20 ± 0.02	0.21 ± 0.02
EC/TG	8.7 ± 1.0	7.7 ± 0.4	2.7 ± 0.5	3.5 ± 2.0
FC/SPH	2.6 ± 0.2	1.9 ± 0.1	2.2 ± 0.1	2.2 ± 0.2
FC/PC	0.29 ± 0.02	0.23 ± 0.01	0.23 ± 0.02	0.24 ± 0.02

Source: Normolipemics, from Kuksis *et al.*, (1981); hyperlipemics, from Kuksis *et al.* (1982a).

[a] TC, total cholesterol; PL, total phospholipid; PC, phosphatidylcholine; SPH, sphingomyelin; FC, free cholesterol; EC, cholesteryl ester; TG, triacylglycerol.

[b] Number of subjects in test group given in parentheses.

HPLC has been used in the analysis of lipids containing sterols on many occasions, but specific applications in free cholesterol assays have been few (Child and Kuksis, 1983a,b) because cholesterol and related compounds have limited UV absorption, which is the most common detection method. However, HPLC has been effective whenever column chromatography is followed by chemical analysis of the collected fractions (Duncan *et al.*, 1979), or whenever the eluate is monitored on-line with other types of detectors, such as refractive-index (Perkins *et al.*, 1981), flame-ionization (Phillips *et al.*, 1982), and laser-infrared (Stolyhwo *et al.*, 1985) or mass-spectrometric (Kuksis *et al.*, 1983a) detectors. Phillips *et al.* (1982) have described a method for direct quantitative analysis of the lipid classes of mammalian lipids, including the sterols and steryl esters, by normal-phase HPLC. Erucyl alcohol was used as an internal standard. More recent work with spectrophotometric-grade solvents has shown that HPLC of sterols can be performed by monitoring at wavelengths as low as 200 nm (Brown, 1987).

C. Composition of Steryl Esters

Since both acyl CoA-cholesterol acyltransferase (ACAT) (Field and Mathu, 1983) and lecithin-cholesterol acyltransferase (LCAT) (Nordby and Norum, 1975) esterify cholesterol and plant sterols and their biosynthetic precursors, a great variety of steryl esters could potentially be present in plasma and plasma lipoproteins. The possibility of quantitative determination of cholesteryl esters without saponification has been demonstrated using argentation TLC (Morris, 1963; Skipski, 1969) and high-temperature GLC (Kuksis, 1964). Conventional TLC allows separations of steryl esters on the basis of fatty acid unsaturation (Morris, 1963), whereas high-performance $AgNO_3$-TLC could also provide a resolution of cis- and trans-isomers of esters differing in degree of unsaturation of sterol moieties. GLC on nonpolar columns provides separations based largely on carbon number, but a partial resolution of saturated and polyunsaturated long-chain esters is also obtained (Kuksis *et al.*, 1969; Smith, 1983). Over the years these techniques have been improved and compared with the estimates obtained by conventional methods, and good agreement has been found (Kuksis *et al.*, 1978b; Mares *et al.*, 1983). High-temperature GLC of steryl esters is applicable to either neutral lipid extracts or dephosphorylated total lipid extracts. The samples are silylated and diluted with tridecanoylglycerol (Kuksis *et al.*, 1975) or cholesteryl butyrate (Mares *et al.*, 1978) as internal standard. In most cases the concentration of the compounds was in the region where the weight correction factor is independent of the amount injected. The possibility of using quantitative GLC for the determination of amounts in the nanogram range has been evaluated by Mares *et al.* (1979), who have made appropriate recommendations.

The separations of steryl esters on polar capillary columns are performed using hydrogen as a carrier gas (Smith, 1982, 1983; Kuksis *et al.*, 1986a; Myher and Kuksis, 1988). It is pertinent to note that certain types of columns apparently contain residual polymerization catalyst that catalyzes the reduction of the steryl esters by the hydrogen carrier gas at the elevated temperatures (Smith, 1982). Work with other polar capillary columns has shown that cholesteryl esters suffer partial breakdown at temperatures exceeding 300°C (Myher and Kuksis, 1988). It is therefore necessary to elute all cholesteryl ester peaks below this temperature in a minimum of time compatible with the desired resolution. Usually, short capillary columns must be used for this purpose. Figure 3 shows the separation of human and rat plasma total cholesteryl ester fraction on a polar capillary GLC column (Myher and Kuksis, 1988).

Smith *et al.* (1980), have shown that reversed-phase HPLC can be used to measure individual cholesteryl esters. For this purpose, the mobile phase was isopropanol:acetonitrile 1:1, and cholesterol and its esters were detected with a variable wavelength UV detector set at 215 nm. Because there was no detectable cholesteryl stearate in the samples, this ester was used as an internal standard in the quantitative studies. Cholesteryl linolenate and cholesteryl palmitoleate were also absent from the profiles.

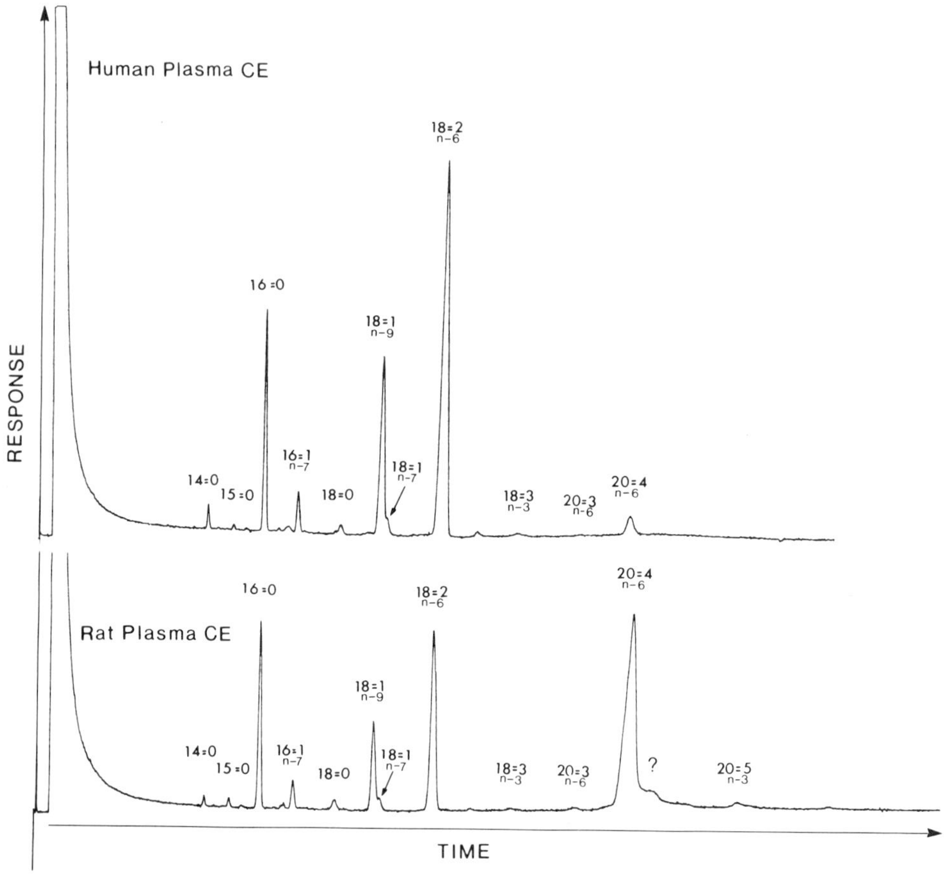

Figure 3 Capillary GLC separation of human and rat plasma total cholesteryl esters on a polar liquid phase. Peak identification by chain length, double-bond number, and location of fatty acids in the cholesteryl esters. GLC conditions: instrument, Hewlett-Packard Model 5880A gas chromatograph equipped with an on-column capillary injector and a flame ionization detector; column, SP-2330 glass capillary (10 m × 0.25 mm i.d.); temperature, 250°C (isothermal); carrier gas, H_2, 8 psi inlet pressure. Sample: intact cholesteryl esters (Myher and Kuksis, 1988).

These esters were only partially resolved from cholesteryl arachidonate and cholesteryl linoleate, respectively. Reproducibility in the range of 4 to 8% was achieved for the extraction and HPLC analysis of four replicate determinations of a control blood sample. A similar method for the separation and quantification of cholesterol and its esters has been described by Carroll and Rudel (1981). It uses a reversed-phase HPLC system to resolve a series of saturated and unsaturated cholesteryl esters and free cholesterol.

Perkins *et al.* (1981) separated cholesterol and cholesteryl esters according to their carbon number and number of double bonds by reversed-phase HPLC using isocratic acetonitrile-chloroform-methanol as mobile phase and detected them by a refractometer. It was found that within the same carbon number, cholesteryl esters with the highest number of double bonds eluted ahead of those with a lower number of double bonds. The cis-isomers were eluted ahead of their trans-partners. Human lipoprotein and rat liver cholesteryl esters were separated by this technique. Helmich *et al.* (1981) have used reversed-phase HPLC to resolve [^{3}H]cholesterol esters.

Kuo and Yeung (1982) have described a reversed-phase HPLC separation of free and esterified human serum cholesterol using an on-line monitoring of the optical rotation of the eluate. The method is suitable for profiling and quantitative analysis. Calculations of the concentrations of free and esterified cholesterol were made using a procedure that eliminates the need for high-purity standards. Because of the uncertainties in the specific rotations (alpha) at the wavelength (514.5) and the solvent (tetrahydrofuran-water) use, a maximum error of $\pm 10\%$ was assessed on the calculated results. The peaks for free cholesterol and its esters were identified on the basis of the retention time, the sign and magnitude of the individual specific rotations, and the anticipated distribution and structural features of the solutes. Five major cholesterol peaks were identified: cholesterol and cholestanol, cholesteryl linolenate and archidonate, cholesteryl palmitoleate and linoleate, cholesteryl palmitate and oleate, and cholesteryl stearate, as already established by Duncan *et al.* (1979). Bernert *et al.* (1982) have used HPLC for a direct determination of the linoleate/oleate ratio in serum cholesteryl esters.

LC/MS methods have been used in the analysis of sterols and steryl esters following adsorption chromatographic isolation (Kuksis *et al.*, 1986a) and in the analysis of crude total lipid extracts of plasma and natural fats (Kuksis *et al.*, 1983a). The free sterols and steryl esters are resolved on a reversed-phase HPLC column, and a preliminary identification is made on the basis of the relative retention time. CI-MS spectra are recorded and used to confirm the presence of the steroid nuclei in each HPLC peak. The system readily distinguishes among cholesteryl and plant steryl esters on the basis of the molecular weight and the sterol nuclei recovered from each HPLC peak.

VI. ANALYSIS OF INDIVIDUAL PLASMA LIPOPROTEIN CLASSES

Complete analysis of sterols and steryl esters in VLDL, LDL, HDL, and their variants requires a major effort, which is not appropriate for many laboratories. In fact, difficulties arise during measurements of total cholesterol in the major lipoprotein classes, and there is good reason to question the accuracy of many of the methods employed for this purpose. Thus, the Lipid Research Clinics' method involves ultracentrifugation for the isolation of VLDL, precipitation with heparin-$MnCl_2$ for isolation of LDL, and measurement of cholesterol in the supernatant to estimate HDL (Lipid Research Clinics Program, 1974). Warnick *et al.* (1979) have shown that the coefficient of variation in an interlaboratory HDL cholesterol determination by this method varied from 9 to 38%. No estimates of variation have been published for the determination of VLDL and LDL cholesterol by the same method, but they also are likely to be high. With Friedewald's formula (Friedewald *et al.*, 1972), the LDL cholesterol is estimated by subtracting from plasma total cholesterol the HDL cholesterol, estimated from precipitation of other proteins by addition of dextran sulfate and manganese chloride (Burstein and Legmann, 1982), and the VLDL cholesterol, estimated as one-fifth of the plasma total triacylglycerol. Variations in the determined values result, depending upon the age, sex and lipoproteinemia type of the subject and the method of lipoprotein separation. A more effective method for the estimation of total cholesterol in individual plasma lipoprotein classes is based on lipoprotein separation in a single vertical spin rotor (Chung *et al.*, 1986). The interrun coefficient of variation for cholesterol concentration in VLDL, LDL, and HDL was 4.8, 2.9, and 2.4%, respectively. Chlorosterol recovery was 98.5($\pm$3.5)%. Conlon *et al.* (1979) have used electrophoresis to quantitate plasma lipoprotein cholesterol, but this method also is not quantitative. Kohl *et al.* (1980) have pointed out that HDL cholesterol measured by this method is poorly reproducible. Marz and Gross (1986) have reassessed the analysis of cholesterol of plasma lipoproteins by quantitative electrophoresis. The concentrations of pre-β-, β-, and α-lipoprotein-cholesterol were computed. Marz and Gross (1986) failed to reproduce the excellent correlation coefficients between lipoprotein electrophoresis and ultracentrifugation observed by Bojanovski *et al.* (1981) and Vogelberg *et al.* (1984). The quantitative lipoprotein electrophoresis, though moderately overestimating HDL cholesterol, proved of acceptable accuracy for pre-β-lipoprotein-cholesterol and particularly β-lipoprotein-cholesterol. HPLC also has shown promise as a fast and large-scale method for lipoprotein separation. Hara *et al.* (1980) and Hara and Okazaki (1986) have found that HDL_2-, HDL_3-, LDL-, and VLDL-cholesterol can be directly analyzed from a small amount of whole serum, without pretreatment, by means of enzymatic reaction after separation by HPLC. The reactor-type detector required as little as 25 μg cholesterol per ml serum, which could be detected using 20 μl of serum for analysis. The respective sensitivities of detection of cholesterol were four times higher than that for protein in the case of HDL_2 and three times higher in the case of HDL_3. The reproducibility of this method was $\pm$0.06 ml for the elution volume and $\pm$0.10 μg for cholesterol quantification (Hara and Okazaki, 1986), Srinivasan *et al.* (1983) have emphasized that the ultracentrifugal, electrophoretic, and precipitation methods of isolation provide independent estimates for lipoprotein cholesterol.

A. Plasma Chylomicrons

Free cholesterol makes up about 35 mol % of the surface components and less than 1% of the neutral lipid core, which, however, contains about 5 mol % of cholesteryl ester (Smith *et al.*, 1983). A detailed discussion of the early determinations of chylomicron sterols and steryl esters of human plasma obtained by ultracentrifugation has been presented by Skipski (1969). Complete analysis of the steryl ester composition was obtained by saponification of the esters and determination of the fatty acid composition by GLC. More recently, the free sterols and steryl esters of plasma chylomicrons have been determined by high-temperature GLC. Griffin *et al.* (1979) and Kuksis *et al.* (1981) have demonstrated quantitative resolution of the free sterols and the steryl esters, based on carbon number using high-temperature GLC, and have obtained good agreement with the results of GLC analyses of their fatty acid methyl esters, prepared following isolation of the steryl esters by TLC. The cholesteryl esters of chylomicrons are synthesized by ACAT in the absorptive cells of the intestine (Norum *et al.*, 1983; Field and Mathur, 1983). The ratio of free to esterified cholesterol in the plasma chylomicrons is significantly higher than in other lipoprotein classes, but the reason for this is not known. Human plasma chylomicrons may gain cholesteryl esters from HDL in exchange for triacylglycerols (Patsch *et al.*, 1984). The plasma chylomicrons of rats (Kuksis *et al.*, 1978a) and mice (Kuksis *et al.*, 1983b) have also been examined for free and esterified cholesterol content and composition. Since rat and mouse plasma do not contain cholesteryl ester transfer protein, esters of these lipoproteins remain largely unchanged.

B. Very-Low-Density Lipoproteins

Human plasma very-low-density lipoprotein (VLDL) is characterized by a significantly higher proportion of total cholesterol than the chylomicrons. Free cholesterol makes up about 43 mol % of the surface components and up to 3% of the neutral lipid core, which also contains about 24 mol % cholesteryl ester (Smith *et al.*, 1983). It has a PC/FC ratio of 1.40 (Kuksis *et al.*, 1981). In normal human liver, the activity of ACAT is low, and nascent VLDL contains few cholesteryl esters. Most of the VLDL cholesteryl ester is acquired by transfer from HDL via a relatively active transferase; hence the cholesteryl esters of human plasma VLDL and HDL are of similar fatty acid composition (Kuksis *et al.*, 1981, 1982a). In the rat, newly synthesized VLDL contains an appreciable complement of cholesteryl esters, synthesized by hepatic ACAT, but acquires little in plasma because it contains little cholesteryl ester transferase (Barter and Lally, 1978). These differences in the biosynthesis of VLDL cholesteryl esters are reflected in the fatty acid composition. Thus, the cholesteryl esters of rat plasma VLDL and HDL remain distinct (Kakis *et al.*, 1988).

Early analyses of free and esterified cholesterol of VLDL were discussed by Skipski (1969), who pointed out the relatively high ratio of free to esterified cholesterol and the preponderance of the oleoyl and linoleoyl esters of cholesterol in human plasma VLDL. More recently, the free and esterified cholesterol ratios and the carbon number distribution of the cholesteryl esters in VLDL from normal subjects (Kuksis *et al.*, 1981, 1982c) and hyperlipemic subjects (Kuksis *et al.*, 1982a) have been obtained by high-temperature GLC on nonpolar packed columns. Subsequently, Kuksis *et al.* (1986b) have demonstrated that high-temperature GLC in combination with short nonpolar capillary columns can also provide separate estimates for the plant sterols and their esters, when present. Capillary GLC on polar columns allows separation of individual cholesteryl and plant steryl esters in mixtures, as shown in Fig. 4 (Kuksis *et al.*, 1986a).

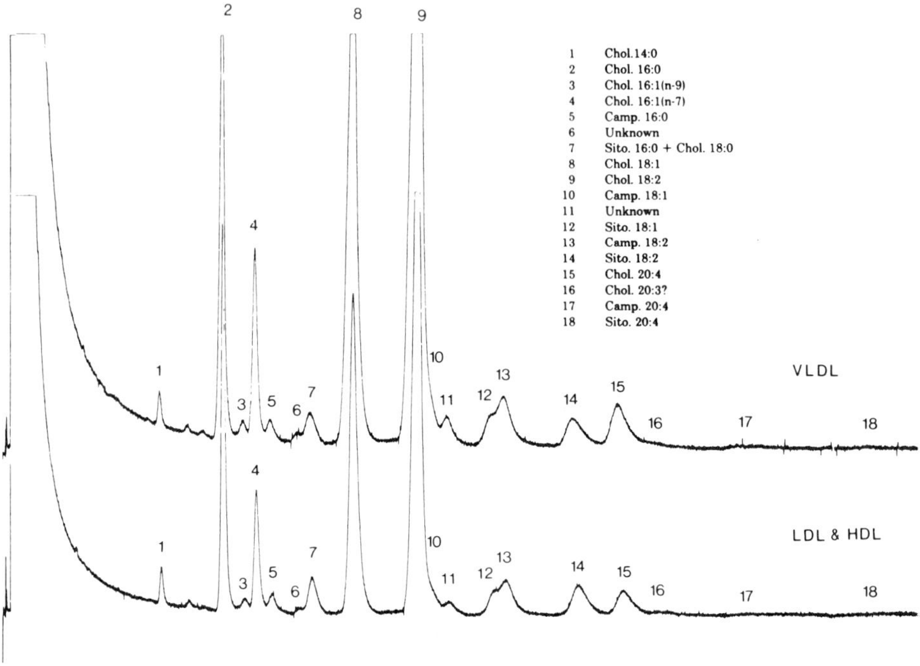

Figure 4 Capillary GLC separation of steryl esters on VLDL and LDL + HDL fractions from a patient with phytosterolemia. Peak identification as given in figure. GLC conditions: as in Fig. 3. Sample: intact steryl esters (Kuksis *et al.*, 1986a).

In some instances, the sterol and steryl ester compositions of VLDL have been compared with those of the LDL and HDL in man (Kuksis *et al.*, 1981, 1982c) and in experimental animals (Kuksis *et al.*, 1978a; Breckenridge *et al.*, 1985). Tong and Kuksis (1988) have quantitated sterols and steryl esters in the mixed VLDL + LDL fraction obtained by Mg^{2+}-phosphotungstic acid precipitation and the HDL recovered from supernatant of human plasma. They obtained significant differences compared with the results from direct ultracentrifugation. Of particular interest were the differences between the ratios of the free cholesterol to other lipid classes.

C. Low-Density Lipoproteins

Both rat and human plasma VLDL gives rise to low-density lipoprotein (LDL), which is characterized by a reduced particle size. Up to 80 mol % of the neutral lipid core of LDL is made up of cholesteryl esters. The free cholesterol content of the surface monolayer accounts for about 42 mol % of the total. It has a PC/FC ratio of nearly 1.0 (Kuksis *et al.*, 1981). The cholesteryl ester compositions of the VLDL and the LDL particles are about the same. The LDL fraction is the major carrier of cholesterol and cholesteryl esters in human plasma. Approximately 60% of the cholesteryl ester is transported as LDL in man and about three-fourths of this is esterified (Smith *et al.*,

1983). Total LDL cholesterol is frequently estimated indirectly, using the Friedewald approximation (Friedewald *et al.*, 1972), as a difference between total plasma cholesterol, HDL cholesterol, and VLDL cholesterol. In many instances, the Friedewald approximation for LDL cholesterol has given good agreement with the values obtained by ultracentrifugation, but in other instances (Marz and Gross, 1986), this formula has underestimated LDL-cholesterol due to an overestimation of VLDL-cholesterol.

The early direct analysis of free and esterified cholesterol content and composition of LDL were discussed by Skipski (1969), who also referred to the early determinations of the fatty acid composition of the cholesteryl esters and the similarity between LDL and HDL, in this respect, in man. More recently, extensive analyses of the free and esterified cholesterol ratios in LDL have been reported for man (Kuksis *et al.*, 1981, 1982a,c), rats (Kuksis *et al.*, 1978a; Ridgway and Dolphin, 1984, 1985; Dolphin *et al.*, 1986), and mice (Breckenridge *et al.*, 1985). The fatty acid compositions of LDL cholesteryl esters of subjects subsisting on free-choice diets (Kuksis *et al.*, 1981) and on controlled experimental diets (Kuksis *et al.*, 1982c) have been tabulated. A consistent finding is the similarity in the steryl ester composition of the LDL_2 and the HDL fractions (Kuksis *et al.*, 1981). Hoffman *et al.* (1985) have compared five methods for measuring total LDL cholesterol in serum.

The free and esterified cholesterol and plant sterols and steryl esters in the LDL of patients with phytosterolemia have been determined by GLC (Bhattacharya and Connor, 1978). Salen *et al.* (1985a,b) have shown that subjects with phytosterolemia and xanthomatosis possessed increased levels of plasma cholestanol and α-saturated plant sterol derivatives. Table 3 shows the saturated and unsaturated sterol concentrations found in the LDL and HDL fractions of such subjects (Salen *et al.*, 1985a) and of another subject (Kuksis *et al.*, 1986a). Detailed analyses of the individual cholesteryl and plant steryl esters in the VLDL and LDL + HDL fractions of a patient with phytosterolemia have been made using LC/MS. Figure 5 shows an LC/MS analysis of the mixed cholesteryl and plant steryl esters recovered from the LDL + HDL fraction (Kuksis *et al.*, 1986a). The steryl esters are identified on the basis of HPLC retention time and the ions characteristic of the sterol nuclei in the mass spectra.

D. High-Density Lipoproteins

The lipids in high-density lipoproteins (HDL) are primarily phosphatidylcholine, free cholesterol, and cholesteryl esters. Free cholesterol makes up about 23 mol % of the surface components, and the cholesteryl esters account for about 82 mol % of the neutral lipid core (Smith *et al.*, 1983). It has a PC/FC ratio of about 4 (Kuksis *et al.*, 1981). Since zonal ultracentrifugation (Patsch and Patsch, 1986) and gel filtration chromatography (Hara and Okazaki, 1986) provide a bimodal distribution, HDL is commonly considered to have two components: HDL_2 and HDL_3. The phosphatidylcholine and free cholesterol in HDL are substrates for LCAT, whereas apoprotein A-I, which is a major apoprotein component, activates the transesterification of the unsaturated fatty acids of phosphatidylcholine to free cholesterol (Glomset *et al.*,

Table 3 Distribution of saturated and unsaturated sterols among lipoprotein classes in subjects with phytosterolemia and xanthomatosis

	Sterols (mol %)					
Source[a]	Cholesterol	Cholestanol	Campesterol	Campestanol	Sitosterol	Sitostanol
LDL (3)	75.2	0.3	6.8	0.1	12.2	0.2
HDL (3)	88.7	1.7	0.01	—	8.6	—
LDL + HDL (1)	79.1	1.3	5.9[b]	0.8	9.5	0.7
VLDL (1)	80.0	1.5	6.5	0.9	10.9	1.0

[a] LDL and HDL data from Salen *et al.* (1985a); LDL + HDL and VLDL data from Kuksis *et al.* (1986a). Number of subjects in test group given in parentheses.

[b] 60% Campesterol (24α-methy) and 40% 22,23-dihydrobrassica sterol (24β-methyl).

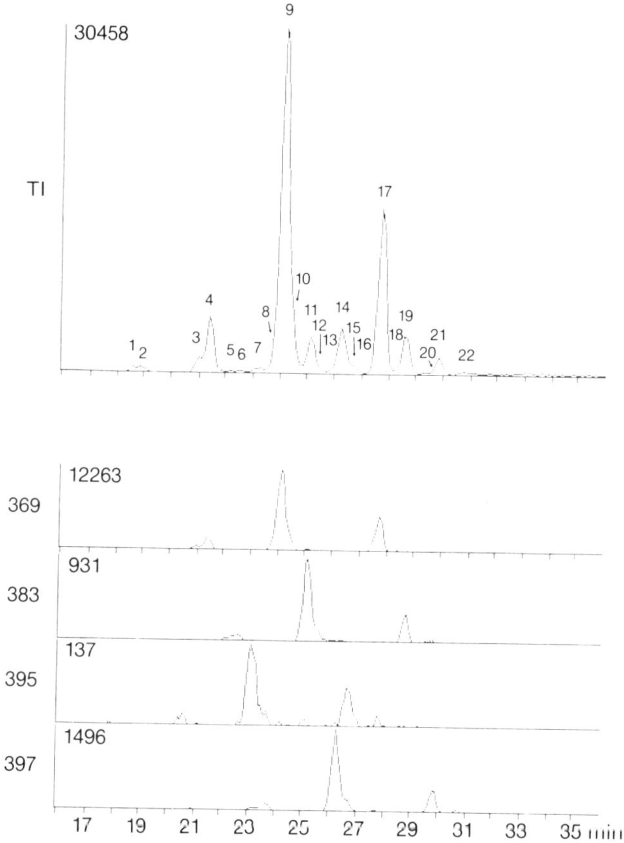

Figure 5 LC/MS elution profile of steryl esters of the LDL + HDL fraction of plasma from a patient with phytosterolemia. TI, total ion current; 369, 383, 395, and 397, fragment ions representing the steroid nuclei of cholesterol, campesterol, stigmasterol and avenasterol, and *β*-sitosterol. Peak identification: 1, cholesteryl docosahexaenoate; 2, cholesteryl eicosapentaenoate; 3, cholesteryl linoleate; 4, cholesteryl arachidonate; 5 and 6, unknown; 7, avenasteryl linoleate; 8, *β*-sitosteryl arachidonate; 9, cholesteryl linoleate; 10, cholesteryl palmitoleate; 11, campesteryl linoleate; 12 and 13, unknown; 14, *β*-sitosteryl lino oleate; 15, avenasteryl oleate; 16, unknown; 17, cholesteryl oleate; 18, unknown; 19, cholesteryl palmitate; 20, unknown; 21, *β*-sitosteryl oleate; 22, unknown. LC/MS conditions: instrument, Hewlett-Packard Model 1084B liquid chromatograph combined with a Hewlett-Packard Model 5985B quadrupole mass spectrometer via a Hewlett-Packard direct liquid inlet interface; column, reversed-phase Supelcosil C_{18} (25 cm × 0.25 cm i.d.); eluant, a linear gradient of 30–90% propionitrile in acetonitrile. Sample: intact steryl esters (Kuksis *et al.*, 1986a).

1983). Hence the cholesteryl esters of HDL reflect to a large extent the fatty acid composition of the corresponding phosphatidylcholines (Aron *et al.*, 1978; Kuksis *et al.*, 1982c). In the absence of LCAT activity, the nascent HDL particles are discoidal and do not contain cholesteryl esters. As noted above, HDL may donate cholesteryl esters to chylomicrons and VLDL in exchange for triacylglycerols. In humans and rabbits, the newly esterified cholesterol is rapidly distributed to other lipoproteins by cholesteryl ester transfer protein (Norum *et al.*, 1983; Hesler *et al.*, 1987; Groener *et al.*, 1987). Glass *et al.* (1983) have determined the plasma clearance of cholesteryl ethers incorporated into HDL as slowly metabolized analogs of cholesteryl esters. The content of free and esterified cholesterol of HDL or its subfractions, HDL_2 and HDL_3, isolated by ultracentifugation, has been obtained by a number of methods including high-temperature GLC (Kuksis *et al.*, 1979). Gavish *et al.* (1987) have used radioactive cholesteryl esters to demonstrate that *in vivo* HDL_3 is a precursor of HDL_2 and of apoE-rich HDL_I, and that lipid transfer proteins delay the conversion process, especially HDL_I.

The determination of cholesterol in the HDL fraction has received nearly as much attention as the determination of plasma total cholesterol (Durrington, 1982; Superko *et al.*, 1986) because of the great importance attached to the HDL level as an indicator of risk for atherosclerosis and the ease of HDL estimation from its cholesterol content; but the clinical significance of assaying HDL subclasses has been questioned (Lippi *et al.*, 1986).

Again, the initial studies of HDL cholesteryl esters were made by TLC/GLC and $AgNO_3$-TLC/GLC (Skipski, 1969), whereas more-recent work has reported on the carbon number distribution of the steryl esters in normal subjects (Kuksis *et al.*, 1981, 1982c) and hyperlipemic subjects (Kuksis *et al.*, 1982a; Skorepa *et al.*, 1979, 1983). The carbon number and fatty acid distribution of cholesteryl esters in normal human HDL, compared with human VLDL and LDL, have been reported by Kuksis *et al.* (1981, 1982c). Detailed analyses, using LC/MS, of cholesterol and plant sterol content and the composition of the individual fatty acid esters of these sterols in the LDL + HDL fraction from a patient with phytosterolemia have been reported by Kuksis *et al.* (1986a). It has recently been observed that tetranitromethane modification of human HDL_3 leads to inhibition of HDL binding, which may be related to cholesteryl ester cross-linking through double bonds to the protein molecule (Chacko *et al.*, 1987), but no specific structures have been identified. This study determined free and total cholesterol by GLC, using coprostanol as internal standard. Esterified cholesterol was obtained by difference from free and total cholesterol. Tam and Breckenridge (1983, 1987) have used high-temperature GLC for the analysis of free and esterified cholesterol in the HDL-like particles obtained during perfusion of rat heart with human VLDL.

E. Lipoprotein (a)

Lipoprotein Lp (a) is a cholesterol-rich lipoprotein that usually makes up less than 15% of total plasma cholesterol. It resembles LDL in several ways but can be distinguished from it by electroimmunoassay (Dahlen *et al.*, 1986). Plasma Lp (a) in white patients appears to be a coronary-risk factor with an importance approaching that of the level of LDL and HDL cholesterol.

VII. ANALYSIS OF LYMPH AND MILK LIPOPROTEINS

Because simple sampling is not feasible, measurements of sterols and steryl esters in lymph have been much less frequent than in plasma. Most of the analyses have been confined to experimental settings in man and to work with experimental animals. Intestinal lymph sterol and steryl ester levels are interesting because of their role in maintaining plasma cholesterol levels. Lymph sterol levels have been generally equated with those of the cholesterol in the chylomicrons, which represent the major lipoprotein fraction of lymph. Reichl *et al.* (1985) determined the cholesterol content of human peripheral lymph, and Julien *et al.* (1984) determined the cholesterol content of cardiac and peripheral lymph of dogs fed cholesterol and saturated fat. Dory *et al.* (1985) examined the composition of dog peripheral lymph and determined its role in reverse cholesterol transport. Differences were found by conventional methods, between plasma and peripheral lymph HDL in cholesterol content. The subject of interstitial fluid lipoproteins has been reviewed by Sloop *et al.* (1987). The milk lipoproteins, though readily accessible, have also received little experimental attention compared with plasma lipoproteins (Lammi–Keefe and Jensen, 1984).

A. Lymph Chylomicrons and VLDL

Early analyses of the sterol and steryl ester content of lymph chylomicrons were reported by Zilversmit (1965) using colorimetric methods and by Kuksis and Huang (1962) and Huang and Kuksis (1967a) using combinations of TLC and GLC. Kuksis and Huang (1962) showed that the C_{24}-methyl plant sterol, campesterol, appeared in dog lymph chylomicrons at a rate intermediate between that of cholesterol and its C_{24}-ethyl derivative, β-sitosterol. Furthermore, although about 30% of the absorbed cholesterol was esterified, the plant sterols were taken up and transported into the lymph largely in the free form. However, even for cholesterol, the ratio of free to esterified sterol far exceeded that seen for plasma lipoproteins, except plasma chylomicrons, which had about the same composition as the lymph chylomicrons.

Marai *et al.* (1988) have used LC/MS to assess the cholesteryl ester content and composition of rat lymph chylomicrons without isolation of cholesteryl esters. With reversed-phase HPLC, the cholesteryl esters are resolved according to their fatty acid composition. LC/MS assay for the steroid nuclei in the elution pattern established the retention times and provided a basis for their quantitation (Fig. 6). There was good agreement between the results of the direct LC/MS analyses and the results based on isolation of the steryl esters by TLC and GLC quantitation of the derived fatty acids.

It is possible to isolate from intestinal lymph a population of lipid particles that float in the density range commonly attributed to plasma VLDL. In several studies the

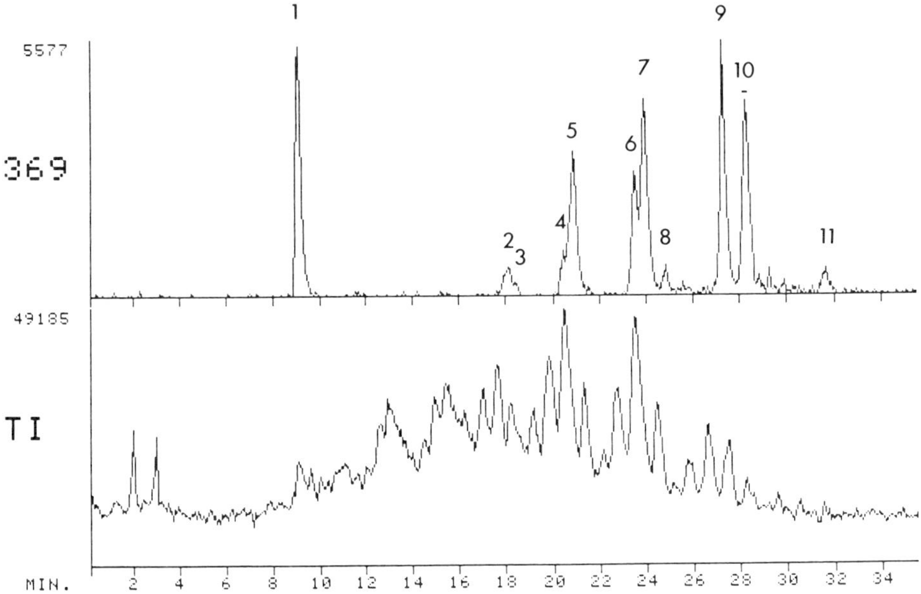

Figure 6 LC/MS profile of cholesteryl esters as obtained by selected ion extraction from the total ion current profile recorded for a total lipid extract of lymph chylomicrons of a rat fed menhaden oil. TI, total ion current; 369, fragment ion representing the steroid nucleus of cholesterol. Peak identification: 1, free cholesterol; 2, cholesteryl docosahexaenoate; 3, cholesteryl eicosapentaenoate; 4, cholesteryl docosapentaenoate; 5, cholesteryl arachidonate; 6, cholesteryl palmitopleate; 7, cholesteryl linoleate; 8, cholesteryl myristate; 9, cholesteryl oleate; 10, cholesteryl palmitate; 11, cholesteryl stearate. LC/MS conditions: as in Fig. 5. Sample: total neutral lipids of lymph chylomicrons (Marai *et al.*, 1988).

cholesterol and cholesteryl ester composition of the lymph VLDL has been characterized separately. Few differences in chemical composition have been observed, including the sterol and steryl ester content, and the separation has been attributed mainly to the size of the particles (Yang *et al.*, 1987). Although the intestine synthesizes also an HDL fraction, the bulk of lymph HDL and LDL is commonly believed to originate by filtration from plasma; the origin of their steryl esters therefore remains uncertain.

B. Milk Fat Globules

The milk triacylglycerols are believed to be secreted from mammary epithelial cells by a budding process in which intracellular fat droplets, presumably enclosed by a free cholesterol-phospholipid monolayer, are further surrounded by a membrane derived largely from the apical cell surface (Patton and Keenan, 1975). This membrane is generally referred to as the milk fat globule membrane. The fat globules are readily separated by centrifugation. The surface membrane and the neutral lipid core of the fat globule can be separated by slow freeze-thawing and centrifugation (Huang and Kuksis, 1967b). Huang and Kuksis (1967b) have described the sterol and steryl ester composition of cow's milk fat globules and milk fat globule membranes. About 80% of the total sterol is present in the free form. Besides cholesterol, cow's milk also contains lanosterol and dihydrolanosterol, which account for about one-sixteenth of the concentration of cholesterol (Schwartz *et al.*, 1968). The sterol esters of milk fat globule membrane contain higher proportions of odd-carbon-number saturated and unsaturated fatty acids than do the milk fat triacylglycerols (Patton and Keenan, 1975). Flanagan and Ferretti (1974) have isolated two steroidal olefins in nonfat dry milk of cows. They were identified as 24-methyl-Δ^2-cholestane (Δ^2-campestane) and 24-ethyl-Δ^2-cholestene (Δ^2-sitostene) by GLC, MS, and synthesis. Parks *et al.* (1966) have reported the presence of Δ^7-cholesten-3-one in bovine milk fat. The sterol composition of the cow's milk fat is surprisingly low in plant sterols despite their abundance in the animal diet.

Mellies *et al.* (1979) have reported that human milk fat contains 460–2640 mg/100 g fat of cholesterol and 90–300 mg/100 g fat of plant sterols. The plant sterol content increased further on feeding the phytosterols (Mellies *et al.*, 1978). Clark *et al.* (1983), however, were unable to detect plant sterols in milk from mothers on normal diets with the methods of Mellies *et al.* (1978) plus sensitive identification by MS. However, Clark *et al.* (1983) have identified desmosterol at about 10% of total human milk fat sterol fraction. Limited amounts of plant sterols in human milk have been reported also by Haug and Harzer (1984), who confirmed the presence of desmosterol but also noted the presence of an unidentified component in the sterol mixture. There exists some controversy regarding the actual amounts of sterol in mature human milk (Lammi–Keefe and Jensen, 1984). Bitman *et al.* (1986) have reported the fatty acid composition of cholesteryl esters of human milk from preterm and term mothers and have noted significant differences. In most instances, the unsaturated fatty acids were associated preferentially with the cholesteryl ester fraction, and their composition differed from that of the total milk lipid. These findings contradict those of Clark *et al.* (1980), who reported very similar patterns of fatty acids in milk triacylglycerols and steryl esters. Bitman *et al.* (1986) have suggested that this is due to an incomplete resolution of the cholesteryl ester fraction (0.03% of total lipid) from the triacylglycerol fraction (98% of total lipid), which runs adjacent to it on TLC. Only trace amounts of cholesterol and cholesteryl esters were found in the colostrum and mature milk from a patient with Type I hyperlipoproteinemia (Myher *et al.*, 1984); Steiner *et al.*, 1985).

VIII. ANALYSIS OF ARTIFICIAL LIPOPROTEINS

The uneven distribution of cholesterol among lipoprotein clssses and cell membranes is of great biochemical, metabolic, and clinical interest, and much effort has been expended in attempts to determine the role of various factors governing this process *in vitro* and *in vivo.* There is evidence that synthetic lipid particles containing neutral lipid cores and phospholipid surface monolayers, faithfully reproduce those metabolic characteristics of the various lipoproteins that are related to size and surface composition, even though they resemble lipoproteins only superficially. Upon *in vivo* infusion, the synthetic particles adsorb apoproteins and sterols and thus further complete the resemblance to natural lipoproteins. Therefore, much effort is currently being made to use various synthetic lipid emulsions to study the metabolism of natural lipoproteins. These studies have provided clues to the sterol composition and distribution among various lipid phases of the lipoprotein particle and have contributed to improved methods of sterol and steryl ester analysis in natural lipoproteins.

A. Triacylglycerol-Rich Particles

It is well established that triacylglycerol-rich emulsions stabilized with phosphatidylcholine and triacylglycerol-rich natural lipoproteins have common structural features (Miller and Small, 1983a,b). Furthermore, the synthetic triacylglycerol emulsions have been shown to absorb, both *in vitro* (Imaizumi *et al.*, 1978) and *in vivo* (Connelly and Kuksis, 1981), those apoproteins generally associated with chylomicrons, except apoprotein B, which is not transferred. Microemulsions of triacylglycerols stabilized with sphingomyelin also exhibit this behavior when injected into the bloodstream of rats (Tong and Kuksis, 1986a), whereas similar microemulsions prepared with other neutral and acidic phospholipids bind much smaller quantities of the apoproteins (Tong and Kuksis, 1986a,b). Connelly and Kuksis (1981) and Tong and Kuksis (1986a,b) have used high-temperature GLC for the estimation of the free and esterified cholesterol and for a resolution of the cholesteryl esters on the basis of carbon number. It was shown that phosphatidylcholine-stabilized particles recovered from rat plasma 10 min after injection had adsorbed free cholesterol and attained a PC/FC ratio of about 1.5 (Connelly and Kuksis, 1981; Tong and Kuksis, 1986a,b). The triacylglycerol microemulsions, stabilized with phosphatidylethanolamine and acidic phospholipids, appeared to take up less free cholesterol than those stabilized with phosphatidylcholine or sphingomyelin (Tong and Kuksis, 1986a,b). The phospholipid class composition of the surface monolayer of the particles also influenced the sterol binding and retention during washing and centrifugation. The synthetic triacylglycerol emulsions recovered from the circulation also contained small amounts of cholesteryl esters, which were shown by GLC to possess a fatty acid composition unlike that of the cholesteryl esters of rat plasma HDL.

Yeagle and Young (1986) have shown that lipid content and composition can play a role in the distribution of cholesterol among the cell membranes and lipoproteins. It was shown that inclusion of small amounts of serine and inositol phosphatides in egg yolk phosphatidylcholine vesicles did not appreciably affect the distribution of cholesterol. Data obtained with vesicles prepared with phosphatidylethanolamine indicated a preference of cholesterol for vesicles composed of phosphatidylcholine. Bovine brain sphingomyelin characteristically showed very slow transfer of cholesterol. A membrane in the gel state was a poor receptor for cholesterol. In these studies cholesterol was assayed enzymatically (Warnick, 1986).

Miller and Small (1982, 1983a) have used radioactive tracers to determine the relative distribution of free and esterified cholesterol between the polar surface monolayer and the neutral lipid core of the synthetic triacylglycerol-rich emulsions. It was found that the percent of total particle cholesterol found in oil phase is a function of the size of the oil droplet. In droplets having a diameter greater than 0.1 μm, over 20% of the total particle cholesterol could be present in the core. Subsequently, Miller and Small (1983b) have prepared lipid emulsions similar to chylomicrons and VLDL and have separated them into pure surface and oil phases by centrifugation. Less than 1% cholesteryl ester was soluble in the surface phase, and less than 2% cholesterol dissolved in the oil at 22°–24°C. In these studies Miller and Small (1982, 1983a,b) used adsorption column chromatography to separate free and esterified cholesterol and determined the cholesterol content of each fraction by the colorimetric method of Rudel and Morris (1973). Earlier, Zilversmit (1965) had used the Liebermann–Burchard reaction and Huang and Kuksis (1967a) a GLC method to report 0.5–0.7% free cholesterol in the oil phase of chylomicrons and less than 1% cholesteryl ester in the surface coating of the particles. Although these results do not support the frequently made assumption that free cholesterol is held exlusively in the surface and cholesteryl esters in the oil phase, they do not seriously invalidate the calculations of the particle size based upon these assumptions.

B. Cholesteryl Ester-Rich Particles

Connelly and Kuksis (1981) also prepared lipid emulsions corresponding in size to chylomicrons and VLDL but containing cholesteryl oleate instead of triacylglycerols as core components and determined the uptake of free cholesterol and apoproteins by these particles following 10 min of circulation in the rat. The particles were found to bind both apoproteins A-I and C like the chylomicron-size emulsions rich in triacylglycerols. Both chylomicron-size and VLDL-size cholesteryl ester emulsions adsorbed free cholesterol in amounts sufficient to approach saturation levels as indicated by the PC/FC ratios. In contrast, the PC/FC ratios of the HDL-size cholesteryl ester emulsions bound only about one-third as much free cholesterol, giving a PC/FC ratio of 4, which is close to that found for natural HDL. In these studies the cholesteryl ester content and composition were determined by high-temperature GLC of the total lipids of the original and the recovered emulsion particles, using the method of Kuksis *et al.* (1975). The cholesteryl ester-rich emulsions of LDL-size after recovery from circulation in the rat contained large amounts of mesophase, with a PC/FC molar ratio of nearly 1.0. Ginsburg *et al.* (1982) prepared microemulsions of LDL-size by sonicating specific phospholipids and specific cholesteryl esters. The cholesteryl ester/phospholipid ratios were determined by measuring the radioactivity recovered in the various fractions prepared with [^{3}H]cholesteryl esters and [^{14}C]phospholipids. The cholesteryl esters were assumed to contribute negligible amounts to the surface area of the particles.

C. Phospholipid-Rich Particles

Extensive analyses of free and esterified sterols have been employed also for the assessment of phospholipid-rich artificial lipid particles. It is well known that an intravenous infusion of phosphatidylcholine liposomes leads to a rapid increase in plasma free cholesterol, which has been attributed to mobilization of tissue cholesterol (Williams *et al.*, 1984). The mobilization of tissue cholesterol can be prevented by infusion of a 1:1 complex of free cholesterol and phosphatidylcholine (Jackoi and Quarfordt, 1974). Similar effects have been obtained during the intravenous infusion of Intralipid, which leads to the formation of LPX due to a transient accumulation of phosphatidycholine liposomes, which attract cholesterol (Kuksis *et al.*, 1978a; Breckenridge *et al.*, 1979; Griffin *et al.*, 1979). Saturation of the Intralipid phosphatidylcholine with plant sterols also prevents the rise in plasma cholesterol to a large extent (Kakis and Kukis, 1984). In these studies, extensive use was made of GLC methods in the identification of free and esterified cholesterol and plant sterols. Total lipid profiles Kuksis *et al.*, 1975) of whole plasma and of individual density classes of lipoproteins and the synthetic emulsions provided data for the quantitation of the sterols and steryl esters.

Bloj and Zilversmit (1977) have shown that nearly all cholesterol in the sonicated vesicles is exchangeable with erythrocyte membranes. The results also indicated that the rate of cholesterol exchange was faster in the presence of unsaturated phosphatidylcholine. The presence of 5% lysophosphatidylcholine in dipalmitoylphosphatidylcholine-cholesterol vesicles did not alter cholesterol exchange rate in large or small vesicles. There is evidence that the transfer of free cholesterol between cells and artificial or natural lipoproteins is bidirectional with the net effect dependent on the relative cholesterol content of each source (Bell, 1984; Johnson *et al.*, 1986). Child and Kuksis (1986) have prepared phosphatidylcholine liposomes containing cholesterol and β-sitosterol and have determined the relative rates of uptake of the two sterols by isolated jejunal villus cells. In comparison with micellar solutions prepared with bile salts, the liposome reduced the absorption of both sterols by the dispersed cells, but promoted a preferential absorption of cholesterol over its 24-ethyl analog, β-sitosterol, in the isolated cell system. The selectivity was determined using radioactive sterols, and the results were confirmed on a mass basis. The greatest absorptive discrimination between sterols occurred when the donor liposomes contained 70 mol % egg yolk phosphatidylcholine and 30 mol % egg yolk phosphatidylethanolamine. A similar degree of selectivity was observed when phospholipids derived from the cells themselves were used. It was concluded that both the composition and the structure of sterol-containing donor particles influence the discrimination between cholesterol and β-sitosterol. Mass analyses of sterols were carried out by TLC and GLC (Child and Kuksis, 1980).

Vaughan *et al.* (1980a,b) have used scintillation counting to measure the distribution of [^{14}C]-cholesterol between the supernatant and pellet after incubation of lipoprotein recombinants prepared by combining synthetic phosphatidylcholine:cholesterol vesicles with purified apoproteins.

Connelly and Kuksis (1983a,b) showed that mixed lysophosphatidylcholine-phosphatidylcholine liposomes and micelles serve as effective acceptors of C and E apolipoproteins from VLDL without demonstrable transfer or triacylglycerols or cholesteryl esters. There was, however, an equilibration of lysophosphatidylcholine and free cholesterol among the VLDL and the synthetic particles, as shown by high-temperature GLC of the total lipids of the two particle types recovered after incubation. Williams and Scanu (1986) have shown that the addition of cholesterol-poor liposomes to canine plasma *in vivo* and *in vitro* selectively alters the distribution of phospholipids, apoproteins, and, especially cholesterol. Intravenously injected phospholipid liposomes remain characteristic particles, which are readily distinguished from the normally occurring lipoproteins by their buoyant density and electrophoretic mobility. They accept unesterified cholesterol from endogenous sources, thereby providing an acute rise in the concentration of the sterol in plasma. Phospholipid liposomes incubated with plasma acquire unesterified cholesterol and apolipoprotein A-I at the expense of high density lipoprotein, the major carrier of cholesterol in normal canine plasma. At sufficiently high concentration, the liposomes nearly completely deplete HDL of its unesterified cholesterol. As a result, two types of particles are generated: one containing mainly esterified cholesterol in its core and the other containing mainly unesterified cholesterol at its surface. Williams and Scanu (1986) analyzed whole plasma and selected fractions from ultracentrifugation or polyanionic precipitation for total and esterified cholesterol using the enzymatic assay (Warnick, 1986), with and without cholesteryl ester hydrolase. Esterified cholesterol was calculated as the difference between total and free cholesterol.

Pittman *et al.* (1987a) have recently prepared phospholipid-rich synthetic lipoproteins resembling HDL in terms of density, particle size, and chemical composition by sonicating apolipoprotein A-I with a microemulsion made with egg yolk lecithin and cholesteryl oleate. These particles, like natural HDL, allowed selective uptake of cholesterol ester moieties by cultured cells without parallel uptake of the particle itself. That uptake was saturable and competed by HDL. Pittman *et al.* (1987a) also prepared synthetic particles containing rat apolipoprotein C or E. These particles, of lower density and larger raddii than those made with apolipoprotein A-I also allowed selective uptake of cholesteryl esters, but with a lower degree of selectivity than in the case of apolipoprotein A-I. It was shown that the selective uptake of cholesteryl esters was a function of particle density or size. In these studies radioactive cholesteryl ether and cholesteryl ester tracers were used as described by Stein *et al.* (1982). In a subsequent study, Pittman *et al.* (1987b) have ruled out both receptor recycling and endocytosis as a mechanism involved in the selective uptake of cholesteryl esters. For this purpose synthetic HDL particles were made to contain two neutral lipid core tracers. One was [^{3}H]cholesteryl ether, which was selectively taken up, and the other was [^{14}C]sucrose octaoleate, which was excluded from selective uptake. Cholesterol and cholesteryl ester mass in the study of Pittman *et al.* (1987b) were measured by the method of Huang *et al.* (1975) as modified by Daniels *et al.* (1981), which makes use of TLC separation and fluorescence measurements. The redistribution of the radiolabeled cholesteryl ether between the synthetic particles and the cells was determined by scintillation counting.

IX. SUMMARY AND INTERPRETATION

The high correlation between the concentration of cholesterol in plasma and the increased or decreased risk for atherosclerotic vascular disease has generated a need for reliable measurements of plasma lipid levels. The need for such measurement has grown in response to the more recent demonstration that a significantly decreased risk accompanies the lowering of plasma total and LDL cholesterol concentrations in a group with primary type II hyperlipoproteinemia (Lipid Research Clinics Program, 1984a,b) and with the finding that the relationship between serum cholesterol and coronary heart disease is a continuously graded, not a threshold one (Stamler *et al.*, 1986). In response to this need, sensitive and accurate methods have been developed for the determination of both free and esterified cholesterol in total plasma and in individual lipoprotein classes. In parallel, improvements have been made in the determination of cholesterol precursors and analogs, and related sterols.

Detailed analyses of total lipoprotein cholesterol on several occasions in the same individual, however, have revealed 7–15% variation in total, LDL, and HDL cholesterol, which remains to be accounted for. According to Friedlander *et al.* (1985), Bachorik (1985), and Superko *et al.* (1986), physiological changes account for more than 50% of the variation in total cholesterol and for less than 50% of the variability of the measurement of cholesterol in LDL and HDL. The physiological sources of variation in plasma cholesterol concentration result from changes in diet and exercise, but these are secondary to the changes caused by diseases and medication, as well as other factors that contribute to the actual concentration and composition of the lipoproteins in the plasma at the time of sampling (Superko *et al.*, 1986; Grundy, 1986). In addition to total levels, these factors can also affect the composition of the cholesteryl esters and the free and esterified sterol ratio in whole plasma and in individual lipoprotein classes. After sampling, other factors come into play that influence the extent to which the measurement reflects the actual levels of cholesterol in the plasma or in the individual lipoprotein classes. Many of these factors, which are related to analytical variability, can be attributed to the methodology employed in the measurement (Bachorik, 1985). However, the conditions of sample handling and storage are also important and can influence profoundly the analytical result. Frequently it may be impossible to obtain an estimate of the magnitude of analytical variability or the intra- and interindividual variability. The problem is most serious in clinical laboratories, where extensive control procedures are not feasible for routine analytical purposes, despite the possibility that the potential sources of both physiological and analytical variability are greater than in control studies, as pointed out by Bachorik (1985). Frequently, the measurements of most interest are subject to the greatest analytical error. Advantage should therefore be taken of the materials available for the standardization and quality control of the meaurements, which can be compared with reference methods of analysis of total and lipoprotein cholesterol (Blank *et al.*, 1986). Both Friedlander *et al.* (1985) and Bachorik (1985) emphasize that clinical decisions should not be made on the basis of a single lipid or lipoprotein measurement and that abnormal results should be confirmed in a subsequent sample. In many laboratories, the more difficult measurements are routinely completed in duplicate, which allows a more reliable initial measurement that can be confirmed by a subsequent analysis.

Finally, studies with synthetic and natural lipoproteins have shown that the cholesterol content of the lipid particles does not remain constant under all conditions and that increases or decreases in the ratio of free cholesterol to other components of the lipoprotein particle can occur under disease conditions. Furthermore, ultracentrifugal, electrophoretic, and the various precipitation methods for isolation of plasma or serum lipoproteins must be considered as independent methods that yield different values for lipoprotein cholesterol. Although the methodology and instrumentation of measuring cholesterol has reached a higher level of sophistication than the measurement of any other metabolite of comparable complexity, the preparative separations of lipoproteins have lagged behind. Hence, the need for standardization of the methodology of both lipoprotein isolation and cholesterol measurement must be emphasized, as must the continued need for vigilance and awareness of the sources and magnitude of both physiological and pathological variation and of analytical error.

ACKNOWLEDGMENTS

The studies by the author and his collaborators that were referred to in this review were supported by the Heart and Stroke Foundation of Ontario, the Medical Research Council of Canada, and the U.S. National Heart, Lung and Blood Institute, NIH, Contract No. NIH-NHLI-72-917, Bethesda, Maryland. I wish to thank Drs. Nina Morley and Philip Connelly for reading the manuscript.

REFERENCES

Abell, L. L., Levy, B. B., Brodie, B. B., and Kendall, F. E. (1952). Simplified method for the estimation of total cholesterol in serum and demonstration of its specificity. *J. Biol. Chem.* **195**, 357–366.

Ambert, J. P., Cahour, A., and Hartmann, L. (1976). A two-step determination of plasma total cholesterol and free cholesterol by gas liquid chromatography. Suggestion for a reference method. *Clin. Chem. (Winston-Salem, N. C.)* **68**, 31–41.

Aron, L., Jones, S., and Fielding, C. J. (1978). Human plasma lecithin-cholesterol acyl transferase. Characterization of cofactor-dependent phospholipase activity. *J. Biol. Chem.* **253**, 7220 7226.

Assmann, G., Schriewer, H., Schmitz, G., and Hagele, E. O. (1983). Quantification of high density lipoprotein cholesterol by precipitation with phosphotungstic acid/$MgCl_2$. *Clin. Chem. (Winston-Salem. N. C.)* **29**, 2026–2030.

Assmann, G., Jabs, H.-U., Kohnert, U., Nolte, W., and Schriewer, H. (1984). LDL-cholesterol determination in blood serum following precipitation of LDL with polyvinylsulfate. *Clin. Chim. Acta* **140**, 77–83.

Bachorik, P. S. (1985). Interpretation of plasma lipid and lipoprotein measurements. *Clin. Chem. (Winston-Salem. N. C.)* **31**, 1107–1108.

Bachorik, P. S., and Albers, J. J. (1986). Precipitation methods for quantification of lipoproteins. *In* "Methods in Enzymology" (J. J. Albers and J. P. Segrest, eds.) Vol. 129, pp. 78–100 Academic Press, Orlando, Florida.

Bachorik, P. S., Wood, P. D. S., Williams, J., Kuchmak, M., Ahmed, S., Lippel, K., and Albers, J. (1979). Automated determination of total plasma cholesterol: A serum calibration technique. *Clin. Chim. Acta* **96**, 145–153.

Barter, P. J., and Lally, J. S. (1978). The activity of an esterified cholesterol transferring factor in human and rat serum. *Biochim. Biophys. Acta* **531**, 233–236.

Bell, F. P. (1984). The dynamic state of membrane lipids: The significance of lipid exchange and transfer reactions to membrane composition, structure, function and cellular lipid metabolism. *Biomembranes* **12**, 543–562.

Bernert, J. T., Akins, J. R., and Miller, D. T. (1982). Direct determination of linoleate/oleate ratio in serum cholesterol esters by liquid chromatography. *Clin. Chem. (Winston-Salem. N. C.)* **28**, 676–680.

Bhattacharyya, A. K., and Connor, W. E. (1978). Familial diseases with storage of sterols other than cholesterol. *In* "The Metabolic Basis of Inherited Disease" (J. B. Stanbury, J. B. Wyngaarden, and D. S. Frederickson, eds.), 4th ed., pp. 656–669. McGraw-Hill, New York.

Bianchini, J.-P., Gaydou, E. M., Sigoillot, J.-C., and Terrom, G. (1985). Determination of sterol and triterpene alcohol acetates in natural products by reversed-phase liquid chromatography and gas-chromatography-mass spectrometry. *J. Chromatogr.* **329**, 231–246.

Billheimer, J. T., Avart, S., and Milani, B. (1983). Separation of steryl esters by reversed-phase liquid chromatography. *J. Lipid Res.* **24**, 1646–1651.

Bitman, J., Wood, D. L., Mehta, N. R., Hamosh, P., and Hamosh, M. (1986). Comparison of the cholesteryl ester composition of human milk from preterm and term mothers. *J. Pediatr. Gastroenterol. Nutr.* **5**, 780–786.

Bjorkhem, I., Blomstrand, R., and Svennson, L. (1974). Serum cholesterol determination by mass fragmentography. *Clin. Chim. Acta* **54**, 185–193.

Bjorkhem, I., Lantto, O., and Svensson, L. (1981). Use of isotope dilution-mass spectrometry as a reference technique in clinical endocrinology. *In* "Quality Control in Clinical Endocrinology" (D. W. Wilson, S. J. Gaskell, and K. Kemp, eds.), pp. 61–66. Alpha Omega Publishing, Cardiff, U.K.

Blank, D. W., Hoeg, J. M., Kroll, M. H., and Ruddel, M. E. (1986). The method of determination must be considered in interpreting blood cholesterol levels. *JAMA, J. Am. Med. Assoc.* **256**, 2867–2870.

Bloj, B., and Zilversmit, D. B. (1977). Complete exchangeability of cholesterol in phosphatidylcholine/cholesterol vesicles of different degrees of unsaturation. *Biochemistry* **16**, 3943–3948.

Bojanovski, D., Wippermann, B., Molinari, E., Schuster, J., and Canzler, H. (1981). Accuracy and reproducibility of a quantitative electrophoresis of plasma lipoproteins: Interlaboratory comparison and verification by ultracentrifugation. *Clin. Chim. Acta* **116**, 381–387.

Bondjers, G., and Bjorkerud, S. (1971). Fluorometric densitometry of cholesterol and cholesteryl esters in tissue on the nanogram level. *Anal. Biochem.* **42**, 363.

Bowyer, D. E., and King, J. P. (1977). Methods for the rapid separation and estimation of the major lipids of arteries and other tissues by thin-layer chromatography on small plates followed by microchemical analysis. *J. Chromatogr. Biomed. Appl.* **143**, 473–490.

Breckenridge, W. C., Kakis, G., and Kuksis, A. (1979). Identification of lipoprotein X-like particles in rat plasma following Intralipid injection. *Can. J. Biochem.* **57**, 72–82.

Breckenridge, W. C., Little, J. A., Aloupovic, P., Wang, C. S., Kuksis, A., Kakis, G., Lindgren, F. T., and Gardiner, G. (1982). Lipoprotein abnormalities associated with a familial deficiency of hepatic lipase. *Atherosclerosis (Shannon, Irel.)* **45**, 161–179.

Breckenridge, W. C., Roberts, A., and Kuksis, A. (1985). Lipoprotein levels in genetically selected mice with increased susceptibility to atherosclerosis. *Arteriosclerosis (Dallas)* **5**, 256–264.

Brown, H. G. (1987). Adaptation of an HPLC system to quantify cholesterol. *J. Am. Oil Chem. Soc.* **64**, 106–108.

Brunnenkreeft, J. W., Boerma, G. J., and Leijnse, B. (1983). Direct determination of total serum cholesterol by on-column gas-liquid chromatographic analysis without previous derivatization compared with the WHO-CDC reference method. *Ann. Clin. Biochem.* **20**, 360–363.

Budzikiewicz, H. (1980). Steroids. *In* "Biochemical Applications of Mass Spectrometry. First Supplementary Volume" (G. R. Waller and O. C. Dermer, eds.), pp. 211–228. Wiley (Interscience), New York.

Burke, R. W., Diamonstone, B. I., Velapoldi, R. A., and Menis, O. (1974). Mechanisms of the Liebermann-Burchard and Zak color reactions for cholesterol. *Clin. Chem. (Winston-Salem. N. C.)* **20**, 794–801.

Burstein, M., and Legmann, P. (1982). Lipoprotein precipitation. *Monogr. Atheroscler.* **11**, 1–131.

Carroll, R. M., and Rudel, L. L. (1981). Evaluation of a high-performance liquid chromatography method for isolation and quantitation of cholesterol and cholesteryl esters. *J. Lipid Res.* **22**, 359–363.

Chacko, G. K., Lund-Katz, S., Johnson, W. J., and Karlin, J. B. (1987). Tetranitromethane modification of human high density lipoprotein (HDL_3): Inactivation of high density lipoprotein binding is not related to cross-linking of phospholipids to apoproteins. *J. Lipid Res.* **28**, 332–337.

Chana, R. S., Cushley, R. J., Wassall, S. R., Smith, I. C. P., and Dufourc, E. J. (1985). Organization of cholesteryl esters in membranes. A deuterium nuclear magnetic resonance study. *Chem. Phys. Lipids* **37**, 345–356.

Chapman, J. R., and Bailey, E. (1974). Determination of plasma testosterone by combined gas chromatography-mass spectrometry. *J. Chromatogr.* **89**, 215–224.

Chapman, M. J. (1980). Animal lipoproteins: chemistry, structure, and comparative aspects. *J. Lipid Res.* **21**, 789–853.

Child, P., and Kuksis, A. (1980). Uptake and transport of sterols by isolated villus cells of rat jejunum. *Can. J. Biochem.* **58**, 1215–1222.

Child, P., and Kuksis, A. (1983a). Uptake of 7-dehydro derivatives of cholesterol, campesterol, and beta-sitosterol by rat erythrocytes, jejunal villus cells, and brush border membranes. *J. Lipid Res.* **24**, 552–565.

Child, P., and Kuksis, A. (1983b). Critical role of ring structure in the differential uptake of cholesterol and plant sterols by membrane preparations in vitro. *J. Lipid Res.* **24**, 1196–1209.

Child, P., and Kuksis, A. (1986). Investigation of the role of micellar phospholipid in the preferential uptake of cholesterol over sitosterol by dispersed rat jejunal villus cells. *Biochem. Cell Biol.* **64**, 847–853.

Christie, W. W., and Hunter, M. L. (1979). Separation of neutral lipids on chromarods. *J. Chromatogr.* **171**, 517–518.

Chung, B. H., Segrest, J. P., Ray, M. J., Brunzell, J. D., Hokanson, J. E., Krauss, R. M., Beandrie, K., and Cone, J. T. (1986). Single vertical spin density gradient ultracentrifugation. *In* "Methods in Enzymology" (J. P. Segrest and J. J. Albers, eds.), Vol. 128, pp. 181–209. Academic Press, Orlando, Florida.

Clark, R. M., Ferris, A. M., Fey, N., Hundrieser, K. E., and Jensen, R. G. (1980). The identity of cholesteryl esters in human milk. *Lipids* **15**, 972–979.

Clark, R. M., Fey, M. B., Jensen, R. G., and Hill, D. W. (1983). Desmosterol in human milk. *Lipids* **18**, 264–266.

Clifton, P. M., MacKinnon, A. M., and Barter, P. J. (1987). Separation and characterization of lipoprotein subpopulation by gel permeation chromatography. *J. Chromatogr. Biomed. Appl.* **414**, 25–34.

Cohen, A., Hertz, H. S., Mandel, J., Paule, R. C., Schafer, R., Sniegoski, L. T., Sun, T., Welch, J. M., and White, E. (1980). Total serum cholesterol by isotope dilution/mass spectrometry: A candidate definitive method. *Clin. Chem.* (*Winston-Salem. N. C.*) **26**, 854–860.

Conlon, D. R., Blankenstein, L. A., Pasakarnis, P. A., Steinberg, C. M., and Damelia, J. E. (1979). Quantitative determination of high density lipoprotein cholesterol by agarose gel electrophoresis. *Clin. Chem.* (*Winston-Salem. N. C.*) **25**, 1965–1969.

Connelly, P. W., and Kuksis, A. (1981). Effect of core composition and particle size of lipid emulsions on apolipoprotein transfer of plasma lipoproteins *in vivo*. *Biochem. Biophys. Acta* **666**, 80–89.

Connelly, P. W., and Kuksis, A. (1983a). Influence of divalent cations on rat apolipoprotein transfer to synthetic lipoprotein-like lipid emulsions *in vitro*. *Can. J. Biochem. Cell Biol.* **61**, 63–71.

Connelly, P. W., and Kuksis, A. (1983b). Differential transfer of C and E apoproteins from very low density lipoproteins to lysophosphatidylcholine-phosphatidylcholine micelles. *Biochim. Biophys. Acta* **752**, 371–382.

Cooper, G. R., Duncan, P. H., Hazelhurst, J. S., Miller, D. T., and Bayse, D. D. (1982). Cholesterol, enzymic method. *In* "Selected Methods in Clinical Chemistry" (W. R. Faulkner and S. Meites, eds.), Vol. 9, pp. 165–174. *Am. Assoc. Clin. Chem.*, Washington, D.C.

Cooper, G. R., Smith, S. J., Duncan, I. W., Mather, A., Fellows, W. D., Foley, T., Frantz, I. D., Jr., Gill, J. B., Grooms, T. A., Hynie, I., Laessig, R., LoBoasso, F. A., Martin, J., Naito, H., Newman, H. A., Sideman, L., Turner, J. H., and D. Williams (1986). Interlaboratory testing of the transferability of a candidate reference method for total cholesterol in serum. *Clin. Chem.* (*Winston-Salem. N. C.*) **32**, 921–929.

Dahlen, G. H., Guyton, J. R., Attar, M., Farmer, J. A., Kautz, J. A., and Gotto, A. M., Jr. (1986). Association of levels of lipoprotein Lp(a), plasma lipids, and other lipoproteins with coronary artery disease documented by angiography. *Circulation* **74**, 758–765.

Daniels, R. J., Guertler, L. S., Parker, T. S., and Steinberg, D. (1981). Studies on the rate of eflux of cholesterol from cultured human skin fibroblasts. *J. Biol. Chem.* **256**, 4978–4983.

De Boever, J., Kohen, F., Vandekerckhove, D., and Van Maele, G. (1984). Solid-phase chemiluminescence immunoassay for progesterone in unextracted serum. *Clin. Chem.* (*Winston-Salem. N. C.*) **30**, 1637–1641.

Deliconstantinos, G. (1983). Free cholesterol not carried by lipoproteins in human serum. *Experientia* **39**, 748–750.

Derks, J. G. M., Van Heiningen, A., and Koedam, H. C. (1985). Gas-chromatographic determination of cholesterol in serium: Candidate reference method. *Clin. Chem.* (*Winston-Salem. N. C.*) **31**, 691–694.

Dhar, T. K., Muller, C., and Schoneshofer, M. (1985). Determination of dehydroepiandrosterone sulfate in plasma by a one-step enzyme immunoassay with a microtitre plate. *Clin. Chem. (Winston-Salem. N. C.)* **31**, 1876–1879.

Dhar, T. K., Voss, E., and Schoneshofer, M. (1986). Enzyme immunoassay of serum cortisol using a new transferable needle lid technique. *Clin. Chim. Acta* **157**, 231–238.

Dolphin, P. J., Forsyth, S. J., and Krul, E. S. (1986). Post secretory acquisition of apoprotein E by nascent rat hepatic very-low density lipoproteins in the absence of cholesteryl ester transfer. *Biochim. Biophys. Acta* **875**, 21–30.

Dory, L., Boquet, L. M., Hamilton, R. L., Sloop, C. H., and Roheim, P. S. (1985). Heterogeneity of dog interstitial fluid (peripheral lymph) high density lipoproteins: Implications for a role in reverse cholesterol transport. *J. Lipid Res.* **26**, 519–527.

Drager, B., Wahlefeld, A. W., and Ziegenhorn, J. A. (1982). A practical method for HDL cholesterol quantitation. *Lab Med.* **6**, 198–202.

Duncan, I. W., Culbreth, P. H., and Burtis, C. A. (1979). Determination of free, total, and esterified cholesterol by high-performance liquid chromatography. *J. Chromatogr. Biomed. Appl.* **162**, 281–292.

Duncan, I. W., Mather, A., and Cooper, G. R. (1982). "The procedure for the Proposed Cholesterol Reference Method." Clinical Chemistry Division, Centers for Disease Control, Atlanta, Georgia.

Dunn, J. F., Nisula, B. C., and Rodbard, D. (1981). Transport of steroid hormone: Binding of 21 endogenous steroids to both testosterone-binding globulin and corticosteroid binding globulin in human plasma. *J. Clin. Endocrinol. Metab.* **53**, 58–68.

Durrington, P. N. (1982). High density lipoprotein cholesterol: Methods and clinical significance. *CRC Crit. Rev. Clin. Lab. Sci.* **18**, 31–78.

Edelstein, C., Kezdy, F. M., Scanu, A. M., and Shen, B. W. (1979). Apolipoproteins and the structural organization of plasma lipoproteins: Human plasma high density lipoprotein-3 *J. Lipid Res.* **20**, 143–153.

Evershed, R. P., and Goad, L. J. (1987). Capillary gas chromatography/mass spectrometry of cholesteryl esters with negative ammonia chemical ionization. *Biomed. Environ. Mass Spectrom.* **14**, 131–140.

Farnworth, E. R., Thompson, B. K., and Kramer, J. K. G. (1982). Quantitative determination of neutral lipids on chromarods. *J. Chromatogr.* **240**, 463–474.

Fears, R. (1985). Lipophilic xenobiotic conjugates: The pharmacological and toxicological consequences of the participation of drugs and other foreign compounds as substrates in lipid biosynthesis. *Prog. Lipid Res.* **24**, 177–195.

Ferreri, L. F. (1984). Fractionation of plasma lipoproteins: Evaluation of preparative methods. *In* "Lipid Research Methodology" (J. A. Story, ed.), pp. 133–156. Alan R. Liss, New York.

Field, E. J., and Mathur, S. N. (1983). Beta-Sitosterol: Esterification by intestinal acylcoenzyme A: Cholesterol acyltransferase (ACAT) and its effect on cholesterol esterification. *J. Lipid Res.* **24**, 409–417.

Fielding, C. J. (1984). The origin and properties of free cholesterol potential gradients in plasma, and their relation to atherogenesis. *J. Lipid Res.* **25**, 1624–1628.

Fielding, C. J., Reaven, G. M., Liu, G., and Fielding, P. E. (1984). Increased free cholesterol in plasma low and very low density lipoproteins in non-insulin-dependent diabetes mellitus: Its role in the inhibition of cholesteryl ester transfer. *Proc. Natl. Acad. Sci. U.S.A.* **81**, 2512–2516.

Flanagan, V. P., and Ferretti, A. (1974). Characterization of two steroidal olefins in nonfat dry milk. *Lipids* **9**, 471–475.

Foreman, J. R., Karlin, J. B., Edelstein, C., Juhn, D. J., Rubinstein, A. H., and Scanu, A. M. (1977). *J. Lipid Res.* **18**, 759–767.

Franzini, C., and Bessozzi, M. (1985). Proposed reference method for serum cholesterol assay. *Ital. Clin. Chim.* **10**, 251–256.

Fredrickson, D. S., Goldstein, J. L., and Brown, M. S. (1978). The familial hyperlipoproteinemias. *In* "The Metabolic Basis of Inherited Disease" (J. B. Stanbury, J. B. Wyngaarden, and D. S. Frederickson, eds.), 4th ed., pp. 604–655. McGraw-Hill, New York.

Freudenthal, J., Derks, H. J. G. M., Gramberg, L. G., ten Hove, G. J., and Klaassen, R. (1981). Isotope dilution mass spectrometry of cholesterol in serum. *Biomed. Mass Spectrom.* **8**, 5–9.

Friedewald, W. T., Levy, R. I., and Fredrickson, D. S. (1972). Estimation of the concentration of low-density lipoprotein cholesterol in plasma, without use of the preparative ultracentrifuge. *Clin. Chem. (Winston-Salem. N. C.)* **18**, 499–502.

Friedlander, Y., Kark, J. D., and Stein, Y. (1985). Variability of plasma lipids and lipoproteins: The Jerusalem lipid research clinic study. *Clin. Chem. (Winston-Salem. N. C.)* **31**, 1121–1126.

Gambert, P., Lallement, C., Archambault, A., Maume, B. F., and Padieu, P. (1979). Assessment of serum cholesterol by two methods: Gas-liquid chromatography on a capillary column and chemical ionization—mass fragmentography with isotopic dilution of [3,4-^{13}C]cholesterol as internal standard. *J. Chromatogr.* **162**, 1–6.

Gartzke, J. (1979). Eine rationelle, quantitative Bestimmungsmethode dunschichtchromatographisch getrennter Lipide des Serums. *J. Chromatogr.* **163**, 86–91.

Gaskell, S. J. and Sieckmann, L. (1986). Mass-spectrometric determination of serum cortisol: Comparison of data from two independent laboratories. *Clin. Chem. (Winston-Salem. N. C.)* **32**, 536–538.

Gaskell, S. J., Brownsey, B. G., and Groom, G. V. (1984). Analysis of progesterone in serum by gas chromatography/mass spectrometry: Target data for external quality assessment of routine assay. *Clin. Chem. (Winston-Salem. N. C.)* **30**, 1696–1700.

Gaskell, S. J., Porter, C. J., and Green, B. N. (1985). Trace analysis by gas-chromatography-mass spectrometry (GC/MS) using a tandem double focusing/quadrupole instrument. *Biomed. Mass Spectrom.* **12**, 139–141.

Gavish, D., Oschry, Y., and Eisenberg, S. (1987). *In vivo* conversion of human HDL_3 to HDL_2 and apoE-rich HDL_1 in the rat: Effects of lipid transfer protein. *J. Lipid Res.* **28**, 257–267.

Gidez, L. I., Miller, G. J., Burstein, M., Slagle, S., and Eder, H. A. (1982). Separation and quantitation of subclasses of human plasma high density lipoprotein by a simple precipitation procedure. *J. Lipid Res.* **23**, 1206–1223.

Ginsburg, G. S., Small, D. M., and Atkinson, D. (1982). Microemulsions of phospholipids and cholesteryl esters. Protein-free models of low density lipoproteins. *J. Biol. Chem.* **257**, 8216–8227.

Glass, C. R., Pittman, R. C., Weinstein, D. B., and Steinberg, D. (1983). Dissociation of tissue uptake of cholesterol ester from that of apoprotein A–I of rat plasma high density lipoprotein: selective delivery of cholesterol ester to liver, adrenal and gonad. *Proc. Natl. Acad. Sci. U.S.A.* **80**, 5435–5439.

Glomset, J. A., Norum, K. R., and Gjone, E. (1983). Familial lecithin-cholesterol acyltransferase deficiency. *In* "The Metabolic Basis of Inherited Disease" (J. B. Stanbury, J. B. Wyngaarden, D. S. Fredrickson, J. L. Goldstein, and M. S. Brown, eds.), 5th ed., pp. 643–654. McGraw-Hill, New York.

Gotto, A. M., Jr., Pownall, H. J., and Havel, R. J. (1986). Introduction to the plasma lipoproteins. "Methods in Enzymology" (J. P. Segrest and J. J. Albers, eds.), Vol. 128, pp. 3–41. Academic Press, Orlando, Florida.

Gray, M. F., Lawrie, T. D. V., and Brooks, C. J. W. (1971). Isolation and identification of cholesterol oxide and other minor sterols in human serum. *Lipids* **6**, 836–843.

Griffin, E., Breckenridge, W. C., Kuksis, A., Bryan, M. H., and Angel, A. (1979). Appearance and characterization of lipoprotein X during continuous Intralipid infusions in the neonate. *J. Clin. Invest.* **64**, 1703–1712.

Groener, J. E. M., Da Col, P. G., and Kostner, G. M. (1987). A hyperalphalipoproteinemic family with normal cholesteryl ester transfer/exchange activity. *Biochem. J.* **242**, 27–32.

Grundy, S. M. (1986). Cholesterol and coronary heart disease. A new era. *JAMA, J. Am. Med. Assoc.* **256**, 2849–2858.

Gyawu, P., and Pope, G. S. (1983). Oestrogens in milk. *J. Steroid Biochem.* **19**, 877–882.

Hamilton, R. L., Williams, M., Fielding, C., and Havel, R. J. (1976). Discoidal bilayer structure of nascent high density lipoproteins from perfused rat liver. *J. Clin. Invest.* **58**, 667–680.

Hansbury, E., and Scallen, T. J. (1980. The separation of sterol intermediates in cholesterol biosynthesis by high pressure liquid chromatography. *J. Lipid Res.* **21**, 921–929.

Hara, I., and Okazaki, M. (1986). High performance liquid chromatography of serum lipoproteins. *In* "Methods in Enzymology" (J. J. Albers and J. P. Segrest, eds.), Vol. 129, pp. 57–78. Academic Press, Orlando, Florida.

Hara, I., Okazaki, M., and Ohno, Y. (1980). Rapid analysis of cholesterol of high density lipoprotein and low density lipoprotein in human serum by high performance liquid chromatography. *J. Biochem. (Tokyo)* **87**, 1863–1865.

Hatch, F. T., and Lees, R. S. (1968). Practical methods for plasma lipoprotein analysis. *Adv. Lipid Res.* **6**, 1–68.

Haug, M., and Harzer, G. (1984). Cholesterol and other sterols in human milk. *J. Pediatr. Gastroenterol. Nutr.* **3**, 816–817.

Haust, H. L., and Beveridge, J. M. R. (1964). The differential photometric estimation of coprostanol in the presence of cholesterol, sitosterol, and other 3β-hydroxysterols. *Can. J. Biochem.* **42**, 251–263.

Haust, H. L., Kuksis, A., and Beveridge, J. M. R. (1966). Quantitative precipitation of various 3β-hydroxysterols with digitonin. *Can. J. Biochem.* **44**, 119–128.

Hedlin, A., Kuksis, A., and Geher, K. (1978). Oral contraceptive estrogen and plasma lipid levels. *Obstet. Gynecol.* **52**, 430–437.

Heider, J. G., and Boyett, R. L. (1978). The picomole determination of free and total cholesterol in cells in culture. *J. Lipid Res.* **19**, 514–518.

Helmich, O., Spacek, P., and Hradec, J. (1981). Separation of [^{3}H]cholesteryl esters by reversed phase high performance liquid chromatography. *J. Chromatogr.* **213**, 105–111.

Hesler, C. B., Swenson, T. L., and Tall, A. R. (1987). Purification and characterization of a human plasma cholesteryl ester transfer protein. *J. Biol. Chem.* **262**, 2275–2282.

Hindricks, F. R., Wolthers, B. G., and Groen, A. (1977). The determination of total cholesterol in serum by gas-liquid chromatography compared with two other methods. *Clin. Chim. Acta* **74**, 207–215.

Hoffmann, G. E., Hiefinger, R., Weiss, L., and Poppe, W. (1985). Five methods for measuring low-density lipoprotein cholesterol concentration in serum compared. *Clin. Chem. (Winston-Salem. N. C.)* **31**, 1729–1730.

Hofman, L. F., Klaniecki, J. E., and Smith, E. K. (1985). Direct solid-phase radioimmunoassay for screening 17alpha-hydroxyprogesterone in whole-blood samples from newborns. *Clin. Chem. (Winston-Salem. N. C.)* **31**, 1127–1130.

Huang, H.-S., Kuan, J.-C. W., and Guilbault, G. G. (1975). Fluorometric enzymatic determination of total cholesterol in serum. *Clin. Chem. (Winston-Salem. N. C.)* **21**, 1605–1608.

Huang, T. C., and Kuksis, A. (1967a). A comparative study of the lipids of chylomicron membrane, fat core, and of the lymph serum of dogs. *Lipids* **2**, 443–452.

Huang, T. C., and Kuksis, A. (1967b). A comparative study of the lipids of globule membrane and fat core, and of the milk serum of cows. *Lipids* **2**, 453–460.

Imaizumi, K., Fainaru, M., and Havel, R. J. (1978). Composition of proteins of mesenteric lymph chylomicrons in the rat and alterations produced upon exposure of chylomicrons to blood serum and serum proteins. *J. Lipid Res.* **19**, 712–722.

Ishikawa, T. T., Brazier, J. B., Stewart, L. F., Fallot, R. W., and Glueck, C. J. (1976). Direct quantitation of cholestanol in plasma by gas-liquid chromatography. *J. Lab. Clin. Med.* **87**, 345–353.

Jackoi, L., and Quarfordt, S. H. (1974). The induction of hepatic cholesterol synthesis in the rat by lecithin mesophase infusions. *J. Biol. Chem.* **249**, 5840–5844.

Jacolot, F., Picart, D., Berthou, F., and Floch, H. H. (1986). Determination of 5α-androstane-3α, 17β-diol and 5α-androstane-3β, 17β-diol in human plasma by selected ion monitoring. *Biomed. Environ. Mass Spectrom.* **13**, 389–394.

Javitt, N. B., Kok, E., Burstein, S., Cohen, B., and Kutscher, J. (1981). 26-Hydroxylcholesterol. Identification and quantitation in human serum. *J. Biol. Chem.* **256**, 12644–12646.

Javitt, N. B., Kok, E., Cohen, B., and Burstein, S. (1982). Cerebrotendinous xanthomatosis: Reduced serum 26-hydroxycholesterol. *J. Lipid Res.* **23**, 627–630.

Jensen, R. G., Clark, R. M., Gerrior, S. A., Fey, M. B., and Gotto, A. M., Jr. (1979). Cholesteryl ester and triacylglycerol fatty acids in Type V hyperlipidemia. *Lipids* **14**, 691–694.

Johnson, W. J., Bamberger, M. J., Latta, R., Rapp, P. E., Phillips, M. C., and Rothblatt, G. H. (1986). The bidirectional flux of cholesterol between cells and lipoproteins. *J. Biol. Chem.* **261**, 5766–5776.

Jonas, A. (1986). Reconstitution of high density lipoproteins. *In* "Methods in Enzymology" (J. P. Segrest and J. J. Albers, eds.), Vol. 128, pp. 553–582. Academic Press, Orlando, Florida.

Jonckheere, J. A., and De Leenheer, A. P. (1983). Candidate definitive method for the determination of cortisol in human serum. *Biomed. Mass Spectrom.* **10**, 197–202.

Julien, P., Fong, B., and Angel, A. (1984). Cardiac and peripheral lymph lipoproteins in dogs fed cholesterol and saturated fat. *Arteriosclerosis (Dallas)* **4**, 435–442.

Kakis, G., and Kuksis, A. (1984). Effect of intravenous infusion of Intralipid, cholesterol and plant sterols on hepatic cholesterogenesis. *Can. J. Biochem. Cell Biol.* **62**, 1–10.

Kakis, G., Kuksis, A., and Breckenridge, W. C. (1988). Redistribution of cholesterol and beta-sitosterol between Intralipid and rat plasma lipoproteins following intravenous infusion. *Biochem. Cell Biol.* (In press).

Kaluzny, M. A., Duncan, L. A., Merritt, M. V., and Epps, D. E. (1985). Rapid separation of lipid classes in high yield and purity using bonded phase columns. *J. Lipid Res.* **26**, 135–140.

Kattermann, R., Kupke, I. R., Borner, K. *et al.* (1983). Candidate selected method for the determination of total cholesterol in serum. *J. Clin. Chem. Clin. Biochem.* **21**, 347–355.

Kohl, H. H., Johnson, W., and Rogers, L. L. (1980). Intercomparison of four precipitation methods and electrophoresis of high density lipoprotein cholesterol determination. *Clin. Chem. (Winston-Salem. N. C.)* **26**, 672–673.

Kostner, G. M., Molinari, E., and Pichler, P. (1985). Evaluation of anew HDL2/HDL3 quantitation method based on precipitation with polyethylene glycol. *Clin. Chim. Acta* **148**, 139–147.

Kuksis, A. (1964). Gas chromatographic fractionation of natural steryl ester mixtures. *Can. J. Biochem.* **42**, 407–417.

Kuksis, A., and Huang, T. C. (1962). Differential absorption of plant sterols in the dog. *Can. J. Biochem.* **40**, 1493–1503.

Kuksis, A., and Myher, J. J. (1986). Lipids and their constituents. *In* "Profiling Body Fluids and Tissues" (C. C. Sweeley and Z. Deyl, eds.). *J. Chromatogr. Biomed. Appl.* **379**, 57–90.

Kuksis, A., Marai, L., and Gornall, D. A. (1967). Direct gas chromatographic examination of total lipid extracts. *J. Lipid Res.* **8**, 352–358.

Kuksis, A., Stachnyk, O., and Holub, B. J. (1969). Improved quantitation of plasma lipids by direct gas-liquid chromatography. *J. Lipid Res.* **10**, 660–667.

Kuksis, A., Myher, J. J., Marai, L. (1975). Determination of plasma lipid profiles by automated gas chromatography and computerized data analysis. *J. Chromatogr. Sci.* **13**, 423–430.

Kuksis, A., Marai, L., Myher, J. J., and Geher, K. (1976). Identification of plant sterols in plasma and red blood cells of man and experimental animals. *Lipids* **11**, 581–586.

Kuksis, A., Breckenridge, W. C., Myher, J. J., and Kakis, G. (1978a). Replacement of endogenous phospholipids in rat plasma lipoproteins during intravenous infusion of an artificial lipid emulsion. *Can J. Biochem.* **56**, 630–639.

Kuksis, A., Myher, J. J., Geher, K., Hoffman, A. G. D., Breckenridge, W. C., Jones, G. J. L., and Little, J. A. (1978b). Comparative determination of plasma cholesterol and triacylglycerol levels by automated gas-liquid chromatographic and Autoanalyzer methods. *J. Chromatogr. Biomed. Appl.* **146**, 393–412.

Kuksis, A., Myher, J. J., Breckenridge, W. C., and Little, J. A. (1979). Lipid profiles of human plasma high density lipoproteins. *In* "Report of the High Density Lipoprotein Methodology Workshop" (K. Lippel, ed.), NIH Publ. No. 79–1661, pp. 142–163. Bethesda, Natl. Inst. Health, Maryland.

Kuksis, A., Myher, J. J., Geher, K., Breckenridge, W. C., Jones, G. J. L., and Little, J. A. (1981). Lipid class and molecular species interrelationships among plasma lipoproteins of normolipemic subjects. *J. Chromatogr. Biomed. Appl.* **224**, 1–23.

Kuksis, A., Myher, J. J., Geher, K., Breckenridge, W. C., Jones, G. J. L., and Little, J. A. (1982a). Lipid class and molecular species interrelationships among plasma lipoproteins of Type III and Type IV hyperlipemic subjects. *J. Chromatogr. Biomed. Appl.* **230**, 231–252.

Kuksis, A., Myher, J. J., Geher, K., Jones, G. J. L., Breckenridge, W. C., Feather, T., Hewitt, D., and Little, J. A. (1982b). Decreased plasma phosphatidylcholine/free cholesterol ratio as an indicator for ischemic vascular disease. *Arteriosclerosis (Dallas)* **2**, 296–302.

Kuksis, A., Myher, J. J., Geher, K., Jones, G. J. L., Shepherd, J., Packard, C. J., Morrisett, J. D., Taunton, O. D., and Gotto, A. M. (1982c). Effect of saturated and unsaturated fat diets on lipid profiles of plasma lipoproteins. *Atherosclerosis (Shannon, Irel.)* **41**, 221–240.

Kuksis, A., Marai, L., and Myher, J. J. (1983a). Strategy of glycerolipid separation and quantitation by complementary analytical techniques. *J. Chromatogr. Biomed. Appl.* **273**, 43–66.

Kuksis, A., Roberts, A., Thompson, J. S., Myher, J. J., and Geher, K. (1983b). Plasma phosphatidylcholine/free cholesterol ratio as an indicator for atherosclerosis. *Arteriosclerosis (Dallas)* **3**, 389–397.

Kuksis, A., Myher, J. J., Marai, L., Little, J. A., McArthur, R. G., and Roncari, D. A. K. (1986a). Fatty acid composition of individual plasma steryl esters in phytosterolemia and xanthomatosis. *Lipids* **21**, 371–377.

Kuksis, A., Myher, J. J., Marai, L., Little, J. A., McArthur, R. G., and Roncari, D. A. K. (1986b). Usefulness of gas chromatographic profiles of plasma total lipids in diagnosis of phytosterolemia. *J. Chromatogr. Biomed. Appl.* **381**, 1–12.

Kuo, J. C., and Yeung, E. S. (1982). Determination of free and esterified cholesterol in human serum by high-performance liquid chromatography and optical activity detection. *J. Chromatogr. Biomed. Appl.* **229**, 293–300.

Kupke, I. R., and Worz-Zeugner, S. (1986). Sequential microultra centrifugation of lipoproteins in 100 ul of serum. *J. Lipid Res.* **27**, 988–995.

Lagana, A., D'Ascenzo, G., Marino, A., and Tarola, A. M. (1986). Liquid-chromatographic determination of progesterone in serum, with spectrophotometric detection. *Clin. Chem. (Winston-Salem. N. C.)* **32**, 508–510.

Lammi-Keefe, C. J., and Jensen, R. G. (1984). Lipids in human milk: A review. 2. Composition and fat-soluble vitamins. *J. Pediatr. Gastroenterol. Nutr.* **3**, 172–198.

Lantto, O. (1982). Radioimmunoassay and liquid chromatographic analysis for free cortisol in urine compared with isotope dilution-mass spectrometry. *Clin. Chem. (Winston-Salem. N. C.)* **28**, 1129–1133.

Lantto, O., Bjorkhem, I., Blomstrand, R., and Kallner, A. (1980). Interlaboratory evaluation of four RIA kits for determination of plasma cortisol, with special reference to accuracy: Influence of matrix in calibration standards. *Clin. Chem. (Winston-Salem. N. C.)* **26**, 1899–1902.

Lillienberg, L., and Svanborg, A. (1976). Determination of plasma cholesterol: Comparison of gas-liquid chromatographic, colorimetric and enzymatic analyses. *Clin. Chim. Acta* **68**, 223–233.

Lin, H.-J., Wang, C., Salen, G., Lam, K.-C., and Chan, T.-K. (1983). Sitosterol and cholesterol metabolism in a patient with coexisting phytosterolemia and cholestanolemia. *Metab., Clin. Exp.* **32**, 126–133.

Lipid Research Clinics Program (1974). Lipid and lipoprotein analysis. *In* "Manual of Laboratory Operations," DHEW Pub. No. (NIH) 75–628, Vol. 1, pp. 1–72. Nat. Heart Lung Inst., Nat. Inst. Health, Bethesda, Maryland.

Lipid Research Clinics Program (1984a). The Lipid research clinics coronary primary prevention trial results. I. Reduction in incidence of coronary heart disease. *JAMA, J. Am. Med. Assoc.* **251**, 351–364.

Lipid Research Clinics Program (1984b). The lipid research clinics coronary primary prevention trial results. II. The relationship of reduction in incidence of coronary heart disease to cholesterol lowering. *JAMA, J. Am. Med. Assoc.* **251**, 365–374.

Lippi, U., D'Angelo, S., and Schinella, M. (1982). Precision and accuracy of a new procedure for HDL separation (PEG-6000) and for the mechanized flow determination of HDL-cholesterol. *Lab. J. Res. Lab. Med.* **9**, 299–303.

Lippi, U., Graziani, M. S., and Manzato, F. (1986). Does assay of cholesterol in high density lipoprotein subclasses give clinically useful information. *Clin. Chem. (Winston-Salem. N. C.)* **32**, 225–226.

Lundberg, B., Hogstrom, S., Pietilainen, P., Suominen, M., and Vikkari, J. (1984). Separation of plasma high-density lipoprotein subclasses by a combined precipitation method using polyethylene glycol 6000 and dextran sulphate. *Scand. J. Clin. Lab. Invest.* **44**, 305–309.

Lusby, W. R., Thompson, M. J., and Kochansky, J. (1984). Analysis of sterol esters by capillary gas chromatography-electron impact and chemical ionization-mass spectrometry. *Lipids* **19**, 888–901.

MacAulay, M. A., Jacklyn, C. L., Mathers, J. M., and Storm, V. A. (1980). Continuous-flow enzymatic determination of total serum cholesterol and method of standardization with CDC-calibrated pool sera. *Clin. Chem. (Winston-Salem. N. C.)* **26**, 896–902.

Marai, L., Kuksis, A., and Mayher, J. J. (1988). Analyses of sterols and steryl esters in crude lipid extracts by LC/MS. *J. Biochem. Biophys. Methods* (submitted for publication).

Mares, P. (1987). The GLC of plasma intact lipids in clinical research. *J. Chromatogr. Libr.* **37**, 128–162.

Mares, P., Tvrzicka, E., and Tamchyna, V. (1978). Automated quantitative-gas liquid chromatography of intact lipids. I. Preparation and calibration of column. *J. Chromatogr. Biomed. Appl.* **146**, 241–251.

Mares, P., Tvrzicka, E., and Skorepa, J. (1979). Automated quantitative gas-liquid chromatography of intact lipids. II. Accuracy, precision and reproducibility of results. *J. Chromatogr. Biomed. Appl.* **164**, 331–343.

Mares, P., Ranny, M., Sedlacek, J., and Skorepa, J. (1983). Chromatographic analysis of blood lipids. Comparison between gas chromatography and thin-layer chromatography with flame ionization detection. *J. Chromatogr. Biomed. Appl.* **275**, 295–305.

Marz, W., and Gross, W. (1986). Analysis of plasma lipoproteins by ultracentrifugation in a new fixed angle rotor: Evaluation of a phosphotungstic acid/$MgCl_2$ precipitation and a quantitative lipoprotein electrophoresis assay. *Clin. Chim. Acta* **160**, 1–18.

Mattson, L. A., Silfverstolpe, G., and Samsioe, G. (1985). Fatty acid composition of serum lecithin and cholesteryl ester in the normal menstrual cycle. Horm. *Metab. Res.* **17**, 414–417.

Mellies, M. J., Ishikawa, T. T., Gartside, P., Burton, K., MacGee, J., Allen, K., Steiner, P. M., Brady, D., and Glueck, C. J. (1978). Effects of varying maternal dietary cholesterol and phytosterol in lactating women and their infants. *Am. J. Clin. Nutr.* **31**, 1347–1354.

Mellies, M. J., Burton, K., Larsen, R., Fixen, D., and Glueck, C. J. (1979). Cholesterol, phytosterols and polyunsaturated, saturated fatty acid ratios during first 12 months of lactation. *Am. J. Clin. Nutr.* **32**, 2383–2389.

Mercer, N. J. H., and Holub, B. J. (1979). Response of free and esterified plasma cholesterol levels in the Mongolian gerbil to the fatty acid composition of dietary lipid. *Lipids* **14**, 1009–1014.

Miettinen, T. A. (1968). Lanosterol and other methyl sterols in serum of fed and fasted human subjects. *Ann. Med. Exp. Fenn.* **46**, 172–176.

Miettinen, T. A. (1971). Serum methyl sterols and their distribution between major lipoprotein fractions in different clinical conditions. *Ann. Clin. Res.* **3**, 264.

Miettinen, T. A. (1980). Phytosterolemia, xanthomatosis and premature atherosclerotic arterial disease: A case with high plant sterol absorption, impaired sterol elimination and low cholesterol synthesis. *Europ. J. Clin. Invest.* **10**, 27–35.

Miller, K. W., and Small, D. M. (1982) The phase behavior of triolein, cholesterol and lecithin emulsions. *J. Colloid Interface Sci.* **89**, 466–478.

Miller, K. W., and Small, D. M. (1983a). Triolein-cholesteryl oleate-cholesterol-lecithin emulsions: Structural models of triglyceride-rich lipoproteins. *Biochemistry* **22**, 443–451.

Miller, K. W., and Small, D. M. (1983b). Surface-to-core and interparticle equilibrium distributions of triglyceride-rich lipoprotein lipids. *J. Biol. Chem.* **258**, 13772–13784.

Mookerjea, S., Park, C. E., and Kuksis, A. (1975). Lipid profiles of plasma lipoproteins of fasted and fed normal and choline deficient rats. *Lipids* **10**, 374–382.

Morris, L. J. (1963). Fractionation of cholesteryl esters by TLC. *J. Lipid Res.* **4**, 357–359.

Murata, T., Takahashi, S., and Takeda, T. (1975). Chemical ionization mass spectrometry. II. Application to analysis of sterol esters. *Anal. Chem.* **47**, 577–580.

Myher, J. J., and Kuksis, A. (1984). Determination of plasma total lipid profiles by capillary gas-liquid chromatography. *J. Biochem. Biophys. Methods* **10**, 13–23.

Myher, J. J. and Kuksis, A. (1987). Facile gas-liquid chromatographic resolution of saturated and unsaturated sterols using a polar capillary column. *J. Biochem. Biophys. Methods* **15**, 111–122.

Myher, J. J. and Kuksis, A. (1988). Improved resolution of saturated and unsaturated steryl esters by gas-liquid chromatography on polar capillary columns. *J. Biochem. Biophys. Methods* (to be submitted for publication).

Myher, J. J., Kuksis, A. and Steiner, G. (1984). Milk fat structure of a patient with Type 1 hyperlipidemia. *Lipids* **19**, 673–682.

Naito, H. K., and David, J. A. (1984). Laboratory Considerations: Determination of cholesterol, triglyceride, phospholipid and other lipids in blood and tissues. *In* "Lipid Research Methodology" (J. A. Story, ed.), pp. 1–76. Alan R. Liss, New York.

Nes, W. R. (1985). A comparison of methods for the identification of sterols. *In* "Methods in Enzymology" (J. H. Law and H. C. Rilling, eds.), Vol. 111, pp. 3–37. Academic Press, Orlando, Florida.

Noel, S. P., Dupras, R., and Filion, A. M. (1983). The activity of cholesterol ester hydrolase in the enzymatic determination of cholesterol: Comparison of five enzymes obtained commercially. *Anal. Biochem.* **129**, 464–471.

Nordby, G., and Norum, K. R. (1975). Substrate specificity of lecithin: cholesterol acyltransferase. Esterification of desmosterol, beta-sitosterol, and cholecalciferol in human plasma. *Scand. J. Clin. Lab. Invest.* **35**, 677–682.

Norum, K. R., Berg, T., Helgerud, P., and Drevon, C. A. (1983). Transport of cholesterol. *Physiol. Rev.* **63**, 1343–1419.

Parks, O. W., Schwartz, D. P., Keeny, M., and Damico, J. N. (1966). Isolation of Δ^7-cholesten-3-one from butterfat. *Nature (London)* **210**, 416–417.

Patsch, J. R., and Patsch, W. (1986). Zonal ultracentrifugation. *In* "Methods in Enzymology" (J. J. Albers and J. P. Segrest, eds.), Vol. 129, pp. 3–26. Academic Press, Orlando, Florida.

Patsch, J. R., Prasad, S., Gotto, A. M., Jr., and Bengtson-Olivecrona, G. (1984). Postprandial lipemia. A key to the conversion of high density lipoprotein 2 into high density lipoprotein 3 by hepatic lipase. *J. Clin. Invest.* **74**, 2017–2023.

Patterson, D. G., Patterson, M. B., Culberth, P. H. *et al.* (1984). Determination of steroid hormones in a human serum Reference Material by isotope dilution-mass spectrometry: A candidate Definitive Method for cortisol. *Clin. Chem. (Winston-Salem. N. C.)* **30**, 619–626.

Patton, S., and Keenan, T. W. (1975). The milk fat globule membrane. *Biochim. Biophys. Acta* **415**, 273–309.

Perkins, E. G., Hendren, D. J., Bauer, J. E., and El-Hamdy, A. H. (1981). High performance reversed phase chromatography of cholesterol and cholesteryl esters of human plasma lipoproteins. *Lipids* **16**, 609–613.

Perret, B. P., Chollet, F., Durand, S., Simard, G., Chap, H., and Douste-Blazy, L. (1987). Distribution of high density lipoprotein 2 and 3 constituents during *in vitro* phospholipid hydrolysis. *Eur. J. Biochem.* **162**, 279–286.

Petty, F., Ragland, J. B., Kuiken, L. B., and Wander, J. D. (1975). Quantitative, multicomponent analysis of fatty acids from cholesteryl esters by chemical ionization reconstructed mass chromatography. *Lipids* **10**, 800–803.

Phillips, F. C., Erdahl, W. L., and Privett, O. S. (1982). Quantitative analysis of lipid classes by liquid chromatography via a flame ionization detector. *Lipids* **17**, 992–997.

Pittman, R. C., Glass, C. K., Atkinson, D., and Small, D. M. (1987a). Synthetic high density lipoprotein particles. Application to studies of the apoprotein specificity for selective uptake of cholesterol esters. *J. Biol. Chem.* **262**, 2435–2442.

Pittman, R. C., Knecht, T. P., Rosenbaum, M. S., and Taylor, C. A., Jr. (1987b). A nonendocytotic mechanism for the selective uptake of high density lipoprotein-associated cholesterol esters. *J. Biol. Chem.* **262**, 2443–2450.

Poll, D. J., Harding, D. R. K., Hancock, W. S., Nye, E. R., Janus, E. D., Hannon, S. F., and Scott, P. J. (1985). The use of reversed phase HPLC to analyze the cholesterol ester profiles present in lipoproteins of patients exhibiting hyperalphalipoproteinemia or hypoalphalipoproteinemia (Tangier disease). *J. Chromatogr.* **343**, 149–154.

Pullinger, C. R., and Gibbons, G. F. (1983). The relationship between the rate of hepatic sterol synthesis and the incorporation of [^{3}H]water. *J. Lipid Res.* **24**, 1321–1328.

Rao, M. K. G., Perkins, E. G., Connor, W. E., and Bhattacharyya, A. K. (1975). Identification of beta-sitosterol, campesterol, and stigmasterol in human serum. *Lipids* **10**, 566–568.

Reichl, D., Forte, T. M., Hong, J. L., Rudra, D. N., and Pflug, J. (1985). Human lymphedema fluid lipoproteins: Particle size, cholesterol and apolipoprotein distributions, and electron microscopic structure. *J. Lipid Res.* **26**, 1399–1411.

Ridgway, N., and Dolphin, P. J. (1984). Lipoprotein lipase-mediated sequestration of long-chain polyunsaturated triacylglycerols in serum LDL from normal and hypothyroid rats. *Biochim. Biophys. Acta* **796**, 64–71.

Ridgway, N., and Dolphin, P. J. (1985). Serum activity and hepatic secretion of lecithin-cholesterol acyltransferase in experimental hypothyroidism and hypercholesterolemia. *J. Lipid Res.* **26**, 1300–1313.

Rodriguez, R. L., and Parks, L. W. (1985). High performance liquid chromatography of sterols: Yeast sterols. *In* "Methods in Enzymology" (J. H. Law and H. C. Rilling, eds.), Vol. 111, pp. 37–51. Academic Press, Orlando, Florida.

Rudel, L. L., and Morris, M. D. (1973). Determination of cholesterol using O-phthalaldehyde. *J. Lipid Res.* **14**, 364–366.

Rudel, L. L., Marzetta, C. A., and Johnson, F. L. (1986). Separation and analysis of lipoproteins by gel filtration. *In* "Methods in Enzymology" (W. J. Albers and J. P. Segrest, eds.), Vol. 129, pp. 45–57. Academic Press, Orlando, Florida.

Salen, G., Shefer, S., and Berginer, V. M. (1983). Familial diseases with storage of sterols other than cholesterol: Cerebrotendinous xanthomatosis and sitosterolemia with xanthomatosis. *In* "The Metabolic Basis of Inherited Disease" (J. B. Stanbury, J. B. Wyngaarden, D. S. Fredrickson, J. L. Goldstein, and M. S. Brown, eds.), 5th ed., pp. 713–730. McGraw-Hill, New York.

Salen, G., Kwiterovich, P. O., Shefer, S., Tint, G. S., Horak, I., Shore, V., Dayal, B., and Horak, E. (1985a). Increased plasma cholestanol and 5-α-saturated plant sterol derivatives in subjects with sitosterolemia and xanthomatosis. *J. Lipid Res.* **26**, 203–209.

Salen, G., Horak, I., Rothkopf, M., Cohen, J. L., Speck, J., Tint, G. S., Shore, V., Dayal, B., Chen, T., and Shefer, S. (1985b). Lethal atherosclerosis associated with abnormal plasma and tissue sterol composition in sitosterolemia with xanthomatosis. *J. Lipid Res.* **26**, 1126–1133.

Scanu, A. M. (1972). Structural studies of serum lipoproteins. *Biochim. Biophys. Acta* **265**, 471–508.

Scanu, A. M. (1981). Plasma lipoproteins: An introduction. *In* "The Biochemistry of Atherosclerosis" (A. M. Scanu, R. Wissler, and G. Gaetz, eds.), pp. 3–8. Dekker, New York.

Schafer, R., Sniegoski, L. T., Welch, M. J. *et al.* (1982). Comparison of two isotope dilution/mass spectrometric methods for determination of total serum cholesterol. *Clin. Chem.* (*Winston-Salem. N. C.*) **28**, 5–8.

Schuh, J., Fairclough, G. F., Jr., and Haschenmeyer, R. H. (1978). Oxygen mediated hetero geneity of apo-low-density lipoprotein. *Proc. Natl. Acad. Sci. U.S.A.* **75**, 3173–3177.

Schwartz, D. P., Burgwald, L. H. Shamey, J. S., and Brewington, C. R. (1968). Identification of lanosterol and dihydrolanosterol in butterfat. *J. Dairy Sci.* **51**, 929.

Serizawa, S., Seyama, Y., Otsuka, H., Kasama, T., and Yamakawa, T. (1981). Simplified determination of cholestanol in serum by gas-liquid chromatography. Biochemical diagnosis of cerebrotendinous xanthomatosis. *J. Biochem.* (*Tokyo*) **90**, 17–21.

Shelburne, F. A., and Quarfordt, S. H. (1977). The interaction of heparin with apoprotein of human very low density lipoprotein. *J. Clin. Invest.* **60**, 944–950.

Siedel, J., Hagele, E. D., Ziegenhorn, J., and Wahlefeld, A. W. (1983). Reagent for the enzymatic determination of serum total cholesterol with improved lipolytic efficiency. *Clin. Chem.* (*Winston-Salem. N. C.*) **29**, 1075–1080.

Siekmann, L., and Breuer, H. (1982). Determination of cortisol in human plasma by isotope dilution-mass spectrometry. Definitive methods in clinical chemistry. I. *J. Clin. Chem. Clin. Biochem.* **20**, 883–892.

Siekmann, L., Huskes, K. P., and Breuer, H. (1976). Determination of cholesterol in serum using mass fragmentography—a reference method in clinical chemistry. *Fresenius Z. Anal. Chem.* **279**, 145–146.

Skipski, V. P. (1969). Lipid composition of lipoproteins in normal and diseased states. *In* "Blood Lipids and Lipoproteins: Quantitation, Composition and Metabolism" (G. J. Nelson, ed.), pp. 471–583. Wiley, New York.

Skorepa, J., Mares, P., Todorovicova, H., and Tvrzicka, E. (1976). New analytical approach to the study of hyperlipidemia. *In* "Phosphatidylcholine: Biochemical and Clinical Aspects of Essential Phospholipids" (H. Peters, ed.), pp. 133–137. Springer-Verlag, New York.

Skorepa, J., Mares, P., Rublicova, J., and Vinogradov, S. (1979). Gas chromatographic evaluation of plasma triglyceride composition in hyperlipidemia. *J. Chromatogr. Biomed. Appl.* **162**, 177–184.

Skorepa, J., Kahudova, V., Kotrlikova, E., Mares, P., and Todorovicova, H. (1983). Gas-liquid chromatography profiling of intact lipids. Observation of differences between triglyceride structure of lipoproteins in type III and type IV hyperlipoproteinemia. *J. Chromatogr. Biomed. Appl.* **273**, 180–186.

Sloop, C. H., Dory, L., and Roheim, P. S. (1987). Interstitial fluid lipoproteins. *J. Lipid Res.* **28**, 225–237.

Smith, L. C., Messey, J. B., Sparrow, J. T., Gotto, A. M., Jr., and Pownall, H. J. (1983). Structure and dynamics of human plasma lipoproteins. *In* "Supramolecular Structure and Function" (G. Pifat and J. N. Herak, eds.), pp. 205–244. Plenum, New York.

Smith, N. B. (1982). Hydrogenation of cholesteryl esters during gas chromatography on a polar fused-silica capillary column. *J. Chromatogr.* **249**, 57–63.

Smith, N. B. (1983). Gas-liquid chromatography of cholesteryl esters on non-polar and polar capillary columns following on-column injection. *J. Chromatogr.* **254**, 195–202.

Smith, S. L., Novotny, M., Moore, S. A., and Felten, D. L. (1980). Studies of hyperlipidemia in drug-induced diabetic rats by high-performance liquid chromatography. *J. Chromatogr. Biomed. Appl.* **221**, 19–26.

Sonnenberg, K., Kuksis, A., and Keystone, E. C. (1987). Effect of MAXEPA on total plasma and lipoprotein lipid profiles of patients with rheumatoid arthritis. *Fed. Proc., Fed. Am. Soc. Exp. Biol.* **46**, 1006. Abs. No. 4022.

Srinivasan, S. R., Webber, L. S., Whitaker, C. F., and Berenson, G. S. (1983). Quantification of lipoprotein cholesterol in serum from children with different lipoprotein profiles: Heparin-calcium precipitation and ultracentrifugation compared. *Clin. Chem.* (*Winston-Salem. N. C.*) **29**, 481–485.

Stamler, J., Wentworth, D., and Neaton, J. D. (1986). Is relationship between serum cholesterol and risk of premature death from coronary heart disease continuous and graded? Findings in 356,222 primary screenees of the multiple risk factor intervention trial (MRFIT). *JAMA, J. Am. Med. Assoc.* **256**, 2823–2828.

Stein, Y., Stein, O., and Halperin, G. (1982). Use of [^{3}H]cholesteryl linoleyl ether for the quantitation of plasma cholesteryl ester influx into the aortic wall in hypercholesterolemic rabbits. *Arteriosclerosis (Dallas)* **2**, 281–289.

Steiner, G., Myher, J. J., and Kuksis, A. (1985). Milk and plasma lipid composition in a lactating patient with Type I hyperlipoproteinemia. *Am. J. Clin. Nutr.* **41**, 121–128.

Stolywho, A., Colin, H., and Guiochon, G. (1985). Analysis of triglycerides in oils and fats by liquid chromatography with the laser light scattering detector. *Anal Chem.* **57**, 1342–1354.

Sugano, M., Morioka, H., Kida, Y., and Ikeda, I. (1978). The distribution of dietary plant sterols in serum lipoproteins and liver subcellular fractions of rats. *Lipids* **13**, 427–432.

Superko, H. R., Bachorik, P. S., and Wood, P. D. (1986). High-density lipoprotein cholesterol measurements. A help or hindrance in practical medicine. *JAMA, J. Am. Med. Assoc.* **256**, 2714–2717.

Svensson, L., Elg, P., Rasmussen, M., Skrede, S., and Bjorkhem, I. A. (1982). A possible model for accuracy control of determination of serum cholesterol with use of reference methods. A Nordkem project. *Scand. J. Clin. Lab. Invest.* **42**, 99–105.

Tam, S. P., and Breckenridge, W. C. (1983). Apolipoprotein and lipid distribution between vesicles and HDL-like fraction formed during lipolysis of human very low density lipoprotein by perfused rat heart. *J. Lipid Res.* **24**, 1343–1357.

Tam, S. P., and Breckenridge, W. C. (1987). The interaction of lipolysis products of very low density lipoprotein with plasma high density lipoprotein (HDL: Perfusate HDL with plasma HDL subfractions. *Biochem. Cell Biol.* **65**, 252–260.

Tel, R. M., and Behrends, G. T. (1980). Incomplete hydrolysis of cholesteryl esters during enzymatic cholesterol determination as evidenced by aqueous cholesteryl ester solutions: Comparison of six enzymatic procedures with the Liebermann-Burchard method. *J. Clin. Chem. Clin. Biochem.* **18**, 595–601.

Thompson, R. H., Jr., Patterson, G. W., Thompson, M. J., and Slower, H. T. (1981). Separation of pairs of C_{24}-epimeric sterols by glass capillary gas-liquid chromatography. *Lipids* **16**, 694–699.

Tong, M.-F., and Kuksis, A. (1986a). Effect of neutral phospholipids on apoliprotein binding by artificial lipid particles *in vivo. Biochem. Cell Biol.* **64**, 826–835.

Tong, M.-F., and Kuksis, A. (1986b). Effect of acidic phospholipids on apolipoprotein binding by artificial lipid particles *in vivo. Biochem. Cell Biol.* **64**, 836–846.

Tong, M.-F., and Kuksis, A. (1988). Total lipid profiles of lipoproteins prepared by polyanionic precipitation methods. *J. Chromatogr. Biomed. Appl.* (to be submitted for publication).

Trinder, P., and Webster, D. (1984). Determination of HDL-cholesterol using 2,4,6-tribromo-3-hydroxybenzoic acid with a commercoal CHOD-PAP reagent. *Ann. Clin. Biochem.* **21**, 430–433.

Vandamme, D., Blaton, V., and Peeters, H. (1978). Screening of plasma lipids by thin-layer chromatography with flame ionization detection on chromarods. *J. Chromatogr. Biomed. Appl.* **145**, 151–154.

Van Doormaal, J. J., Muskiet, F. A. J., Jansen, G., Walthers, B. G., Sluiter, W. J., and Doorenbos, H. (1986). Increase of plasma and red cell cholesterol sulfate levels in induced hypothyroidism in man. *Clin. Chim. Acta* **155**, 195–200.

Vaughan, D. J., Breckenridge, W. C., and Stanacev, N. Z. (1980a). Reconstitution of lipoproteins. I. Lipid-protein interaction of high density apoproteins, purified apo A–I and apoA–II with dimyristoyl-lecithin and dimyristoyl-lecithin: cholesterol vesicles studied by isomeric spin-labelled lecithins. *Can. J. Biochem.* **53**, 581–591.

Vaughan, D. J., Breckenridge, W. C., and Stanacev, N. Z. (1980b). Reconstitution of lipoproteins. II. Lipid-protein interaction between dimyristoyl-lecithin and dimyristoyl-lecithin: cholesterol vesicles and purified apolipoprotein C-I and C-III$_2$ studied by isomeric spin-labelled lecithins. *Can. J. Biochem.* **58**, 592–598.

Vogelberg, K. H., Dannehl, K., and Heggen, E. M. (1984). Quantitative lipoprotein electrophoresis and preparative ultracentrifugation. A comparison of methods for lipoprotein cholesterol determination. *Aertzl. Lab.* **30**, 75–79.

Wakeham, S. G., and Frew, N. M. (1982). Glass capillary gas chromatography-mass spectrometry of wax esters, steryl esters and triacylglycerols. *Lipids* **17**, 831–843.

Wang, S. T., and Peter, F. (1983). Gas-liquid chromatographic determination of fatty acid composition of cholesteryl esters in human serum using silica Sep-Pak cartridges. *J. Chromatogr. Biomed. Appl.* **276**, 249–256.

Warnick, G. W. (1986). Enzymatic methods for quantification of lipoprotein lipids. *In* "Methods in Enzymology" (J. J. Albers and J. P. Segrest, eds.), Vol. 129, pp. 101–123. Academic Press, Orlando, Florida.

Warnick, G. R., Benderson, J. and Albers, J. J. (1982). Dextran sulfate-Mg^{2+} precipitation procedure for quantitation of high-density-lipoprotein cholesterol. *Clin. Chem.* **28**, 1379–1388.

Warnick, G. R., Cheung, M. C., and Albers, J. J. (1979). Comparison of current methods for high-density lipoprotein cholesterol quantitation. *Clin. Chem.* **25**, 596–604.

Watson, D., Taylor, G. W., Laird, S., and Vinson, G. P. (1987). Identification of steroids in rat adrenal glands by liquid chromatography-thermospray mass spectrometry. *Biochem. J.* **242**, 109–114.

Weisgraber, K. H., and Mahley, R. W. (1986). Characterization of apolipoprotein E-containing lipoproteins. *In* "Methods in Enzymology" (J. J. Albers and J. P. Segrest, eds.), Vol. 129, pp. 145–166. Academic Press, Orlando, Florida.

Wiebe, D. A., and Bernert, J. T., Jr. (1984). Influence of incomplete cholesteryl ester hydrolysis on enzymic measurements of cholesterol. *Clin. Chem. (Winston-Salem. N. C.)* **30**, 352–356.

Williams, K. J., and Scanu, A. M. (1986). Uptake of endogenous cholesterol by a synthetic lipoprotein. *Biochim. Biophys. Acta* **875**, 183–194.

Williams, K. J., Werth, V. P., and Wolff, J. A. (1984). Intravenously administered lecithin liposomes: A synthetic antiatherogenic lipid particle. *Perspect. Biol. Med.* **27**, 417–431.

Wolthers, B. G., Hindriks, F. R., Muskiet, F. A., and Groe, A. (1980). A mass fragmentographic method for the determination of total cholesterol in serum using heptadeuterated internal standards. *Clin. Chim. Acta* **103**, 305–315.

Yang, Y.-L., and Kuksis, A. (1987). Size and composition of lymph chylomicrons following feeding corn oil or its fatty acid methyl esters. *Biochem. Cell Biol.* **65**, 514–524.

Yang, Y.-L., Myher, J. J., and Kuksis, A. (1987). Intestinal digestion and absorption of fatty acid methyl and ethyl esters in the rat. *Fed. Proc., Am. Soc. Exp. Biol.* **46**, 1469. Abs. No. 6724.

Yeagle, P. L., and Young, J. E. (1986). Factors contributing to the distribution of cholesterol among phospholipid vesicles. *J. Biol. Chem.* **261**, 8175–8181.

Zilversmit, D. B. (1965). The composition and structure of lymph chylomicrons in dog, rat and man. *J. Clin. Invest.* **44**, 1610–1622.

Zilversmit, D. B. (1969). Chylomicrons. *In* "Structural and Functional Aspects of Lipoproteins in Living Systems" (E. Tria and A. M. Scanu, eds.), pp. 329–368. Academic Press, New York.

10

Steroid Conformational Analyses Based on X-Ray Crystal Structure Determination

W. L. Duax and J. F. Griffin
Medical Foundation of Buffalo, Inc.
Buffalo, New York

Clair Cheer
Department of Chemistry
University of Rhode Island
Kingston, Rhode Island

I. INTRODUCTION

The three-dimensional structure of steroids plays a primary role in governing their interactions and activities. X-ray crystallographic studies provide the most reliable and precise data concerning molecular structure. By combining solid state data with physical chemical data on structures in solution and with molecular energy calculations, a reasonable picture of dynamic properties of steroids can be constructed. This information, examined together with biochemical, pharmacological, and physiological data, can give a better understanding of the molecular mechanisms of biosynthesis, metabolism, membrane transport, receptor binding, and nuclear interaction.

The three-dimensional structural details of hormones, drugs, and antibiotics determined by X-ray crystallographic techniques provide reliable information on the global minimum-energy conformations of these molecules or local minimum-energy conformations that are within a few kilocalories per mole of the global minimum (Duax *et al.*, 1982a). Consequently, X-ray data can be used to define the most stable conformations of molecules (Duax *et al.*, 1984), to gain insight into the relative stability of low-energy forms, to detect the characteristic influence of specific substitution on conformation (Duax *et al.*, 1981), to aid in the interpretation of solution spectra (Ly *et al.*, 1983), and to improve parametrization of molecular mechanics programs.

This review will include (1) summaries of the conformational analyses of the progesterone side chain, the cholesterol side chain, and the steroid A-ring based upon crystallographic observations and (2) discussion of correlations with physical data from other sources.

II. PROGESTERONE SIDE-CHAIN CONFORMATION

A. Background

A number of steroid hormones including progestins and corticoids have a two-carbon keto side chain. It is highly probable that the 17β-side-chain conformation influences the interaction of these hormones with metabolizing, binding, and receptor proteins. For this reason, the preferred conformation of the side chain, the change in energy during rotation about the C(17)—C(20) bond (Fig. 1), and the influence of substitution upon side-chain conformation have been the subject of numerous investigations.

Wellman and Djerassi (1965) concluded that for steroids having the D-ring and side chain of progesterone, the two most stable side-chain conformations are those shown in Fig. 1. Modeling studies and circular dichroism (CD) spectra indicated that the conformer with a C(16)-C(17)-C(20)-O(20) torsion angle ϕ of approximately $-30°$ (Fig. 1a) was 1.1 kcal/mol lower in energy than the conformer for which ϕ is $-90°$ (Fig. 1b). In the case of the 16β-methyl-substituted structures, double maxima in the CD spectra suggested an equilibrium between the two conformers.

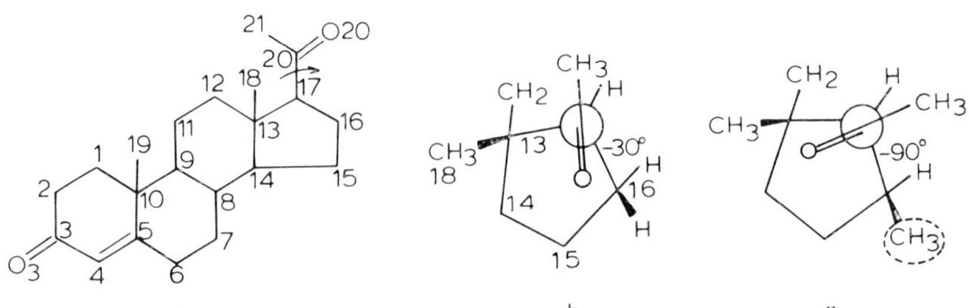

Figure 1 (a) Chemical formula for progesterone; Newman projections C(20) → C(17) illustrating two conformations of the progesterone side chain C(16)-C(17)-C(20)-O(20): (b) $-30°$ and (c) $-90°$.

B. Results from Crystallographic Observations

The 50,000 crystallographic studies of organic structures in the Cambridge Structural Database provide ample evidence that variation in torsional energy as a function of rotation about an sp^2-sp^3 carbon-carbon bond should have six minima with approximate values of $\pm 30°$, $\pm 90°$, $\pm 150°$ relative to an orientation in which substitutents on the sp^2 carbon and the sp^3 carbon are eclipsed. The side-chain conformation of progesterone-like steroids represents a special case of the sp^2-sp^3 bond for which a substantial amount of crystallographic data are available (Duax *et al.*, 1981).

There are 148 steroid crystal structures having C(17β) substituted with the two-carbon keto group, the side chain on progesterone. In these structures three of the six most probable conformers are entirely forbidden due to steric hindrance between the methyl groups on C(13) and C(20), and one conformer is highly preferred in the absence of a bulky 16β-substituent. In 138 of these structures the C(16)-C(17)-C(20)-O(20) torsion angle ϕ is in the range of 0° to $-50°$ (Fig. 2). The conformations appear to be normally distributed about the average value of $-21°$. These observations suggest that this orientation of the side chain represents a well-defined minimum energy conformation that is significantly lower than any other minimum, and that the barrier to rotation about the C(17)-C(20) bond is high enough to hold the side group within this minimum at normal temperatures.

The distribution of observed conformations of the eight 16β-substituted analogs is somewhat different (Duax *et al.*, 1981). Four of these structures have 17β-side-group orientations at the low extreme in the range of the unsubstituted analogs (mean $\phi = -43 \pm 3°$, conformer ϕ_1, see Fig. 2), but in three other structures the mean value of ϕ is $-115 \pm 11°$ (conformer ϕ_2), and in one case $\phi = \pm 162°$ (conformer ϕ_3). Although the number of observations is limited, the addition of the 16β substituent seems to shift the location of the lowest minimum energy orientation and reduce the difference between minima so that additional orientations have significant populations. This is consistent with the earlier proposal by Wellman and Djerassi

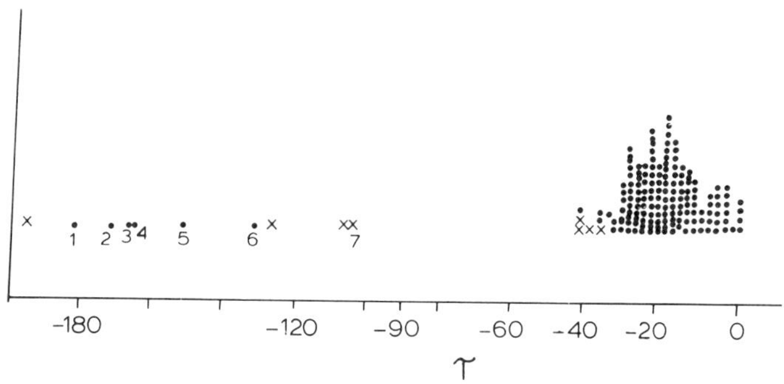

Figure 2 Observed values of the C(16)-C(17)-C(20)-O(20) torsion angles τ in the 148 crystal-structure determinations of pregnanes having a 20-one substituent (x = 16β-substituent other than hydrogen).

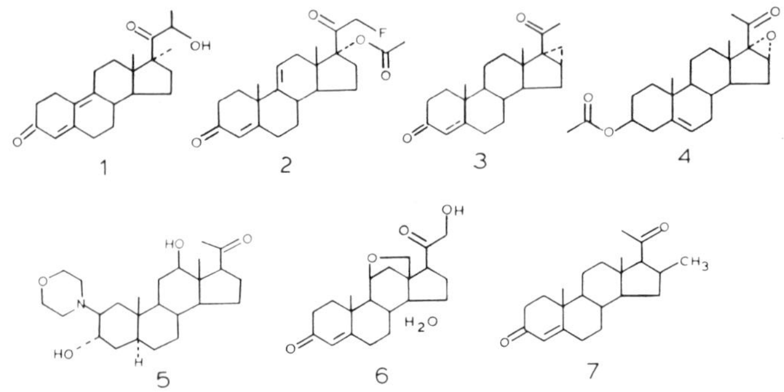

Figure 3 Structures in which intramolecular factors stabilize an unusual conformation of the progesterone side chain.

(1965) from CD spectra that two conformations of the 17β side group were present in solutions of 16β-substituted progesterone compounds. Although the actual conformations predicted may not have been correct, conformers ϕ_1 and ϕ_2 are probably the forms responsible for spectral observations. The other six structures having side-chain conformations that lie outside the range $-50° < \phi < 0°$ are illustrated in Fig. 3. Each of these structures contains an unusual feature not present in the other 142 steroids. Those unusual features appear to be responsible for stabilizing a conformation that would not otherwise be preferred. The introduction of a cyclopropyl ring at the C(16)—C(17) positions in steroids 3 and 4 (Kamernitzky *et al.*, 1982) stabilizes a conformation in which the carbonyl is nearly trans to the C(16)—C(17) bond.

An intramolecular hydrogen bond donated by the 12β-hydroxyl to the 20-carbonyl stabilizes the conformation $\phi = -150°$, observed in steroid 5 (Wawrzak *et al.*, 1987). This suggests that the energy difference between the conformations $\phi = -20°$ and $\phi = -150°$ is less than the energy of a single hydrogen bond. Current estimates of the energy of a hydrogen bond range from 1 to 10 kcal/mol (Newton, 1987; Wells *et al.*, 1987; Weiner *et al.*, 1984). The epoxide formation in steroid 6 draws the C(18) away from the D-ring (Duax *et al.*, 1982b). This reduces steric hindrance so that the position in which $\phi \simeq -130°$ is as stable as the position in which $\phi \simeq -30°$. Consequently, the two conformers are present in high concentration in solution, and single crystals grown from such a solution contain an equal mixture of the two conformers (Fig. 4). In the case of steroid 2, the combination of the C(9)-C(11) double bond in the C-ring and the 21-fluoro substituent apparently alter the balance of intramolecular interaction in favor of a conformation in which $\phi = -173°$ (Wawrzak *et al.*, 1987). Finally, in steroid 1 (RU27988, the 21R enantiomer), steric hindrance associated with the methyl substituent on C(21) is calculated to cause the normal conformation ($\phi \simeq -30°$) to be 12 kcal/mol higher in energy than the crystallographically observed conformation (Raynaud *et al.*, 1980). Compound 1 (Fig. 3) has very low affinity for all steroid receptors (Raynaud *et al.*, 1980). The low affinity and unusual observed conformation of steroid 1 (RU27988)

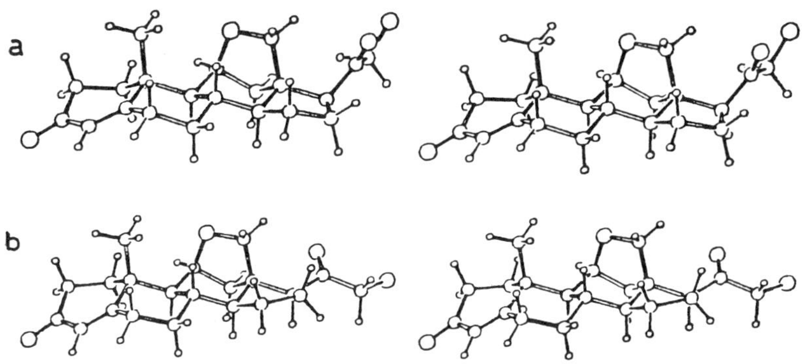

Figure 4 Stereo ORTEP views of the two conformers of 18-deoxyaldosterone observed in the crystal structure illustrating the difference in 17β-side chain orientation: (a) $\phi = -28°$ and (b) $\phi = -132°$.

support the contention that the minimum-energy conformation of the progesterone side chain ($\phi \simeq -30°$) is the biologically active conformation.

C. Results from Energy Calculations

1. Molecular Mechanics

Molecular mechanics calculations provide information concerning variation in potential energy as a function of variation in molecular structure. The accuracy with which a given program successfully identifies the global minimum-energy conformation, the relative energies of local minimum conformations, and the height and shape of barriers to conformational transition is difficult for the average user of these programs to estimate.

The molecular mechanics program MM2p (Allinger and Yuh, 1981) has been used to minimize the energy of 17 progesterone-related structures, starting with the crystallographic observations (Duax *et al.*, 1982a). With the exception of conformers in the ϕ_2 and ϕ_3 ranges ($\phi = -120°$ and $180°$), the C(17)-side chains in the minimized structures are rotated an average of 15° toward the point at which the carbonyl eclipses the C(17)-C(16) bond ($\phi = 0°$). The published calculations (Profeta *et al.*, 1982) on a smaller subset of steroid data reveal similar systematic differences of smaller magnitude. The systematic difference between observed and calculated conformations of the O=C—C—C torsion angle must be due to a pattern in the intermolecular interactions in the crystal or to inaccuracy in the relative weighting of various components in the MM2p program. A careful examination of the crystal packing in 80 of the pregna-20-one analogs revealed no obvious pattern in intermolecular interactions. There is no apparent correlation between the presence or directionality of hydrogen bonding involving side-chain substitutions and the observed conformation (Duax *et al.*, 1981).

The curves relating torsional energy to rotation about sp^2-sp^3 bonds in the MM2p calculation is a summation over six curves having three maxima and minima. Minor variations in the relative scaling of these curves and variation in the types and combinations of torsional angle profiles radically alters the relative heights and locations of predicted minima. Inaccuracies in these torsional energy curves and the relative weight assigned to them versus the nonbonding interactions could easily account for the systematic 5°–30° discrepancy between the crystallographically observed and calculated values of ϕ.

2. *Ab initio* Calculations

Data from a variety of sources are taken into consideration in the development of parameters that influence the results of molecular mechanics calculations. *Ab initio* calculations (Wiberg and Martin, 1985) on 2-butanone and microwave data on propionaldehyde (Butcher and Wilson, 1964) indicate a preference for eclipsing of the C—C single bond and the C=O bond. These data were taken into consideration in the development of parameters for the MM2p programs that predict the most stable progesterone side-chain orientation is one in which the C(16)-C(17)-C(20)-O(20) angle is 0°. Recent *ab initio* calculations on methylisopropylketone, a slightly larger fragment model for the progesterone side chain, indicate the presence of intrinsic steric/dipole effects (K. B. Wiberg, private communication, 1986). These calculations of relative energies of conformers of isopropylketone as a function of the C—C—C=O angle (Fig. 5) demonstrate that the minimum-energy conformations are those in which one of the methyls is 30° from eclipsing the carbonyl. This result is consistent with the X-ray data on the progesterone side chain. It is highly probable that when *ab initio* calculations are made on a larger fragment that incorporates a chiral element analogous to that present in progesterone, they will produce an energy curve that

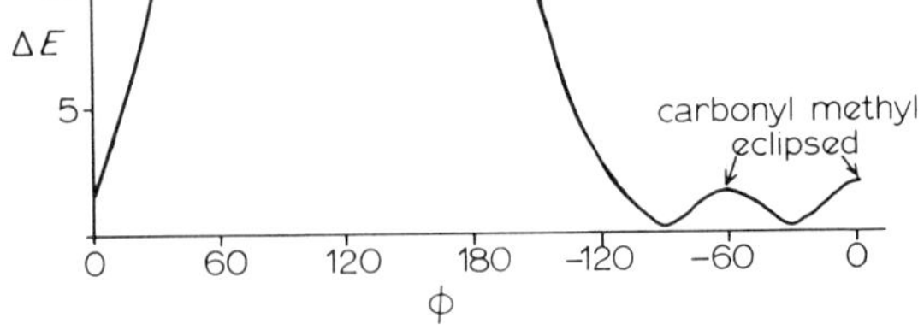

Figure 5 Relative energies of the conformation of isopropylketone as a function of ϕ calculated with Gaussian 80 using a 6–31G* basis set (S. Profeta, Jr., private communication).

mirrors the distribution of side-chain conformations observed in the crystal structures of progesterone and its derivatives. Taken together, all of these results demonstrate that the solid state conformations are dominated by intramolecular interactions and largely are independent of crystal packing forces.

III. CHOLESTEROL CONFORMATION

A. Cholestane Side-Chain Conformation from Crystallographic Observations

Cholesterol plays a vital role in cell growth and development, but the accumulation of cholesterol in certain tissues can be lethal. The key to understanding the diverse properties of cholesterol lies in determining the nature of its molecular-level associations with other bioactive molecules (lipids, proteins, hormones, and drugs). Since these interactions take place on a submicroscopic level and usually in fluid media, the desired details of molecular interaction are often difficult to obtain. A variety of physical techniques have been developed to determine the three-dimensional structures of individual components and aggregates and to probe the nature of these interactions.

Crystal and molecular structure determinations have been reported for single crystals of 111 cholestanes, 28 ergostanes, and 24 lanostanes. Many of these crystal forms contain more than one crystallographically independent molecule in the asymmetric unit, thus providing information on the flexibility of the molecule and low-energy aggregation states. Polymorphs and solvated crystal forms also provide independent observations of molecular geometry that offer insight into the conformational flexibility and relative stability of different conformers of the sterols.

An example of the overall shape of one crystallographically observed cholestane molecule is illustrated in Fig. 6. The conformation of the side chain can be unambiguously defined by six torsion angles:

$$\omega_1 = \text{C(13)-C(17)-C(20)-C(22)}$$

$$\omega_2 = \text{C(17)-C(20)-C(22)-C(23)}$$

$$\omega_3 = \text{C(20)-C(22)-C(23)-C(24)}$$

$$\omega_4 = \text{C(22)-C(23)-C(24)-C(25)}$$

$$\omega_5 = \text{C(23)-C(24)-C(25)-C(26)}$$

$$\omega_6 = \text{C(23)-C(24)-C(25)-C(27)}$$

1. Factor Analysis

The conformation of the cholesterol side chain was analyzed using the factor analysis routines in Version II of the software for the Cambridge Structural Database (CSD) (Allen *et al.*, 1979). A search of the CSD using a fragment composed of the steroid

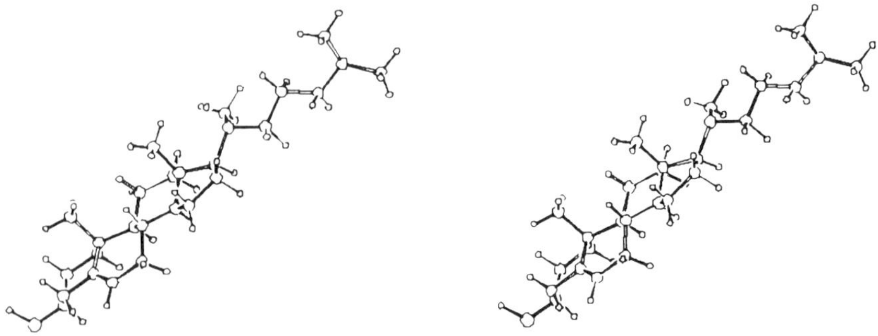

Figure 6 Stereo views of a cholesterol molecule observed in the solid state with a fully extended side-chain conformation (Shieh *et al.*, 1981).

D-ring and the seven-atom cholesterol side chain (Fig. 7) found 123 molecules containing the fragment. Factor analysis was applied directly to the atomic positions themselves and not to geometric parameters derived from those positions. Two primary factors account for 44% of the variation in the set. A two-dimensional plot of those factors separated the 123 structures into four classes (Fig. 8). The classes included 87 structures having fully extended side chains (class A), 11 structures in which the major variation was due to the fact that the ω_4 torsion angle was $\pm$gauche (class B), 10 structures in which the major variation was due to the fact that the ω_3 torsion angle is $+$gauche (class C), and 15 structures in which the major variation was due to the fact that the ω_2 torsion angle is $\pm$gauche (class D).

Structures in class A form a dense cluster of spots on the scatter diagram. Class C is somewhat more diffuse. Members of classes B and D are far more diverse and mutually overlapping because of the existence of conformers with both $\pm$gauche conformations and additional flexibility associated with rotation about more than one of the side-chain bonds.

In the majority of structures, one of the terminal carbons [C(26) or C(27)] is observed to be trans to C(23), and the other is either $+$gauche or $-$gauche in conformation. These two distinct conformations of the extended chain occur with a relative frequency of 2:1. The average values of the ω_4 torsion angles in these two subsets differ by 10°. This population difference indicates that the conformer in which the C(21) and C(27) atoms are on opposite sides of the plane of the rest of the carbon atoms of the side chain is more stable than the conformer in which these methyls are on the same side of the plane.

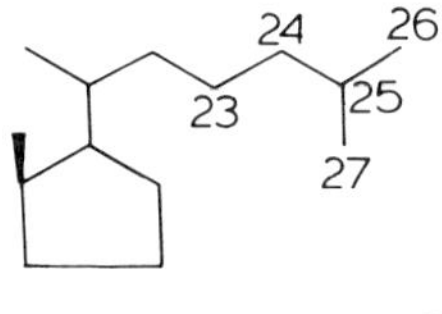

Figure 7 The fragment used in the search of the Cambridge Structural Database that produced 123 hits.

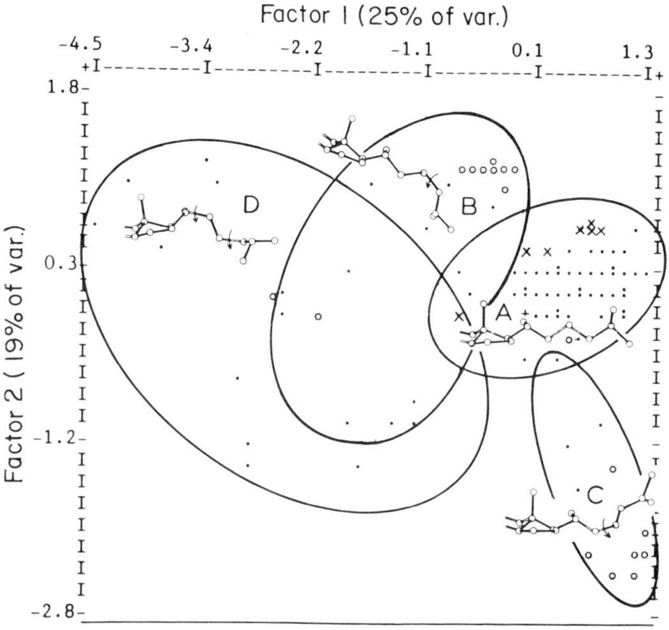

Figure 8 Scatter plot of 123 structural fragments as a function of two factors governing 44 % of the variance. The domains occupied by the four principal conformers (A, B, C, and D), defined on the basis of rotation about three critical bonds in the side chain, are identified. Arrows refer to gauche angles. Sample A is the all-trans conformation. Cholesterol molecules in anhydrous (x) and solvated (O) crystal forms are designated accordingly.

2. Molecular Mechanics Calculations

The molecules in each of the major conformations observed crystallographically were subjected to energy minimization calculations (Allinger and Yuh, 1981). Twelve distinct conformers have energies within 1 kcal/mol of the global minimum. The calculated energies for the most stable conformer in each of the four subgroups are listed in Table 1. A comparison between the observed and calculated values for the six torsion angles that define the side-chain conformation in the two subdivisions of conformer A is presented in Table 2. The calculations confirm that in most cases the

Table 1 Calculated energies ranked in increasing order

Conformer	Frequency	*E* Total (kcal/mol)
D	15	47.5
A	87	47.8
B	11	48.0
C	10	48.2

Note: Classes are defined in the text.

Table 2 Comparison of observed and calculated conformation of the cholesterol side chain

	C(26) trans[a]		C(27) trans[b]	
	Obs.	Calc.	Obs.	Calc.
ω_1	180	180	180	180
ω_2	−169	−171	−167	−170
ω_3	177	172	179	173
ω_4	175	174	−175	−176
ω_5	−172	−174	−55	−64
ω_6	58	63	172	173

[a] The average geometry for 57 side chains having the terminal methyls in the trans, +gauche conformation [C(26) trans] is compared with the geometry generated by full energy minimization of a model having that conformation.

[b] The average geometry of 29 side chains having the −gauche, trans conformation [C(27) trans] is compared with the energy-minimized conformation. The calculations indicate that the observed difference in ω_4 is due to intramolecular factors.

observed structures are local minimum-energy confirmations and reproduce conformational features in some detail. However, there is no correlation between the frequency of observations and the relative energies of the conformers. The energy calculations appear to be insensitive to intramolecular factors that account for the prevalence of the extended form and the unequal distribution of subsets of that form.

B. Cholesterol Data Analysis

1. Crystallographic Observations

For cholesterol itself, single crystal X-ray diffraction determinations of five different crystal forms have been reported: four at room temperature, which include

an anhydrous crystal form (I) (Shieh *et al.*, 1981),

a monohydrate (II) (Craven, 1976),

triclinic (III) (Shieh *et al.*, 1982) and monoclinic (IV) (Shieh *et al.*, 1982) forms containing ethanol,

and an anhydrous form (V) (Nordman and Hsu, 1983) studied at 37° which shows the conformational and structural changes associated with a phase transition at 31.6°.

An example of the overall shape of one cholesterol molecule derived from these studies is illustrated in Fig. 6. All of the crystallographic determinations have more than one molecule in the asymmetric unit, that is, the molecular structure of more than one molecule is determined in each experiment. The number of independent molecules determined in five crystal structures is 48; eight each in I, II, III, and IV and 16 in V. This means that units of 8 (or 16) molecules of cholesterol are repeated to form the molecular crystals and must represent a low-energy aggregation state.

a. Side-Chain Conformation Crystal and molecular structure data for four of these crystal form (I, II, III, and IV) are included in the Cambridge Structural Database. The observed distribution of side-chain conformation in these 24 molecules is significantly different from the distribution in the complete sample, particularly in the case of the solvated crystals. The cholesterol structures displayed in the scatter diagram as a function of the two principal factors are identified in Fig. 8. In the anhydrous crystal form, six of the eight crystallographically independent molecules are in the extended low-energy conformation. In the crystals containing solvent, where the molecules form bilayers with solvent, forming chains of hydrogen bonds on the polar surface, *none* of the sixteen molecules is in the extended conformation. The significant difference in the conformations of the side chains in the solvated crystal forms of cholesterol is almost certainly a result of the formation of these well-defined solvated bilayers in the solid state. To maximize the hydrogen bonding at the A-ring end of the molecule, adjustments are made in the side chain to improve the van der Walls contacts between side chains.

b. Aggregation, Solvation, and Bilayer Formation The various crystal forms of cholesterol itself differ from those of the derivatives in having eight or more crystallographically independent molecules in the asymmetric unit and in exhibiting a bilayer-like structure. The aggregates found in the anhydrous forms of cholesterol differ from those found in the solvated forms. In the solvated forms the infinite bilayer results when the solvent links the aggregates together to generate well-defined polar surfaces in the bilayer (Fig. 9). In the anhydrous forms the 8- (and 16-) member

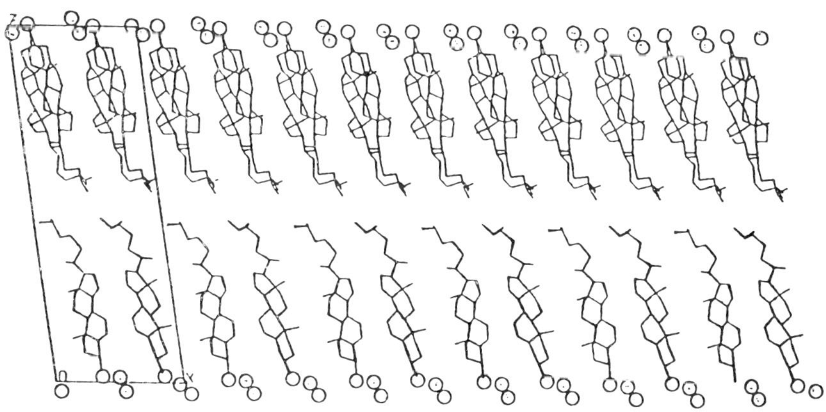

Figure 9 Bilayer structure found in the hydrated forms of cholesterol. Oxygen atoms of the water molecules and the 3β-hydroxyl substituents are indicated by open circles.

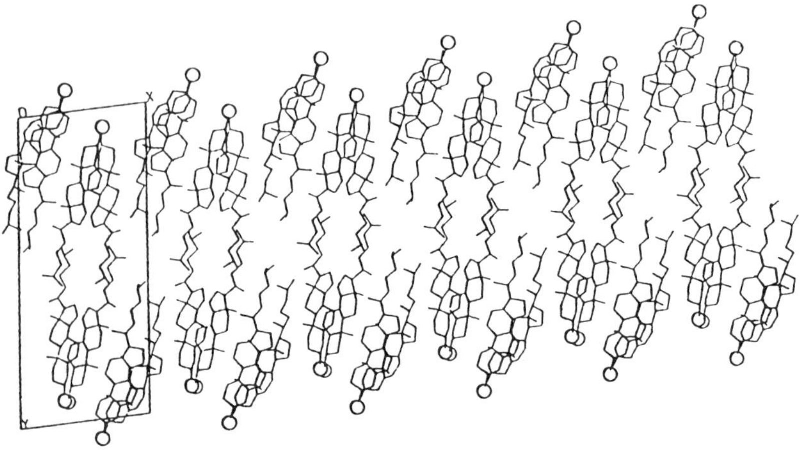

Figure 10 Cholesterol aggregates found in the anhydrous forms of cholesterol do not form the infinite bilayers found in solvated forms. Oxygen atoms of the 3β-hydroxyl substituents are indicated by open circles.

"blocks" stack together in a slightly staggered fashion that disrupts the formation of infinite bilayers (Fig. 10). In this staggered form the side chains are interdigitated in such a way as to permit most of them to adopt the fully extended low-energy form. A comment on the 37° form should be added here. In the solvated crystals the formation of infinite bilayers could lead to an inefficient packing of the cholesterol chains in the aggregates if they were to take up the low-energy extended form. Consequently the side chains take up kinked forms and derive stabilization energy from intermolecular interaction. It may be that this conflict between the inefficiency of packing of the stable extended form and the instability of the observed kinked form relative to the extended form sets the stage for a dynamic equilibrium in cholesterol domains in membranes that has a direct bearing on the mobility, permeability, and function of those domains.

c. *Fatty Acid Derivatives of Cholesterol* Craven and co-workers have reported a series of crystallographic studies of fatty acid derivatives of cholesterol that illustrate a variety of types of interaction between the steroid ring system and the hydrocarbon chains. In most cases, the fatty acid chains are fully extended. In the myristate (Craven and DeTitta, 1976) and heptadecanoate derivatives of cholesterol (Abrahamsson and Dahlen, 1977), the steroid rings are packed adjacent to one another, the fatty acid chains are packed together, and the cholesterol side chains are at the surfaces of bilayers, where thermal motion is highest. In the oleate (Craven and Guerina, 1979a) and octanoate (Craven and Guerina, 1979b) derivatives, the steroids are again packed adjacent to one another, but the fatty acid chains and the cholesterol side chains are packed together. In the laurate (Dahlen, 1979; Sawzik and Craven, 1979) decanoate (Pattabhi and Craven, 1979), undecanoate (Sawzik and Craven, 1980), and nonanoate (Guerina and Craven, 1979) derivatives, the fatty acid chains pack with the cholesterol tetracyclic systems and not with themselves.

IV. 4-EN-3-ONE A-RING CONFORMATION

A. Description of Ring Conformations

The 4-en-3-one A-ring, characteristic of many endogeneous steroid hormones, has conformational flexibility that appears to influence the selectivity of receptor interaction. Generally, the 4-en-3-one A-ring is observed in a conformation in the range from an ideal 1α,2β half-chair (Fig. 11a) to an ideal 1α sofa (Fig. 11b). A significantly different A-ring conformation (Fig. 11c) has been observed in 2β-acetoxy derivatives of testosterone (Duax *et al.*, 1971). In 191 of 237 steroid structures having 4-en-3-one composition (Duax and Norton, 1975; Griffin *et al.*, 1984), the A-rings have normal conformations in which C(1) is below and C(2) is above or in the plane of the conjugated double bonds (Figures 11a, b). In Fig. 12, the displacement of the C(2) atom from the plane is plotted versus a measure of 4-ene-3-one conjugation, the O(3)-C(3)-C(4)-C(5) torsion angle. The conformations of the A-rings of structures that have no other substituents on the all-trans steroid backbone vary in a range centered about the point of perfect conjugation of the 4-en-3-one (180°), as shown in the ellipse of Fig. 12. In 46 of the 4-en-3-one steroids studied crystallographically, the A-ring is observed in the inverted conformation. In this conformation C(1) is above and C(2) below the plane of the en-one group (Fig. 11c). In general there are three main groups of steroids possessing the inverted A-ring: those having an additional double bond at the C(9)-C(10) position, those with nonstandard 9α,10β configuration, and those having a bulky 2β-substituent (Duax *et al.*, 1978, 1985).

B. Conformational Transmission to A-Ring: The Effect of 6α-Methyl and 17α-Ester Substitution

The relative stabilities of the two principal conformations of the A-ring (the normal 1α,2β conformer and the inverted 1β,2α conformer) appear to be sensitive to subtle structural variations. Quite unexpectedly, the A-ring of medroxyprogesterone acetate (MPA, 6α-methyl-3,20-dioxo-4-pregen-17-yl acetate) is observed in a crystal structure

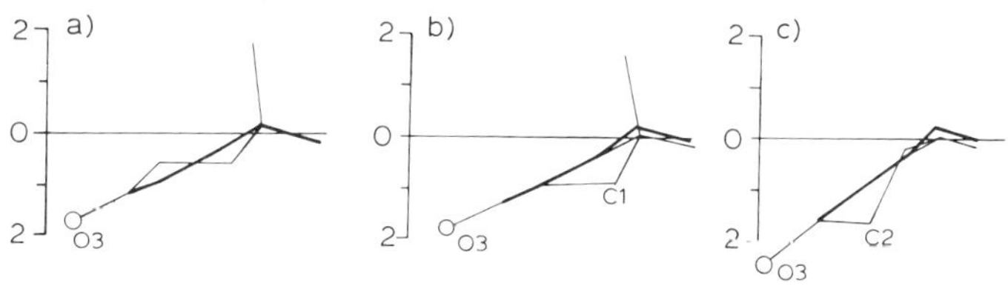

Figure 11 Of 237 steroids having 4-en-3-one composition, the A-rings of 191 range between two conformations: (a) the 1α,2β half-chair and (b) the 1α sofa. Only 46 have the unusual 1β,2α (inverted) half-chair conformation (c).

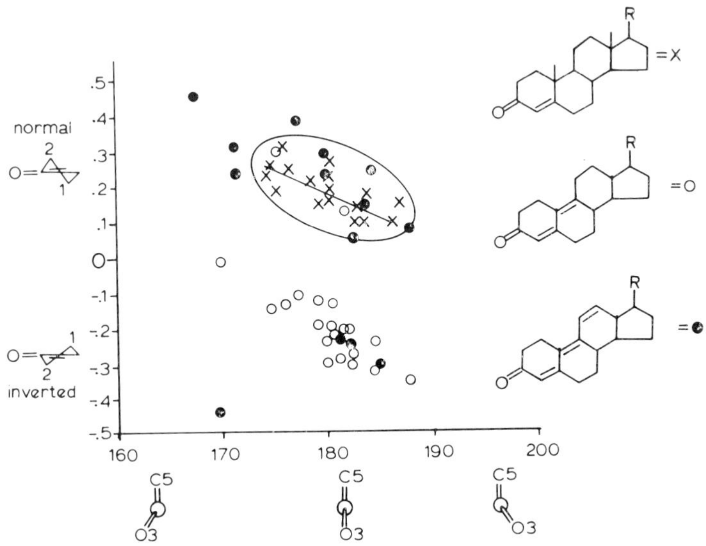

Figure 12 A-ring conformation as a function of the distance of the C(2) atom from the plane of the atoms C(3), C(4), C(5), and C(10) versus the conjugation of the 4-en-3-one system as measured by the torsion angle τ [O(3)-C(3)-C(4)-C(5)]. The distinct conformational patterns of the 4-en-3-one (**X**), 4,9-diene-3-one (○), and 4,9,11-trien-3-one (●) structures are compared.

determination (Duax *et al.*, 1978) to be in the inverted form (Fig. 13a). On the basis of this observation and the consistently high affinity shown by 4,9-diene-3-one compounds for the progesterone receptor, we proposed that ring inversion is responsible for the high affinity of this clinically useful antifertility agent for the progesterone receptor (Duax *et al.*, 1978).

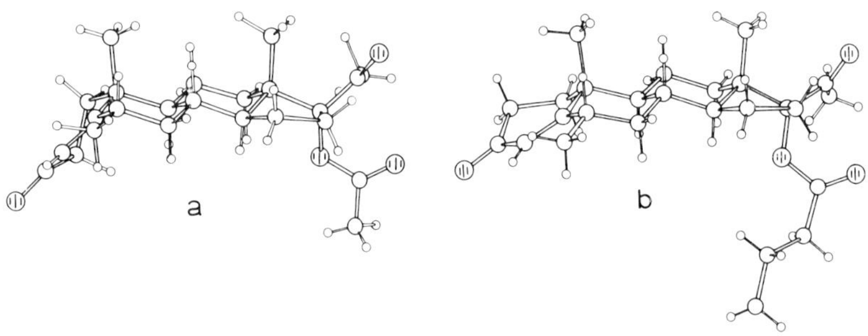

Figure 13 The crystallographically observed conformation of (a) MPA and (b) MPB, illustrating the differences between the inverted and normal conformation of the A-rings . The illustrations were prepared using the program ORTEP.

1. Analysis of Crystallographic Observations

We have proposed that in the case of MPA, the A-ring inversion involves long-range conformational transmission effects associated with the 17α substituent combined with the proximal influence of the 6α-methyl group (Duax *et al.*, 1978). X-ray studies have demonstrated that the presence of the 17α-acetoxy group (Duax *et al.*, 1977) or the 6α-methyl group (Duax and Strong, 1979) alone do not stabilize the inverted A-ring, but the presence of both the 17α-acetate and the 6α-methyl (Duax *et al.*, 1978) appears to have that capability. To explore the influence of other 17α-substituents on A-ring conformation and the relative stability of normal and inverted conformers, the X-ray analyses of the propionate, butyrate, and pivolate analogs of MPA were undertaken. The A-rings of the 17α-pivolate (MPPv) and 17α-butyrate (MPB) derivatives were observed in the normal conformation (Fig. 13b), and the A-ring of the 17α-propionate (MPP) was found to be a disordered mixture of the normal and the inverted forms in the solid state. To determine whether the disorder in the propionate derivative is static or dynamic, full intensity data on a single crystal of MPP were collected at 85, 264, and 323 K. The percentage occupancy of the *inverted* form was found to be 72 % at 85 K, 52 % at 264 K, and 48 % at 323 K.

The observed conformations of MPB and MPP are illustrated in Fig. 14. When the MPP structure having the inverted A-ring conformation is compared with that of MPA, the overall conformations are seen to be nearly identical (Fig. 14a). In contrast, when the MPP structure having the normal conformation is compared with the

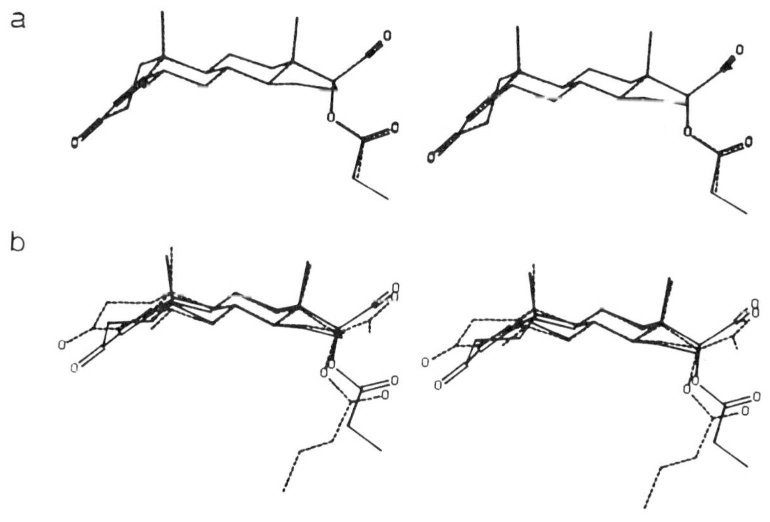

Figure 14 Stereo views of (a) the superposition of MPP with the inverted A-ring (solid line) and MPA (dashed line) and (b) the superposition of MPP with the normal A-ring (solid line) and MPB (dashed line). The least-squares fit is calculated from atoms of the B-, C-, and D-rings. Note that even though in (b) both A-rings are in the 1α,2β-conformation, the overall shapes are significantly different.

butyrate derivative, the orientation of the A-rings is seen to be quite different (Fig. 14b), even though both have A-rings with 1α,2β half-chair conformations. This difference in orientation of the A-ring is influenced by the relationship between the 6α-methyl substituent and the plane of the 4-ene-3-one.

2. Molecular Mechanics Calculations

The crystallographically observed structures of MP and its acetate, butyrate, and propionate derivatives were subjected to energy minimization using the program MM2p (Allinger and Yuh, 1981). The energy minimized structures for MP and MPB (in which the A-ring has the normal conformation) are in reasonably good agreement with the X-ray results (Fig. 15a). The C(4)-C(5)-C(6)-C(6Me) torsion angles ϕ_1 in the minimized structures are 8° and 7° for MP and MPB, respectively, and the crystallographically observed angles are 8.5° and 1.1°. The energy-minimized

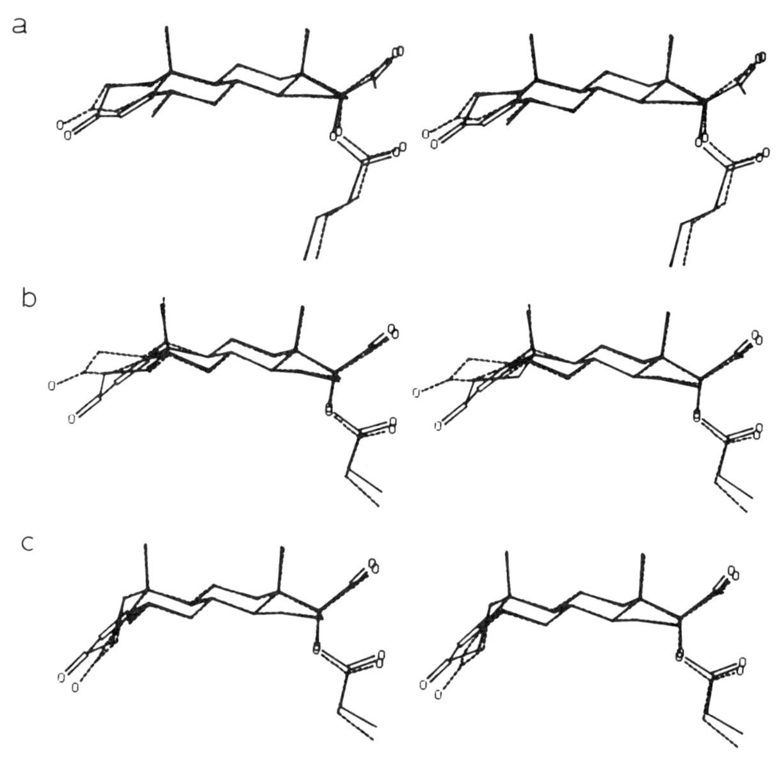

Figure 15 Stereoviews of the superposition of molcules obtained from X-ray data (solid line) and molecular mechanics calculations (dashed line) for (a) MPB, (b) MPP with normal A-ring, and (c) MPP with inverted A-ring. Note that the energy-minimized structures in (b) and (c) differ significantly from the observed structures. The minimized MPP structure (b) resembles the conformation observed in MPB (Figure 13b). The fit is calculated from atoms of the C- and D-rings.

structures for MPA and both conformers of MPP differ significantly from the crystallographically observed forms (Figs. 15b and 15c). The ϕ_1 torsion angles in the minimized structure of MPA and the inverted A-ring conformer of MPP are much more negative (-20°) than the crystallographically observed angles (-11° and -9°). The minimized structure of the normal A-ring conformation of MPP has a ϕ_1 torsion angle of $+6^\circ$ rather than the observed -9°, and the A-ring is in the conformation observed for MPB. The X-ray determination and the energy calculations suggest that it is energetically unfavorable for the 6α methyl group to be coplanar with the C(4)-C(5) double bond. When the A-ring has the normal 1α,2β conformation, the ϕ_1 torsion angle is in the range $+4^\circ$ to $+9^\circ$. Ester substitution at O(17α) introduces subtle shifts in the orientation of the 17β-side chain and certain backbone torsion angles. These changes appear to induce the near eclipsing of the ϕ_1 angle. The strain associated with the eclipsed relationship can be relieved by a shift of the 4-ene-3-one plane so that the ϕ_1 torsion angle is negative and the plane of the A-ring is sharply tilted relative to the plane of the rest of the steroid. This shift in 4-ene-3-one orientation destabilizes the normal A-ring relative to the inverted A-ring in the MPA and MPP structures.

Analysis of the change in population as a function of temperature and a careful examination of close contacts in the crystal suggest that the conformer having the normal A-ring conformation is the lower-energy form and that unfavorable crystal packing interactions involving this form induce a conformational transition to the higher-energy inverted form that does not have such unfavorable interactions. This conclusion is consistent with interpretation of nuclear magnetic resonance data on MPA (Barrett *et al.*, 1982) and the energies calculated using MM2p. Nevertheless, it should be stressed that although the relative energies calculated by MM2p are consistent with the other data, the conformations resulting from energy minimization differ significantly from those observed crystallographically.

ACKNOWLEDGMENTS

Research supported in part by NIAAMDD Grant No. AM-26546, DRR Grant No. RR-05716, and the Richard W. Goode and Mae Stone Goode Gift. The organization and analysis of the data base associated with the investigation, and some of the illustrations, were carried out using the PROPHET system, a unique national computer resource sponsored by the NIH.

The authors wish to express their appreciation to G. Del Bel, J. Gallmeyer, P. Strong, and M. Tugac for assistance in the organization and preparation of the manuscript.

REFERENCES

Abrahamsson, S., and Dahlen, B. (1977). The crystal structure of cholesteryl 17-bromoheptadecanoate. *Chem. Phys. Lipids* **20**, 43.

Allen, F. H., Bellard, S., Brice, M. D., Cartwright, B. A., Doubleday, A., Higgs, H., Hummelink, T., Hummelink-Peters, B. G., Kennard, O., Motherwell, W. D. S., Rodgers, J. R., and Watson, D. G. (1979). The Cambridge Crystallographic Data Centre: Computer-based search, retrieval, analysis and display of information. *Acta Crystallogr.* **35**, 2331–2339.

Allinger, N. A., and Yuh, V. H. (1981). *Quantum Chem. Program Exch.* **13**, 394.

Barrett, M. W., Farrant, R. D., Kirk, D. N., Mersh, J. D., Sanders, J. K. M., and Duax, W. L. (1982). The solution conformation of 17α-acetoxy-6α-methylprogesterone ('medroxyprogesterone acetate'): Use of circular dichroism, nuclear overhauser effect difference and two-dimensional J. spectroscopy. *J. Chem. Soc., Perkin Trans. 2* pp. 105–110.

Butcher, S. S., and Wilson, E. B., Jr. (1964). Microwave spectrum of propionaldehyde. *J. Chem. Phys.* **40** , 1671–1678.

Craven, B. M. (1976). Crystal structure of cholesterol monohydrate. *Nature* (*London*) **260**, 728.

Craven, B. M., and DeTitta, G. T. (1976). Cholesteryl myristate: Structure of the crystalline solid and mesophases. *J. Chem. Soc., Perkin Trans. 2* p. 814.

Craven, B. M., and Guerina, N. G. (1979a). The crystal structure of cholesteryl oleate. *Chem. Phys. Lipids* **29**, 91.

Craven, B. M., and Guerina, N. G. (1979b). The crystal structure of cholesteryl octanoate. *Chem. Phys. Lipids* **24**, 157–166.

Dahlen, B. (1979). The crystal structure of cholesteryl dodecanoate: Copacking of steroid skeleta and hydrocarbon chains. *Chem. Phys. Lipids* **23**, 179.

Duax, W. L., and Norton, D. A. (1975). "Atlas of Steroid Structure," Vol. 1. Plenum, New York.

Duax, W. L., and Strong, P. D. (1979). A-Ring conformation in 17-hydroxy-6c-methylpregenolone. *Steroids* **34**, 501–508.

Duax, W. L., Eger, C., Pokrywiecki, S. A., and Osawa, Y. (1971). Crystalline molecular structures of two derivatives of 2β-hydroxytestosterone having an unusual A-ring conformation. *J. Med. Chem.* **14**, 295–300.

Duax, W. L., Cody, V., and Hazel, J. (1977). Steroid structure and function. I. Conformational transmission in 17α-acetoxy progesterone. *Steroids* **30**, 471–480.

Duax, W. L., Cody, V., Griffin, J., Hazel, J., and Weeks, C. M. (1978). Steroid structure and function. II. Conformational transmission and receptor binding of medroxyprogesterone acetate. *J. Steroid Biochem.* **9**, 901–907.

Duax, W. L., Griffin, J. F., and Rohrer, D. C. (1981). Conformation of the progesterone side chain: Conflict between X-ray data and force field calculations. *J. Am. Chem. Soc.* **103**, 6705–6712.

Duax, W. L., Fronckowiak, M. D., Griffin, J. F., and Rohrer, D. C. (1982a). A comparison between crystallographic data and molecular mechanics calculations on the side chain and backbone conformations of steroids. *In* "Intramolecular Dynamics" (J. Jortner and B. Pullman, eds.), pp. 505–524. Reidel Publ., Dordrecht, The Netherlands.

Duax, W. L., Griffin, J. F., Strong, P. D., Funder, J. W., and Ulick, S. (1982b). Molecular structure of 18-deoxyaldosterone and its relationships to receptor binding and activity. *J. Am. Chem. Soc.* **104**, 7291–7293.

Duax, W. L., Smith, G. D., Griffin, J. F., Strong, P. D., and Portoghese, P. S. (1984). The crystal structure and molecular conformation of threo-5-methylmethadone in relation to opioid receptor binding. *Tetrahedron* **40**, 467–471.

Duax, W. L., Griffin, J. F., and Weeks, C. M. (1985). Models for steroid-receptor interactions derived from X-ray crystallographic investigations. *In* "Interaction of Steroid Hormone Receptors with DNA" (M. Sluyser, ed.), pp. 58–83. Ellis Horwood, Ltd., Chichester, England.

Griffin, J. F., Duax, W. L., and Weeks, C. M. (1984). "Atlas of Steroid Structure," Vol. 2. Plenum, New York.

Guerina, N. G., and Craven, B. M. (1979). Crystal structure of cholesteryl nonanoate. *J. Chem. Soc., Perkin Trans. 2* pp. 1414–1419.

Kamernitzky, A. V., Turuta, A. M., Fundlieler, I. N., Pavlov, V. A., Antipin A. Yu., Struckhov, Yu. T., and Polishchuk, A. P. (1982). α-Epithioketosteroids: Conformation and reactivity. *Tetrahedron* **38**, 165–168.

Ly, Y., Barth, G., Kieslich, K., Strong, P. D., Duax, W. L., and Djerassi, K. (1983). Optical rotatory dispersion studies. 136. The enzymatic reduction of 2-methyl-2-(trideuteriomethyl)-cyclohexane-1,3-dione. An unusual conformation of 2,2-dimethyl-3-hydroxycyclohexane. *J. Org. Chem.* **48**, 4549–4554.

Newton, M. D. (1987). Current views of hydrogen bonding from theory and experiment—structure, energetics, and control of chemical behavior. *Trans. Am. Crystallogr. Assoc.* **22**, 1–17.

Nordman, C. E., and Hsu, L.-Y. (1983). Phase transition and crystal structure of the 37° form of cholesterol. *Science* **220**, 604.

Pattabhi, V., and Craven, B. M. (1979). Crystal structure of cholesteryl decanoate. *J. Lipid Res.* **20**, 753.

Profeta, S., Jr., Kollman, P. A., and Wolfe, M. E. (1982). Conformation of the progesterone side chain: Resolution of the apparent conflict between X-ray data and force field calculations using MM2. *J. Am. Chem. Soc.* **104**, 3745.

Raynaud, J. P., Brown, N. L., Coussedieri, C., Pottier, J., Delettre, J., and Mornon, J. P. (1980). Role of receptor binding and metabolism in progestin-induced responses in the uterus. *In* "Steroid Induced Uterine Proteins" (M. Beato, ed.), pp. 217–236. Elsevier/North-Holland Biomedical Press, Amsterdam.

Sawzik, P., and Craven, B. M. (1979). The structure of cholesteryl laurate at 98°. *Acta Crystallogr. Sect. B* **B35**, 789.

Sawzik, P., and Craven, B. M. (1980). Structure of cholesteryl undecanoate. *Acta Crystallog., Sect. B* **B36**, 215.

Shieh, H.-S., Hoard, L. G., and Nordman, C. E. (1981). The structure of cholesterol. *Acta Crystallogr. Sect. B* **B38**, 2411–2419.

Shieh, H.-S., Hoard, L. G., and Nordman, C. E. (1982). Structures of triclinic and monoclinic cholesterol hemiethanolate. *Acta Crystallogr., Sect. B* **B38**, 2411–2419.

Wawrzak, Z., Duax, W. L., and Strong, P. D. (1987). The conformation of the progesterone side chain. X-ray observations and molecular mechanics calculations. *Am. Crystallogr. Assoc., Program Abstr.* p. 58.

Weiner, S. J., Kollman, P. A., Case, D. A., Singh, U. C., Ghio, C., Alagona, G., Profeta, S., and Weiner, P. (1984). A new force field for molecular mechanical simulation of nucleic acids and proteins. *J. Am. Chem. Soc.* **106**, 765–784.

Wellman, K. M., and Djerassi, C. (1965). Optical rotatory dispersion studies. XCVIII. The conformation of the 17-acetyl group in steroids and its correlation with variable-temperature circular dichroism. *J. Am. Chem. Soc.* **87**, 60–66.

Wells, T. N. C., Leatherbarrow, R. J., and Fersht, A. R. (1987). Hydrogen bonding in enzyme catalysis studied by protein engineering. *Am. Crystallogr. Assoc.* **22**, 63–72.

Wiberg, K. B., and Martin, E. (1985). Barriers to rotation adjacent to double bonds. *J. Am. Chem. Soc.* **107**, 5035–5041.

11

Mass Spectral Identification of Phytosterols

Alain Rahier and Pierre Benveniste
Laboratoire de Biochimie Végétale, CNRS UA 1182
67083 Strasbourg Cédex, France

INTRODUCTION

Mass spectrometry (MS) and particularly the combination of mass spectrometry with gas chromatography (GC/MS) has become an indispensable method for studying plant sterols and their biosynthesis. Vascular plants generally contain a complex mixture of sterols, which in most cases (Nes, 1977; Benveniste, 1986), include large amounts of three 4-desmethyl sterols: 24-methyl cholesterol (2B), sitosterol (2C), and stigmasterol (2D). Thus, plant sterols differ from animal sterols in having either one or two extra carbons at C-24. Besides these major sterols, plants contain a great variety of minor 4-desmethyl-, 4α-methyl-, and 4,4-dimethyl-sterols that can be precursors of 2B, 2C, and 2D. More recently the use of sterol biosynthesis inhibitors (SBI) (Benveniste, 1986; Schmitt *et al.*, 1982; Taton *et al.*, 1987), have permitted the control of several key enzymes involved in sterol biosynthesis *in vitro* and *in vivo*. SBIs, when

Analysis of Sterols and Other Biologically Significant Steroids

used *in vivo*, have been very useful in revealing hidden metabolic pathways. They led to the accumulation of sterols other than those normally found in nontreated plant cells, some having been discovered in organisms (fungi, algae) other than higher plants, but many of them being new, to the best of our knowledge. Moreover, some of these new compounds were recognized as intermediates of higher-plant biosynthesis, not being detected in the absence of SBI because of their high turnover. Thus, the use of SBIs gives rise to complex mixtures of sterols, the separation and structure determination of which is greatly facilited by the use of GC/MS, which permits the analysis of small quantities. Moreover, in the most favorable cases, the use of a specific SBI gives rise to the accumulation of successive members of a series characterized by a common structural feature (e.g., presence of a 9β,19-cyclopropyl ring or of a Δ^8 double bond) and leads to interesting sets of MS data, which can be correlated with the presence of a specific structural feature. See the following structures:

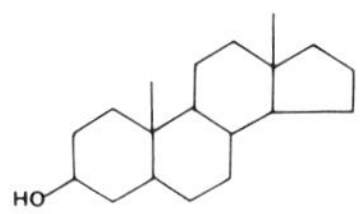
1

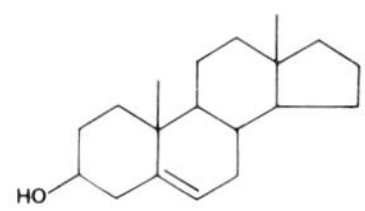
2

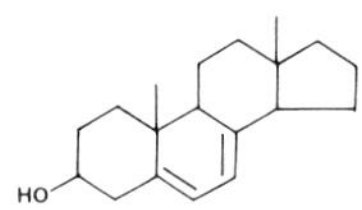
3

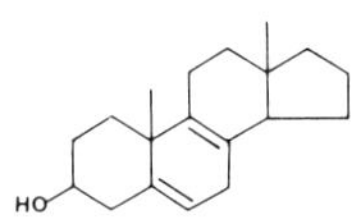
4

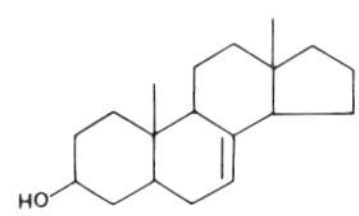
5

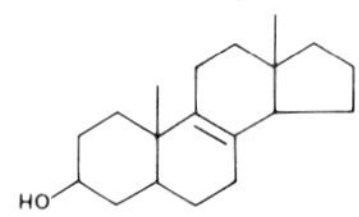
6

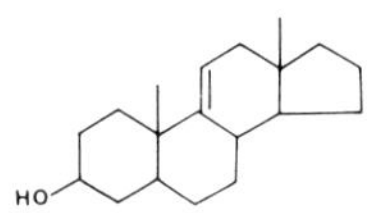
7

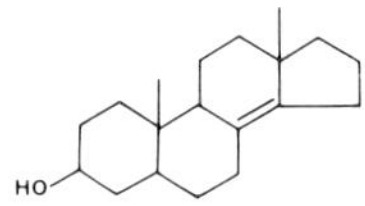
8

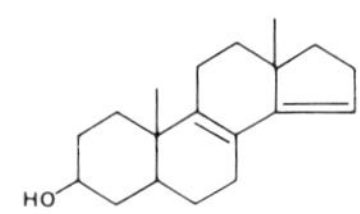
9

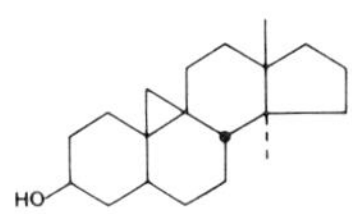
10

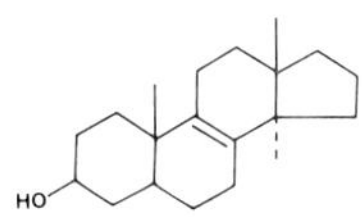
11

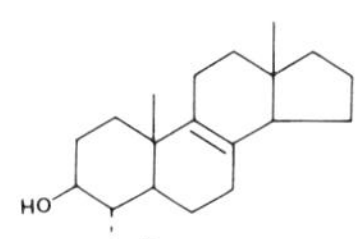
12

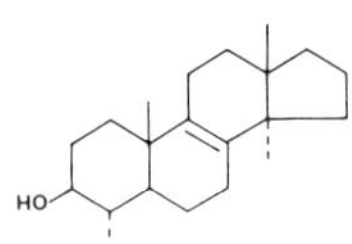
13

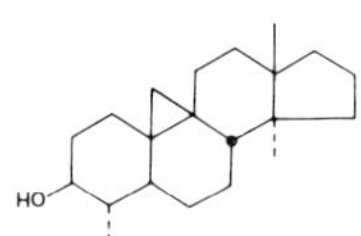
14

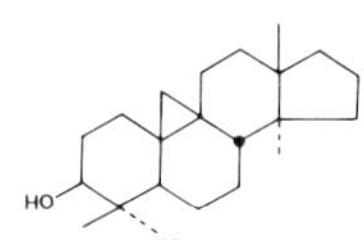
15

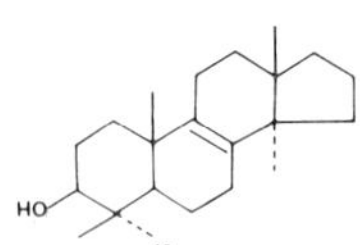
16

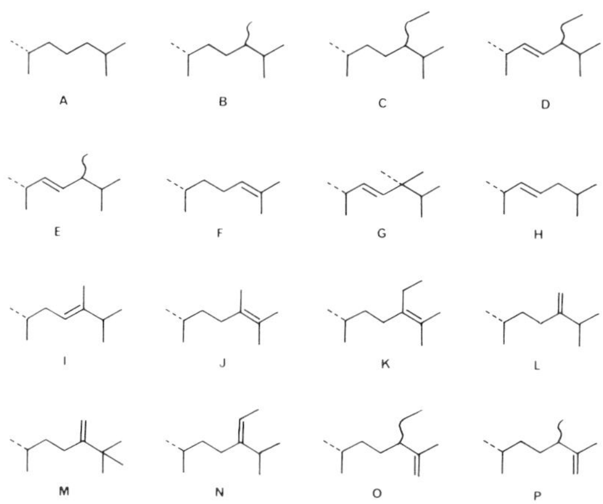

This chapter deals with the MS identification of sterols in vascular plants and fungi, an area that has already been the subject of publications (Knights, 1967; Brooks *et al.*, 1968; Patterson, 1984); and a few recent papers have dealt with MS identification of animal sterols (Nes, 1985; Dumazer *et al.*, 1986). Sterols from marine organisms will not be considered here because this area has been reviewed in detail recently in different papers (Caarlson *et al.*, 1978; Djerassi, 1981).

The aim of this chapter is to provide information for identifying plant and fungi sterols by MS or GC/MS in the light of our experience in isolating and analyzing numerous sterol structures in our laboratory by the use of SBIs *in vivo*. We shall restrict our discussion to 3β-hydroxy sterols and their acetate or trimethylsilyl (TMS) derivatives at this position. After some general comments, we shall consider the important characteristic fragmentations of the various possible sterol nuclei and the various possible side chains.

I. GENERAL COMMENTS

A. Ionization Methods and Analysis Conditions

The most commonly used method of ionization for MS of sterols is electron impact, in which positively charged ions are produced during the collision of sample molecules with a beam of energetic electrons in the ionization chamber. This process generally extracts an electron from the molecule, leading to a molecular ion with an odd number of electrons (a radical ion) that is denoted by a plus sign and a dot. If this positively charged radical ion has sufficient energy, it will fragment the molecule. The abundance of ions is thus directly dependent on the energy of the processes involved. An ionizing voltage of approximately 15 eV usually produces an intact ionized molecule whereas higher electron energy gives more fragmentation. Most of the analyses described herein (when not otherwise specified) have been obtained with an ionizing voltage of 70 eV, which produces a high level of ions from fragmentation of chemical bonds. Although the mass-to-charge ratio is now referred to as *m/z*, in this review we will use the older nomenclature *m/e*.

The temperature of the ion source also affects the mass spectra of thermally labile molecules; in particular, the 3β-hydroxy groups of sterols can dehydrate at high ion-source temperature. Most of the data described in this chapter (if not otherwise specified) have been obtained in our laboratory using a computerized gas chromatography/mass spectrometer LKB 9000 S. The operating conditions were

Ion-source temperature	250°C
Electron energy	70 eV (or 15 eV, if specified)
Acceleration voltage	3500 V
Trap current	60 μA

and the GC/MS analysis used the following:

Column	SE30 CAP15 Q Greff/220–290°C
Molecular separator	250°C

In spite of the wide use of electron-impact mass spectroscopy (EIMS) for identification, proof of structure, and elucidation of fragmentation processes in the sterol field, chemical-ionization mass spectroscopy (CIMS) has been used complementarily in a few cases to establish more rapidly the molecular weights of some sterols (Lin and Smith, 1984). We shall not discuss CIMS here, because it is used routinely only in structure studies of highly oxidized sterols, for which CI spectra give fast information on molecular weight and functional groups (Lin and Smith, 1984).

B. Fragmentation Process: Generalities

The relative intensities of the molecular-ion responses and the fragment responses depend on various parameters, among which two important ones are the stability of the molecular ion and the structural features of the molecule. We shall see that many fragments can be correlated with distinct structural features, which gives us, in many cases, a "finger print" of a particular sterol structure. There are thus three major uses and applications of MS in the sterol field: (1) determination of the molecular weight, which often permits us to choose among various postulated structures, (2) empirical identification by comparison of the MS spectra with an authentic standard that is recorded under the same conditions, and (3) elucidation of structural features by interpretation of the fragmentation patterns. In addition, in some cases the use of high-resolution techniques leads to the determination of the emprical formula of the molecular ion or of some fragments.

Interpretation of mass spectra of sterols can be very complicated, and the elucidation of the fragmentation processes of the sterols and steroids can be considered to be a well-defined field of research. Djerassi's laboratory has made the most significant contribution to the field of sterols (Budzikiewicz *et al.*, 1964; Djerassi, 1979; Massey and Djerassi, 1979; Li *et al.*, 1981); but some other important contributions to the steroid field are also very useful (Zaretskii, 1976; Galli and Maroni, 1967).

Table 1 Correlation between the relative abundance of M^+ versus $|M\text{-AcoH}|^+$ ions and the presence of a Δ^5 double bond for various classes of 4-desmethyl sterols

Sterol	M^+	M^+-ACOH
Cholestanol acetate **1A**	430(25)	370(58)
Campestanol acetate **1B** (24β)	444(20)	384(34)
Stigmastanol acetate **1C** (24β)	458(20)	398(31)
22-dehydrostigmastanol acetate 1D (24α)	456(27)	396(13)
Cholesteryl acetate **2A**	428 —	368(100)
Campesteryl acetate **2B** (24α)	442 —	382(100)
Sitosteryl acetate **2C** (24α)	456 —	396(100)
Stigmasteryl acetate **2D** (24α)	454 —	394(100)
Cholesta-5,7-diene acetate **3A**	426 —	366(100)
Ergosteryl-acetate **3E** (24β)	438(9)	378(100)
Δ^7-cholestenyl acetate **5A**	428(72)	368(84)
Δ^7-campestenyl acetate **5B** (24α)	442(72)	382(36)
Δ^7-stigmastenyl acetate **5C** (24α)	456(75)	396(31)
Δ^8-campesteryl acetate **6B** (24α)	442(100)	382(53)
Δ^8-sitosteryl acetate **6C** (24α)	456(100)	396(61)
Δ^8-stigmasteryl acetate **6D** (24α)	454(14)	394(20)
Pollinastanol acetate **10A**	442(10)	382(100)
24ξ-24 methyl-pollinastanol acetate **10B**	456(7)	396(86)
24ξ-24 ethyl-pollinastanol acetate **10C**	470(6)	410(100)

Notation for Tables 1–18: **1A**, cholestanol; **1B**, 24ξ-ergostanol; **1C**, 24ξ-stigmastanol; **1D**, 24ξ-Δ^{22}-stigmastenol; **2A**, cholesterol; **2B**, 24ξ-Δ^5-ergostenol: *campesterol* (24α); **2C**, 24ξ-Δ^5-stigmastenol: *sitosterol* (24α) + *dihydroporiferasterol* (24β) (*clionasterol*); **2D**, 24ξ-$\Delta^{5,22}$-stigmastadienol: *stigmasterol* (24α); **2E**, 24ξ-$\Delta^{5,22}$-ergostadienol: *brassicasterol* (24α); **2F**, $\Delta^{5,24}$-cholestadiene: *desmosterol*; **2I**, $\Delta^{5,23}$-ergostadienol; **2J**, $\Delta^{5,24}$-ergostadienol; **2K**, $\Delta^{5,24}$-stigmastadienol; **2L**, $\Delta^{5,24(28)}$-ergostadienol; **2M**, 25-methyl-$\Delta^{5,24(28)}$-ergostadienol; **2N**, $\Delta^{5,24(28)}$-stigmastadienol: *isofucosterol* (Z) = Δ^5-*avenasterol, fucosterol* (E); **2O**, $\Delta^{5,25(27)}$-stigmastadienol: *cleroasterol* (24β); **2P**, $\Delta^{5,25(27)}$-ergostadienol; **3A**, $\Delta^{5,7}$-cholestadienol; **3B**, 24ξ-$\Delta^{5,7}$-ergostadienol: 7-dehydro-campesterol (24α); **3C**, 24ξ-$\Delta^{5,7}$-stigmastadienol: 7-dehydro-sitosterol (24α); **3D**, 24ξ-$\Delta^{5,7,22}$-stigmastatrienol: 7-dehydro-stigmasterol (24α); **3E**, 24ξ-$\Delta^{5,7,22}$-ergostatrienol: *ergosterol* (24β); **3H**, $\Delta^{5,7,22}$-cholestrienol; **4A**, $\Delta^{5,8}$-cholestadienol; **4B**, 24ξ,$\Delta^{5,8}$-ergostadienol; **4E**, 24ξ,$\Delta^{5,8,22}$-ergostatrienol: *lichesterol* (24β); **5A**, Δ^7-cholestenol: *lathosterol*; **5B**, 24ξ-Δ^7-ergostenol: *24ξ-methyl lathosterol, fungisterol* (24β); **5C**, 24ξ-Δ^7-stigmastenol; **5D**, 24ξ-$\Delta^{7,22}$-stigmastadienol: *spinasterol* (24α)-*chondrillasterol* (24β); **5E**, 24ξ-$\Delta^{7,22}$-ergostadienol; **5G**, 24-methyl-$\Delta^{7,22}$-ergostadienol: *stellasterol* (24α); **5I**, $\Delta^{7,23}$-ergostadienol; **5N**, $\Delta^{7,24(28)}$-stigmastadienol: Δ^7-*isofucosterol* (Z) = Δ^7-*avenasterol* (Z); **5O**, $\Delta^{7,25(27)}$-stigmastadienol; **6A**, Δ^8-cholestenol; **6B**, 24ξ-Δ^8-ergostenol: Δ^8-*campesterol* (24α); **6C**, 24ξ-Δ^8-stigmastenol: Δ^8-*sitosterol* (24α); **6D**, 24ξ-$\Delta^{8,22}$-stigmastadienol: Δ^8-*stigmasterol* (24α); **6E**, 24ξ-$\Delta^{8,22}$-ergostadienol; **6F**, $\Delta^{8,24}$-cholestadienol: *zymosterol*; **6L**, $\Delta^{8,24(28)}$-ergostadienol: *fecosterol*; **6N**, $\Delta^{8,24(28)}$-stigmastadienol: Δ^8-*isofucosterol* (Z) = Δ^8-*avenasterol* (Z); **7C**, 24ξ,$\Delta^{9(11)}$-stigmastenol; **8A**, $\Delta^{8(14)}$-cholestenol; **8B**, 24ξ-$\Delta^{8(14)}$-ergostenol; **9A**, $\Delta^{8,14}$-cholestadienol; **9B**, 24ξ-$\Delta^{8,14}$-ergostadienol: *ignosterol*; **9C**, $\Delta^{8,14}$-stigmastadienol; **9N**, $\Delta^{8,14,22,(28)}$-stigmastatrienol; **10A**, 14α-methyl-9β,19-cyclo-cholestanol: *pollinastanol*; **10B**, 24ξ-14α-methyl-9β, 19-cyclo-ergostanol: *24-methyl pollinastanol*; **10C**, 24ξ-14α-ethyl-9β,19-cyclo-stigmastanol: *24-ethyl pollinastanol*; **10L**, 14α-methyl-9β,19cyclo-$\Delta^{24(28)}$-ergostenol: *24-methylene-pollinastanol*; **10N**, 14α-methyl-9β,19-cyclo-$\Delta^{24(28)}$-stigmastenol: *24-ethylidene-pollinastanol*; **11L**, 14α-methyl-$\Delta^{8,24(28)}$-ergostadienol: *14α-methyl fecosterol*; **12L**, 4α-methyl-$\Delta^{8,24(28)}$-ergostadienol: *4α-methyl fecosterol*; **13L**, 4α,14α-dimethyl-$\Delta^{8,24(28)}$-ergostadienol: *obtusifoliol*; **14L**, 4α,14α-dimethyl-9β,19-cyclo-$\Delta^{24(28)}$-ergostenol: *cycloeucalenol*; **15L**, 4,4,14α-trimethyl-9β,19-cyclo-$\Delta^{24(28)}$-ergostenol: *24 methylene-cycloartanol*; **16L**, 4,4,14α-trimethyl-$\Delta^{8,24(28)}$-ergostadienol: *24-methylene-lanostenol.*

C. Determination of the Molecular Weight of Sterols

Before surveying the fragmentation induced by the various structural features of the sterol molecule, we shall examine some criteria that influence the abundance of the molecular ion of 3β-hydroxy-sterols and their 3β-acetoxy or trimethylsilyl ether derivatives.

Besides the effects of the ionizing voltage and the temperature of the ion source, the abundance of the molecular ions is also influenced by (1) the presence or absence of a Δ^5 double bond, which stabilizes the diene produced by dehydration, deacetylation, or desilylation of the 3β oxygenated function by conjugation, and (2) the nature of this 3β oxygenated substituent.

Table 1 illustrates the first point and emphasizes the absence of molecular ions to the profit of the deacetylated fragment for 3β-acetoxy-Δ5-sterols. The case of the 9β,19-cyclopropyl-sterol will be discussed later. These results are in accordance with those already published (Galli and Maroni, 1967).

Table 2 shows that Δ^5-sterol derivatives, which produce the larger molecular ions, are the free sterols whereas 3β-acetoxy and 3β-trifluoroacetoxy sterols show no molecular ions. In the case of trimethylsilyl ethers, a peak due to the molecular ion is always observed, even if it is not the base peak. Thus, these derivatives as well as the free sterols appear useful for defining the molecular weight of Δ^5-sterols. With a few

Table 2 Influence of the 3β-derivatives of Δ^5-sterol on the abundance of the molecular ion M^+ versus $(M\text{-}ROH)^+$ (R=H, CH_3CO, CF_3CO, Me_3Si)

Sterol	M^+	$(M\text{-}ROH)^+$	References
Cholesterol **2A**	386(98)	368(64)	Knights (1967)
Cholesteryl acetate	428 —	368(100)	Knights (1967)
Cholesteryl trifluoroacetate	482(2)	368(100)	Knights (1967)
Cholesteryl trimethylsilyl ether	458(22)	368(52)	Knights (1967)
Campesterol **2B** (24α)	400(100)	382(62)	Knights (1967)
Campesteryl acetate	442 —	382(100)	
Campesteryl trimethylsilyl ether	472(32)	382(77)	Brooks *et al.* (1968)
Sitosterol **2C** (24α)	414(100)	396(54)	Knights (1967)
Sitosteryl acetate	456 —	396(100)	
Sitosteryl trimethylsilylether	486(37)	396(80)	Brooks *et al.* (1968)
Stigmasterol **2D** (24α)			
Stigmasteryl acetate	454 —	394(100)	
Stigmasteryl trimethylsilyl ether	484(42)	394(52)	Brooks *et al.* (1968)
Desmosterol **2F**	384(30)	366(8)	Brooks *et al.* (1968)
Desmosteryl acetate	426 —	366(100)	Brooks *et al.* (1968)
Desmosteryl trimethylsilyl ether	456(32)	366(44)	Brooks *et al.* (1968)
Ergosterol **3E** (24β)	396(72)	378 —	
Ergosteryl acetate	438(9)	378(100)	
Ergosteryl trimethylsilyl ether	468(58)	378(30)	Knights (1967)

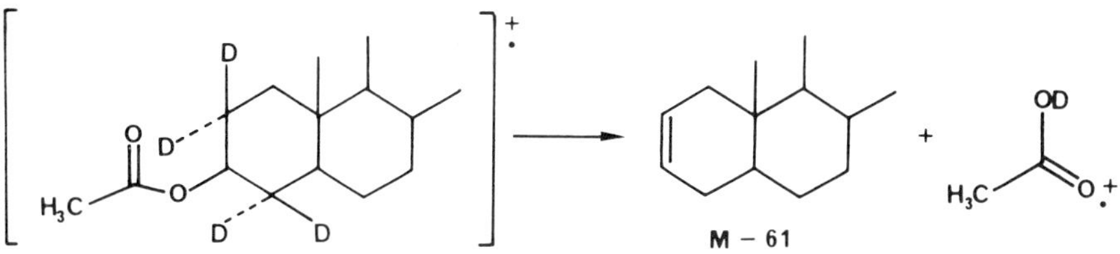

Figure 1 Fragmentation of deutero steryl acetate (data from Budzikiewicz *et al.*, 1964).

exceptions, in the case of other 4-desmethyls-sterols, even when well-defined fragmentations are favored, the above considerations still apply, especially the easier elimination of acetic acid in the case of acetoxy derivatives (Fig. 1). This is the case even for 4α-methyl and 4,4-dimethyls-sterols (Budzikiewicz *et al.*, 1964).

II. FRAGMENTATION OF THE STEROID NUCLEUS

A. Mass Spectra of Stanols

Table 3 shows the principal fragments obtained for stanols without any unsaturation with *m/e* above 210. In all tables R′ denotes the substituent at C-24, and R denotes the derivatives attached to the oxygen at C-3. In these tables, figures in parentheses indicate relative abundances for ions measured in the range *m/e* 210 to the molecular ion. The origin of most fragments is made clear by Fig. 2.

The most important characteristic of these completely saturated homologs is the presence of the base peak at *m/e* 215. The origin of this ion resulting from the loss of the side chain and part of the D-cycle has been discussed in detail elsewhere (Budzikiewicz *et al.*, 1964; Zaretskii, 1976). Besides this, it is notable that all stanols exhibit a molecular ion.

Table 3 Molecular ion and most characteristic ions resulting from the fragmentation of stanols

Sterol R	**1A** Ac	**1B**(24α) Ac	**1C**(24α) Ac
M^+	430(25)	444(35)	458(38)
M^+-Me	415(9)	429(7)	443(6)
M^+-ROH	370(58)	384(34)	398(31)
M^+-ROH-Me	355(23)	369(23)	383(21)
M^+-SC	317(6)	317 —	317 —
M^+-SC-42	275(30)	275(28)	275(24)
M^+-SC-ROH	257(37)	257(16)	257(17)
M^+-SC-42-ROH	215(100)	215(100)	215(100)

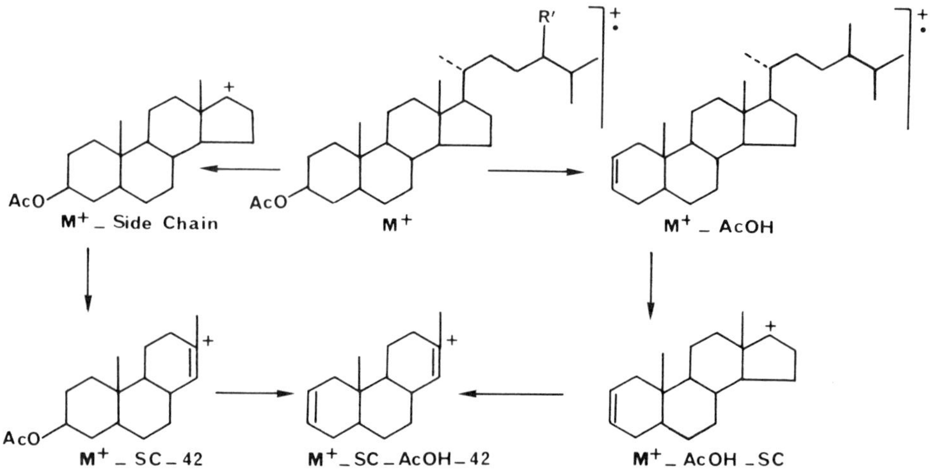

Figure 2 Major fragments of stanols.

B. Δ^5-Unsaturated Sterols

The origins of most ions are clear from Fig. 3. Table 4 summarizes the relative abundances of the principal fragments above *m/e* 210 for the most common Δ^5-sterols with no other unsaturation. Some general characteristics can be pointed out:

- As noted before, 3β-acetoxy derivatives exhibit neither a molecular ion nor a $|M\text{-}Me|^+$ fragment.

- Ions $|M\text{-}ROH|^+$ and $|M\text{-}Me\text{-}ROH|^+$ are common features of these sterol spectra.

- Ion $|M\text{-}ROH\text{-}67|^+$ is intense only in the case of free sterols (R=H). This peak is the most characteristic indication of the presence of a Δ^5-double bond in the steroid nucleus and can serve to distinguish this class of sterol. The mechanism of formation of this fragment has been discussed elsewhere (Zaretskii, 1976).

- Ion $|M\text{-}129|^+$ is the characteristic base peak of 3β-hydroxy-Δ^5-sterol trimethylsilyl ether derivatives and can serve to distinguish monounsaturated Δ^5-sterols from corresponding diunsaturated sterols and Δ^7-sterols (Brooks *et al.*, 1968; Patterson, 1984). The origin of this fragment has been discussed in detail elsewhere (Brooks *et al.*, 1968; Massey and Djerassi, 1979).

- The Δ^5-double bond initiates another intense decomposition process in TMS sterols, that is, the elimination of $(CH_3)_3SiOH$ (90 mass units) from the molecular ion (Zaretskii, 1976).

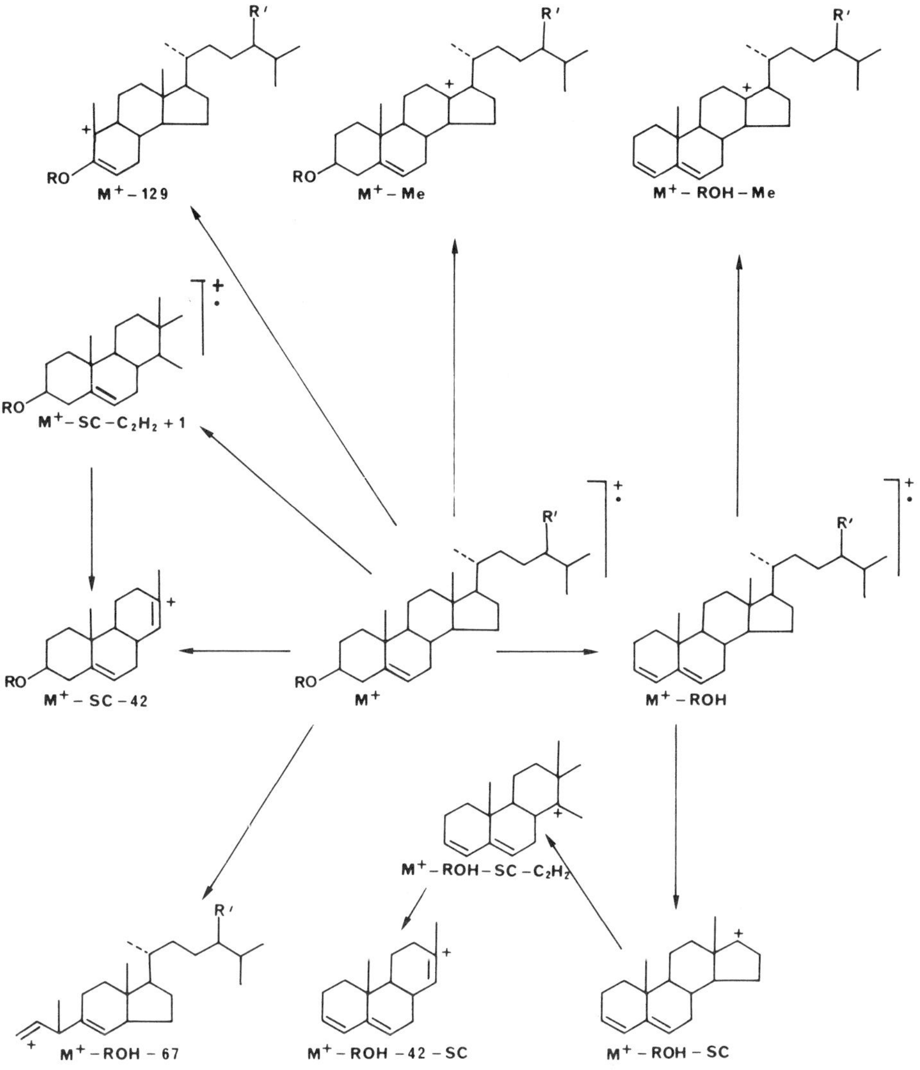

Figure 3 Major fragments of Δ^5-sterols.

C. $\Delta^{5,7}$-Unsaturated Sterols

Although $\Delta^{5,7}$-diene-sterols are not common in higher plants, they are found in fungi or may result from the metabolism of Δ^5-sterols in phytophagous insects. Galli and Maroni (1967) studied the mass spectra of 3β-acetoxycholesta-5,7-diene (3A) and 3β-acetoxycholesta-5,7,24-triene (3F).

Table 5 summarizes the principal fragments of several other $\Delta^{5,7}$-sterols. Besides the fact, already mentioned, that acetoxy-derivatives do not exhibit a molecular ion,

Table 4 Molecular ion and most characteristic ions resulting from the fragmentation of Δ^5-sterols without other unsaturation

Sterol R	**2A** Ac	**2B**(24α) Ac	**2C**(24α) Ac	**2A** H	**2B**(24α) H	**2C**(24α) H	**2A** TMS	**2B**(24α) TMS	**2C**(24α) TMS
M^+	428 —	442 —	456 —	386(98)	400(100)	414(100)	458(22)	472(32)	486(37
M^+-Me	413 —	427 —	441 —	371(46)	385(50)	399(45)	443(20)		
M^+-ROH	368(100)	382(100)	396(100)	368(64)	382(62)	396(54)	368(52)	382(77)	396(80)
M^+-Me-ROH	353(28)	367(19)	381(18)	353(52)	367(50)	381(42)	353(30)	367(31)	381(30)
M^+-ROH-67	301 —	315 —	329 —	301(56)	315(60)	329(50)	301(4)		
M^+-129	299 —	313 —	327 —	257 —	271 —	285 —	329(100)	343(94)	357(93)
M^+-SC	315 —	315 —	315 —	273(36)	273(50)	273(54)	345 —		
M^+-SC-42	273 —	273 —	273 —	231(42)	231(42)	231(58)	303 —		
M^+-SC-ROH	255(37)	255(45)	255(40)	255(50)	255(82)	255(60)	255(16)		255(16)
M^+-SC-ROH-42	213(30)	213(29)	213(30)	213(68)	213(74)	213(78)	213(10)		

Sources: Data for **2A** (H), **2B** (24α) (H), **2C** (24α) (H), and **2A** (TMS) Patterson (1984); data for **2B** (24α) (TMS) and **2C** (24α) (TMS) Brooks *et al.* (1968).

Table 5 Molecular ion and most important fragments of some $\Delta^{5,7}$-sterols and derivatives

Sterol R	**3A** Ac	**3B**(24α) Ac	**3C**(24α) Ac	**3D**(24α) Ac	**3E**(24β) Ac	**3E** H	**3A** TMS	**3E**(24β) TMS
M^+	426 —	440(2)	454(4)	452(10)	438(9)	396(72)	456(37)	468(58)
M^+-Me	411 —	425 —	439 —	437 —	423 —	381(7)		
M^+-ROH	366(100)	380(100)	394(100)	392(76)	378(100)	378 —	366(10)	378(30)
M^+-Me-ROH	351(50)	365(40)	379(40)	377(60)	363(34)	363(100)	351(37)	363(58)
M^+-SC	313 —	313 —	313 —	313 —	313 —	271(18)		
M^+-SC-42	271 —	271 —	271 —	271 —		229(6)		
M^+-SC-ROH	253(28)	253(35)	253(37)	253(100)	253(60)	253(67)	253(10)	253(29)
M^+-ROH-SC-C_2H_2	227 —	227(30)	227(43)	227(36)		227(13)		211(12)
M^+-SC-42-ROH	211(18)	211(19)	211(17)	211(14)	211(14)	211(33)		
Fragment A	158(30)	158(25)	158(40)	158(30)		158(16)		
Fragment B	143(24)	143(50)	143(55)	143(75)	143(42)	143(50)		

Sources: Data for **3A** (TMS) and **3E** (24β) (TMS) from Brooks *et al.* (1968); data for **3E** (24β) (AC) from Raederstorff (1985).

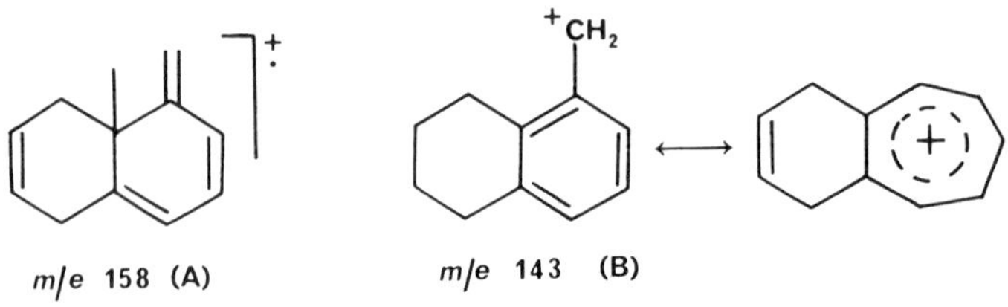

Figure 4 Characteristic fragments of $\Delta^{5,7}$-sterols.

which is present in the free alcohol or TMS derivatives, the only characteristic intense peaks for such sterols are *m/e* 158 and 143 (Galli and Maroni, 1967). The structure of these ions is shown in Fig. 4.

D. $\Delta^{5,8}$-Unsaturated Sterols

The $\Delta^{5,8}$-sterols (Table 6) are rare, but are present in the fungus *Gibberella fujikuroi* (Nes *et al.*, 1985), the fungal component of lichens (Lenton *et al.*, 1973), and in a very few green plants (*Chlorella ellipsoidea*, for example) (Patterson *et al.*, 1974). The fragmentation at *m/e* 363 (100%) is chracteristic for the $\Delta^{5,8}$ system. The general fragmentation resembles that of a Δ^{5}-sterol with two mass units less than for the corresponding fragment due to the supplementary Δ^{8}-unsaturation. However, the fragmentation pattern is sensitive to the temperature of the ion source. For instance, at elevated temperatures, the cracking pattern for a $\Delta^{5,7}$- and a $\Delta^{5,8}$-system may appear similar (W. D. Nes, personal communication).

E. Δ^{7}-Unsaturated Sterols

The Δ^{7}-sterols (Table 7) are the major sterols of a few plant families such as Cucurbitaceae, Chenopodiaceae, Cactaceae, and Caryophilaceae (Nes, 1977). In

Table 6 Molecular ion and prominent fragments of $\Delta^{5,8}$-sterols

Sterol R	**4A** H	**4B**(24β) H	**4E**(24β) Ac	**4E**(24β) H
M^+	384(100)	398(60)	438(7)	396(67)
M^+-Me	369(5)		423 —	381(1)
M^+-ROH	366(5)	378(6)	378(70)	
M^+-Me-ROH	351(61)	363(100)	363(100)	363(100)
M^+-SC	271(7)		313 —	271(22)
M^+-SC-ROH	253(2)	253(10)	253(48)	
M^+-SC-ROH-42	211 —	211(20)	211(18)	
Other prominent ions	217(7)		337(10)	253(65)

Sources: Data for **4B** (24β) from Ziogas *et al.* (1983); data for **4E** (24β) (H) from Nes *et al.* (1985).

Table 7 Molecular ion and prominent fragments of Δ^7-unsaturated sterols

Sterol R	**5A** Ac	**5B**(24β) Ac	**5B**(24α) Ac	**5C**(24α) Ac	**5G** Ac	**5A** TMS	**5B**(24α) TMS	**5C**(24α) TMS
M^+	428(100)	442(100)	442(78)	456(81)	456(100)	458(100)	472(100)	486(100)
M^+-Me	413(23)	427(21)	427(15)	441(18)	441(17)	443(18)	457(18)	471(20)
M^+-ROH	368(13)	382(14)	382(31)	396(21)	396(58)		382(9)	396(6)
M^+-Me-ROH	353(15)	353(15)	353(8)	381(13)	381(12)	353(10)		
M^+-SC	315(12)	315(14)	315(11)	315(11)	315(11)		345(12)	345(9)
M^+-SC-42	273(11)	273(15	273(16)	273(13)	273(9)			
M^+-SC-ROH	255(75)	255(83)	255(100)	255(84)	255(67)	255(60)	255(89)	255(87)
M^+-SC-ROH-C_2H_2	229(29)	229(30)	229(26)	229(27)	229(19)	229(18)	229(25)	229(25)
M^+-SC-ROH-42	213(35)	213(40)	213(67)	213(40)	213(19)	213(14)	213(36)	213(39)
Other prominent ions								
M^+-SC-C_2H_2 + 1	288(8)	288(8)	288(8)	288(9)	288(8)			

Sources: Data for **5A** (TMS) Brooks *et al.* (1968); data for **5B**(24α) (TMS) and **5C**(24α) (TMS) from Smith *et al.* (1973); data for **5G** from Akilusa *et al.* (1986); cata for **5B** (24β) Raederstorff (1985).

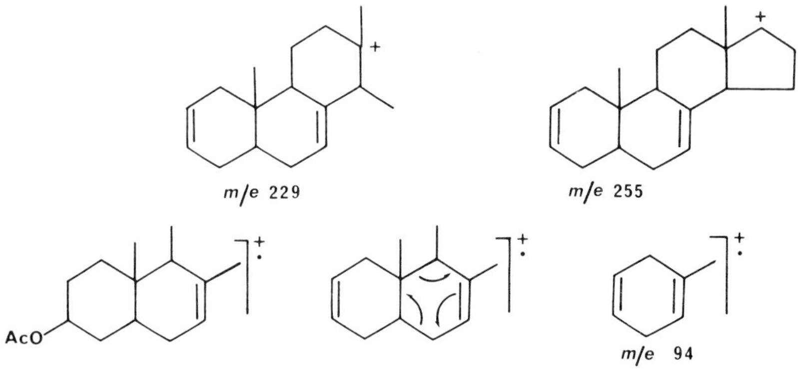

Figure 5 Characteristic fragments of Δ^7-sterols.

contrast to the Δ^5-sterols, Δ^7-unsaturated sterols without other unsaturation always present a strong molecular ion. They also lose their lateral chain much more easily, leading to a characteristic intense peak at *m/e* 255. Moreover, the intensity of the peak at *m/e* 229 (and *m/e* 243 in the case of 4α-methyl sterols) is much higher in these sterols than in Δ^5-sterols; this peak represents the fragments shown in Fig. 5 (Zaretskii, 1976). Δ^7-Sterols, like Δ^8-sterols but unlike Δ^5-sterols, fail to induce a significant M^+-H_2O (W. D. Nes, personal communication). Galli and Maroni (1967) assume that a diagnostic fragment for Δ^7-unsaturated sterols is the retro-Diels-Alder reaction, resulting in an ion *m/e* 94 (*m/e* 108 for a 4α-methyl sterol) as shown in Fig. 5.

F. Δ^8-Unsaturated Sterols

The Δ^8-sterols (Table 8) are known to be intermediates during sterol biosynthesis but are only minor constituents of undisturbed plants due to their high turnover. However, these compounds can accumulate in plant cells treated with an inhibitor of

Table 8 Molecular ion and prominent fragments of Δ^8-unsaturated sterols

Sterol R	**6A** H	**6B**(24α) Ac	**6B**(24β) Ac	**6C**(24α) Ac	**6C**(24β) Ac
M^+	386(100)	442(100)	442(100)	456(100)	456(100)
M^+-Me	371(37)	427 —	427(22)	441 —	441(26)
M^+-ROH	368(14)	382(27)	382(33)	396(15)	396(40)
M^+-Me-ROH	353(11)	367 —	367(31)	381 —	381(27)
M^+-SC-42	273(19)	273(13)	273(13)	273(9)	273(10)
M^+-SC-ROH	255(14)	255(46)	255(24)	255(40)	255(31)
M^+-SC-ROH-42		213(65)	213(43)	213(65)	213(40)
Other prominent ions					
M^+-SC-C_2H_2 + 1			288(7)		288(12)

Source: Data for **6B** (24β) and **6C** (24β) from Raederstorff (1985).

Table 9 MS of 24ξ,$\Delta^{9(11)}$-stigmastenol 7C

Sterol R	**7C** H	**7C** Ac
M^+	414(16)	456(4)
M^+-Me	399(27)	441(3)
M^+-ROH	396(39)	396(28)
M^+-ROH-Me	381(34)	381(33)
M^+-SC	273(9)	315 —
M^+-SC-42	231(5)	273(5)
M^+-SC-42-ROH	213(4)	213(4)
Other prominent ions	288(4)	288(8)

Source: Data from Gupta *et al.* (1981).

the Δ^8-Δ^7-isomerase (Schmitt and Benveniste, 1979). The mass spectra of these sterols do not display a characteristic peak (Galli and Mavoni, 1967), which characterizes the location of the double bond. However, these sterols always show a strong molecular peak.

G. $\Delta^{9(11)}$-*Unsaturated Sterols*

The $\Delta^{9(11)}$-sterols (Table 9) are rare compounds of plants and fungi. However, in some cases they have been identified by MS (Gupta *et al.*, 1981). As in the case of Δ^8-sterols, these sterols do not display a characteristic peak that permits location of the $\Delta^{9(11)}$ double bond.

H. $\Delta^{8(14)}$-*Unsaturated Sterols*

The occurrence in nature of a sterol with $\Delta^{8(14)}$ unsaturation is rare (Table 10). However, for example, 5α-stigmasta-8(14), 22-dien-3β-ol has been isolated from

Table 10 Molecular ion and prominent fragments of $\Delta^{8(14)}$-unsaturated sterols

Sterol R	**8A** Ac	**8B** H
M^+	428(100)	400(100)
M^+-Me	413(26)	385(32)
M^+-ROH	368(10)	382(13)
M^+-ROH-Me	353(16)	367(6)
M^+-SC	315(14)	273(21)
M^+-SC-42	273(6)	231(15)
M^+-SC-ROH	255(24)	255(15)
M^+-SC-ROH-42	213(44)	213(18)
Other prominent ions		
M^+-SC-ROH-C_2H_2	229(44)	229(29)

Source: Data for **8A** from Bouvier *et al.* (1976).

Table 11 Molecular ion and prominent fragments of $\Delta^{8,14}$ diunsaturated sterols with saturated side chain

Sterol R	**9A** Ac	**9B**(24α) Ac	**9C** Ac
M^+	426(36)	440(100)	454(100)
M^+-Me	411(9)	425(28)	439(26)
M^+-ROH	366(8)	380(23)	394(15)
M^+-Me-ACOH	351(100)	365(98)	379(95)
M^+-SC	313(16)	313(27)	313(26)
M^+-SC-ROH	253(5)	253(23)	253(20)
M^+-SC-ROH-Me	238(25)	238(36)	238(26)
Other prominent ions			
M^+-SC-ROH-Me + 1		239(28)	239(22)

Sources: Data for **9A** from Campbell and Kirchen (1980); data for **9B**(24α) from Schmitt *et al.* (1980).

a higher plant *Haplopappus heterophyllus* (Zalkow *et al.*, 1968) and a 4α-methyl-$\Delta^{8(14)}$-sterol from *Capsicum annum* (Matsumoto *et al.*, 1983). As in both preceding cases, the $\Delta^{8(14)}$-double bond does not induce a specific fragmentation that permits location in the nucleus.

I. $\Delta^{8,14}$-Diunsaturated Sterols

The $\Delta^{8,14}$-sterols (Table 11) are well known as transitory intermediates during cholesterol and ergosterol biosynthesis (Benveniste, 1986) and have been reported only a very few times as constituents of undisturbed plants, such as *Senita cactus*, for example (Campbell and Kirchen, 1980). However, these compounds have been shown to accumulate dramatically in plant cells treated with an inhibitor of the sterol Δ^{14}-reductase (Schmitt *et al.*, 1980).

The mass spectrum of $\Delta^{8,14}$-sterols displays typical fragments. First, it shows unambiguously the presence of two cyclic double bonds (fragments $|M\text{-}SC|^+$ and

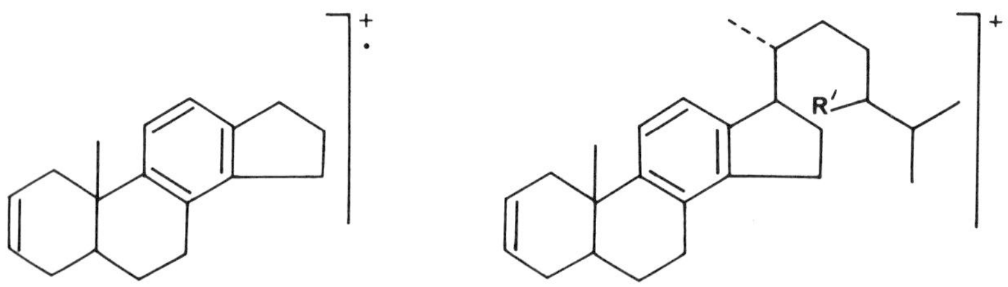

m/e 238 *m/e* 351 (R′=H)

Figure 6 Characteristic fragments of $\Delta^{8,14}$-sterols.

Table 12 MS of 9β,19-cyclopropyl sterols without other unsaturation

Sterol R	**10A** Ac	**10B** Ac	**10C** Ac
M^+	442(10)	456(7)	470(6)
M^+-Me	427(10)	441 —	455 —
M^+-ROH	382(100)	396(86)	410(100)
M^+-ROH-Me	367(90)	381(100)	395(94)
M^+-A	288(10)	302(9)	316(10)
M^+-SC-ROH	269(65)	269(89)	269(93)
M^+-SC-ROH-42		227(11)	227(16)

$|M\text{-SC-ROH}|^+$). Second, the fragment $|M\text{-SC-ROH-Me}|^+$ at *m/e* 238 can be considered as characteristic of the $\Delta^{8,14}$-diene system (as well as the fragment $|M\text{-Me-ROH}|^+$). These fragments probably result from the aromatization of the C cycle, as shown in Fig. 6.

J. 9β,19-Cyclopropyl Sterols

The 9β,19-cyclopropyl sterols (Table 12) are known to be intermediates during phytosterol biosynthesis. Thus, they are not detected in mammals or fungi and could be biochemical markers of photosynthetic eukaryotic phyla (Benveniste, 1986). These 9β,19-cyclopropyl sterols always possess the additional C14α methyl group since the C14α elimination does not work on a steroid skeleton with the 9β,19-cyclopropyl ring (Benveniste, 1986).

The presence of the 19β,19-cyclopropyl ring in the sterol molecule induces a characteristic fragmentation denoted as in Fig. 7. The mechanism of the fragmentation of the B-ring has been studied in detail in the case of cycloartenol, and two mechanisms have been proposed in the literature (Fig. 8) (Audier *et al.*, 1966; Aplin

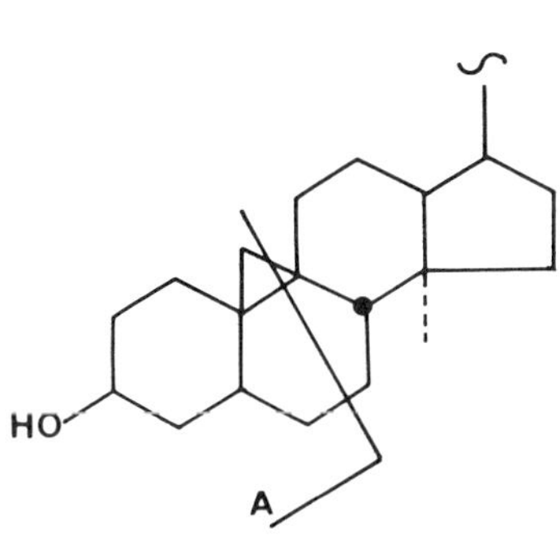

Figure 7 Typical fragmentation of 9β,19-cyclopropyl sterols.

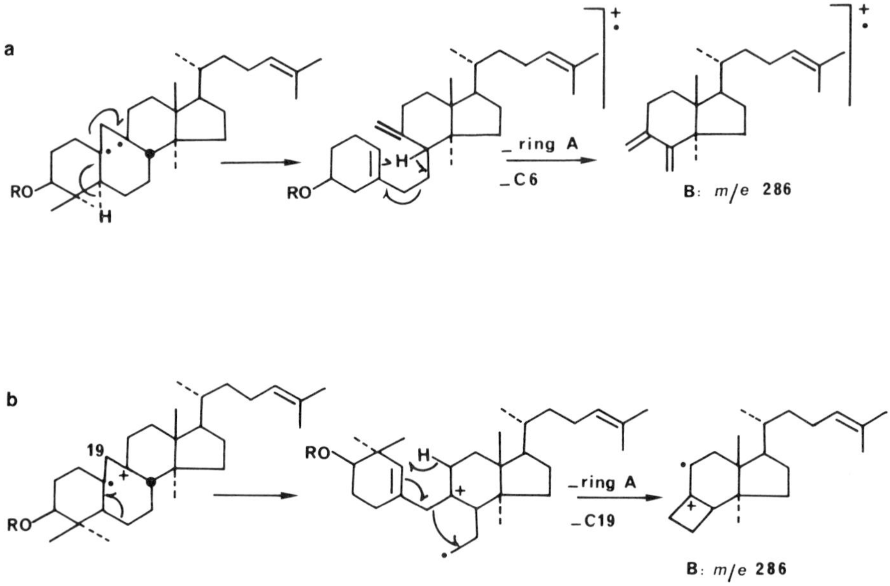

Figure 8 Mechanism of fragmentation of 9β,19-cyclopropyl sterols: (a) mechanism 1 and (b) mechanism 2.

and Hornby, 1966). However, MS spectra recorded on a sample of cycloartanol specifically deuterated at C-19 loses the label in fragment B, thus giving strong support to mechanism 2 (Blattler, 1978).

Another characteristic of 9β,19-cyclopropyl sterols is the low relative intensity of the molecular-ion peak with respect to the $|M\text{-}ROH|^+$ peak (Table 12). A reverse situation is observed in the case of Δ^8- or Δ^7-sterols (Tables 7 and 8).

III. FRAGMENTATION OF THE SIDE CHAIN: STEROLS WITH UNSATURATED SIDE CHAINS

In Section II of this chapter, we gave an overview of the MS characteristic peaks that permit the location of the unsaturation in the steroid nucleus. We shall now examine the various possible side chains.

In many cases, when it is not too weak, the cleavage of the entire side chain leading to fragments $|M\text{-}SC|^+$ and $|M\text{-}SC\text{-}ROH|^+$ usually permits the determination of the structure of the side chain. In addition both these fragments usually give good information about the degree of unsaturation of the sterol nucleus. For example, the formation of an ion corresponding to the elimination of the side chain with the loss of two hydrogen atoms by the charged fragment is an important characteristic of all sterols with an unsaturated side chain (Wyllie and Djerassi, 1968). This can be used as a diagnostic because in sterols with saturated side chains, this fragmentation is absent.

Moreover, the relative intensity of the MS peak associated with this fragmentation is modulated by the position of the double bond in the side chain, and each particular unsaturated side-chain isomer gives rise to a number of other characteristic fragments, which usually permits the location of the side-chain double bond, as we shall see now in more detail.

A. Δ^{22}-Unsaturated Sterols

Table 13 shows prominent MS fragments of Δ^{22}-unsaturated sterols with various steroid nuclei. These sterols easily lose the side chain. In most cases, in addition to elimination of the side chain with the loss of two hydrogen atoms $|M\text{-SC-2H}|^+$, these derivatives also show an intense $|M\text{-SC-ROH}|^+$ peak that corresponds simply to the elimination of the side chain and 3β substituant; but in some cases, peaks due to the elimination of only part of the side chain $|\text{-}C_3H_7\text{-ROH}|^+$ are found. However, the most characteristic peaks are found in the case of $\Delta^{7,22}$-diunsaturated sterols (5D, 5E), which, in addition to the already mentioned characteristic intense peak at *m/e* 255 (Table 7), generally display a base peak *m/e* 313 that corresponds to the fragment $|M\text{-SC-2H}|^+$, already mentioned as a characteristic of a sterol with an unsaturated side chain.

B. Δ^{23}-Unsaturated Sterols

The intermediacy of 24-methyl Δ^{23}-sterols (Table 14) in the biosynthesis of sterols in maize has been demonstrated recently (Benveniste, 1986). In $\Delta^{5,23}$-sterols the intense peak corresponding to the fragment $|M\text{-ROH}|^+$, which is representative of a Δ^5 double bond, is accompanied by another intense fragment $|M\text{-ROH-a}|^+$ that is due to allylic cleavage of the 20-22 bond (Wyllie and Djerassi, 1968), whereas in $\Delta^{7,23}$-sterols the base peak corresponds to the fragment $|M\text{-SC-2H}|^+$, which is characteristic of a Δ^7 double bond in addition to a double bond in the side chain (Wyllie and Djerassi, 1968) (Fig. 9). $\Delta^{5,23}$- and $\Delta^{5,24}$-24-methyl sterols have been prepared by

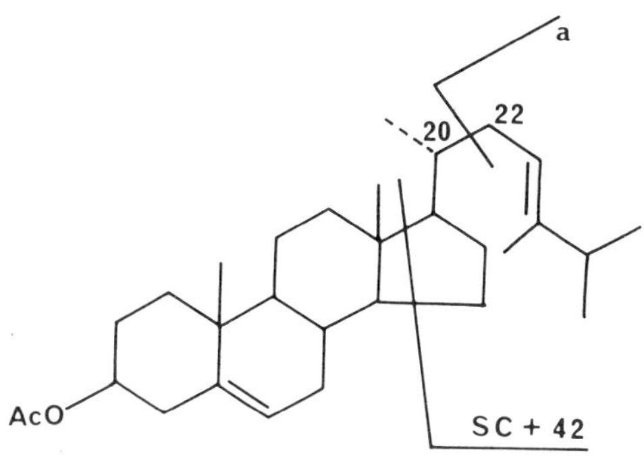

Figure 9 Fragmentation of Δ^{23}-sterols.

Table 13 Molecular ion and prominent fragments of Δ^{22}-unsaturated sterols with various nuclei

Sterol R	**1D**(24α) Ac	**2D** Ac	**3D**(24α) Ac	**5D** Ac	**6D** Ac	**2E**(24β) Ac	**3E**(24β) Ac	**4E**(24β) Ac	**5E**(24β) Ac	**6E**(24β) Ac	**3H** Ac	**5G** Ac
M^+	456(27)	454(0)	452(10)	454(39)	454(24)	440 —	438(9)	438(7)	440(60)	440(45)	424(6)	454(8)
M^+-C_3H_7	413 —	411 —	409 —	411 —	411 —	397 —	395 —	395 —	397 —	397 —	381 —	411(100)
M^+-Me	441 —	439 —	437 —	439(10)	439(8)	425 —	423 —	423 —	425(15)	425(16)	409 —	439 —
M^+-ROH	396(13)	394(100)	392(76)	394(9)	394(12)	380(100)	378(100)	378(70)	380(9)	380(10)	364(100)	394 —
M^+-Me-ROH	381 —	379(8)	377(60)	379(6)	379(10)	365(7)	363(34)	363(100)	365(9)	365(9)	349(44)	379 —
M^+-ROH-C_3H_7	353 —	351(15)	349 —	351(12)	351 —	337 —	335 —	335(10)	337 —	337 —	321 —	351(27)
M^+-SC	317(23)	315 —	313 —	315 —	315(11)	315 —	313 —	313 —	315 —	315(24)	313 —	315 —
M^+-SC-2H	315(32)	313 —	311 —	313(100)	313(16)	313 —	311 —	311 —	313(100)	313(43)	311 —	313(59)
M^+-SC-42	275 —	273 —	271 —	273(10)	273(4)	273 —	271 —	271(—)	273(12)	273(7)	271 —	273(18)
M^+-SC-ROH	257(100)	255(95)	253(100)	255(67)	255(35)	255(47)	253(60)	253(48)	255(81)	255(46)	253(72)	255(33)
M^+-SC-ROH-2H	255(50)	253(25)	251 —	253(16)	253 —	253 —	251 —	251(10)	253(15)	253 —	251 —	253 —
M^+-SC-42-ROH	215(29)	213(24)	211(14)	213(21)	213(12)	213(13)	211(14)	211(18)	213(23)	213(19)	211 —	213(7)
Other prominent fragments												
M^+-ROH-42 + H							337(6)					
M^+-SC-C_2H_2 — H				288(20)	288(16)				288(31)	288(33)		
M^+-SC-C_2H_2 — ROH			227(36)	229(28)	229(40)							229(5)
Fragment A (Fig. 4)			158(30)								158(47)	
Fragment B (Fig. 4)			143(75)				143(42)		143(42)		143(12)	

Sources: Data for **6D** and **3H** from Raederstorff (1985); data for **5G** from Akilusa *et al.* (1986).

Table 14 Molecular ion and prominent fragments of Δ^{23}-unsaturated sterols

Sterols R	**21** Ac	**51** Ac
M^+	440 —	440(15)
M^+-Me	425 —	425 —
M^+-ROH	380(100)	380(11)
M^+-Me-ROH	365 —	365 —
M^+-a	343 —	343(19)
M^+-SC-2H	313 —	313(100)
M^+-a-ROH	283(100)	283(60)
M^+-SC-42	273(3)	273 —
M^+-SC-ROH	255(10)	255(12)
M^+-SC-2H-ROH	253(35)	253(22)
M^+-SC-42-ROH	213(10)	213(21)

iodine-promoted isomerization of 24(28)-methylenecholesterol (Nes *et al.*, 1981). The presence of a base peak in the mass spectrum at *m/e*, 296 for the C-3 acetate derivative confirmed the 24-methyldesmosterol structure.

C. $\Delta^{24(25)}$- and $\Delta^{24(28)}$-Unsaturated Sterols

The presence of a $\Delta^{24(25)}$ or $\Delta^{24(28)}$ double bond in the sterol side chain generally gives rise to an intense peak corresponding to the allylic cleavage of the 22-23 bond due to the McLafferty-type rearrangement (Gilpin and McLafferty, 1957), $|M\text{-a-ROH}|^+$ or $|M\text{-a-H-ROH-Me}|^+$ (Fig. 10).

In this case also the Δ^7-sterols show the strong tendency to lose the unsaturated side chain with two hydrogen atoms from the nucleus. Moreover, as in the case of

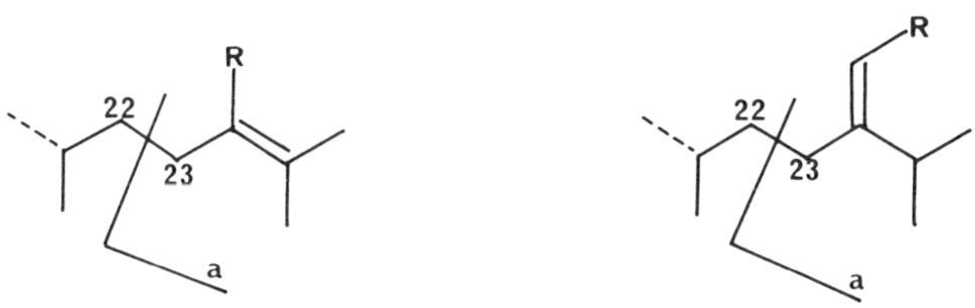

Figure 10 Fragmentation of $\Delta^{24(25)}$- and $\Delta^{24(28)}$-sterols.

Table 15 Molecular ion and prominent fragments of $\Delta^{24(25)}$-unsaturated sterols

Sterols R	**2F** Ac	**6F** Ac	**2J** Ac	**2K** Ac
M^+	426 —	426(100)	440 —	454 —
M^+-Me	411 —	411(41)	425 —	439 —
M^+-ROH	366(100)	366(19)	380(72)	394(27)
M^+-Me-ROH	351(14)	351(24)	365(18)	379(5)
M^+-a	356 —		356 —	
M^+-SC	315 —		315 —	
M^+-SC-2H	313 —	313(16)	313 —	
M^+-a-ROH	296(4)		296(100)	296(75)
M^+-a-ROH-Me	281 —		281(30)	281(15)
M^+-SC-42	273 —		273 —	
M^+-SC-ROH	255(8)		255(16)	255(8)
M^+-SC-2H-ROH	253(36)		253(36)	253(19)
M^+-SC-42-ROH	213(16)		213(32)	213(16)
Other prominent fragments	259(6)		259(18)	
	229(3)		229(20)	228(10)

Sources: Data for **2K** from Misso and Goad (1984); data for **6F** from Taylor *et al.* (1981).

other unsaturated side chains, the presence and location of the double bond in the steroid rings may modulate the intensity ratio of the fragments induced by the side-chain double bond, as shown in Tables 15 and 16 (see fragments $|M\text{-SC}|^+$, $|M\text{-SC-2H}|^+$, or $|M\text{-SC-2H-ROH}|^+$, for example). $\Delta^{8,24}$-Sterols show a much stronger fragment at *m/e* 213 than Δ^8-sterols; this fragment corresponds to the loss of the side chain and the D-cycle. In the case of $\Delta^{24(28)}$-ethylidene compounds, it has been proposed that in the mass spectra from acetate derivatives, the McLafferty rearrangement is slightly hindered in the E-series compared with the Z-series (Brooks *et al.*, 1972).

D. $\Delta^{25(27)}$-Unsaturated Sterols

The 24-methyl and 24-ethyl-25(27) methylene sterols (Table 17) are not so widely found in nature as the 24-methylene and 24-ethylidene sterols. Their MS do not display strong characteristics that enable location of the double bond in the side chain. However, to differentiate between $\Delta^{24(25)}$, $\Delta^{24(28)}$, and $\Delta^{25(27)}$ side chains, one possible diagnosis is the generally weaker intensity, in the case of $\Delta^{25(27)}$-sterol, of the peak $|M\text{-a}|^+$, $|M\text{-a-ROH}|^+$, or $|M\text{-a-ROH-Me}|^+$ corresponding to allylic cleavage of the 23-24 bond (compare 2J and 2L with 2P and 2O).

In the case of $\Delta^{25(27)}$-unsaturation, fragment *m/e* 296 could be attributed to the allylic cleavage of the 23-24 bond with the loss of an extra carbon atom, as proposed in the next mechanism (Zaretskii, 1976) (Fig. 11).

Table 16 Molecular ion and prominent fragments of $\Delta^{24(28)}$-unsaturated sterols

Sterol R	**2L** Ac	**2M** Ac	**6L** Ac	**10L** Ac	**2N** Ac	**3N** Ac	**6N** Ac	**9N** Ac	**10N** Ac
M^+	440 —	454 —	440(100)	454(8)	454 —	454(5)	454(100)	452(100)	468(11)
M^+-Me	425 —	439 —	425 —	439(6)	439 —	439 —	439 —	437(50)	453(6)
M^+-ROH	380(100)	394(80)	380(64)	394(100)	394(15)	394(5)	394(40)	392(17)	408(100)
M^+-Me-ROH	365 —	379(18)	365 —	379(98)	379 —	379 —	379 —	377(38)	393(88)
M^+-a	356 —		356(7)	356 —	356 —	356(40)	356(59)	354 —	370(8)
M^+-a-Me	341 —		341 —	341 —	341 —	341 —	341 —	339(91)	355 —
M^+-SC	315 —		315(10)	329(6)	315 —	315 —	315 —	313(35)	329 —
M^+-SC-2H (or H)	313 —		313(49)	327 —	313 —	313(100)	313(90)	312(47)	327 —
M^+-a-ROH	296(46)	296(100)	296(3)	310(10)	296(100)	296(45)	296(13)	294 —	310(58)
M^+-a-ROH-Me	281 —	281(30)	281 —	295 —	281 —	281 —	281 —	279(31)	295 —
M^+-SC-42	273 —		273(32)	287 —	273 —	273 —	273(25)	271 —	287 —
M^+-SC-ROH	255(15)		255(31)	269(60)	255(5)	255(18)	255(45)	253(30)	269(63)
M^+-SC-2H (or-H)-ROH	253(30)	253(31)	253(30)	267(19)	253(10)	253(45)	253(35)	252(21)	267 —
M^+-SC-42-ROH	213(25)	213(19)	213(100)	227(20)	213(27)	213(25)	213(100)	211 —	227(29)
Other prominent fragments								409(41)	
				300(11)				238(47)	314(5)
		228(15)						327(21)	
		211(12)						267(20)	

Source: Data for **2M** from Matsumoto *et al.* (1983a).

Table 17 Molecular ion and prominent fragments of $\Delta^{25(27)}$-unsaturated sterols

Sterols R	**2P** Ac	**2O** Ac	**5O** H
M^{+}	440 —	454 —	412(11)
M^{+}-Me	425 —	439 —	397(9)
M^{+}-ROH	380(100)	394(98)	379(3)
M^{+}-ROH-Me	365(12)	379(7)	
M^{+}-a-Me	356 —	356 —	314(17)
M^{+}-SC	315 —	315(3)	273(7)
M^{+}-SC-H			272(23)
M^{+}-SC-2H	313 —	313 —	271(100)
M^{+}-a-Me-ROH	296(11)	296(5)	296(5)
M^{+}-SC-42	273 —	273 —	231(13)
M^{+}-SC-ROH	255(12)	255(13)	255(17)
M^{+}-SC-2H-ROH	253 —	253(16)	253(5)
M^{+}-SC-2H-42	271 —	271 —	229(11)
M^{+}-SC-42-ROH	213(16)	213(16)	213(12)
Other prominent fragments	228(7)	281(6)	299(7)

Sources: Data for **2P** and **2O** from Misso and Goad (1984); data for **5O** from Garg and Nes (1984).

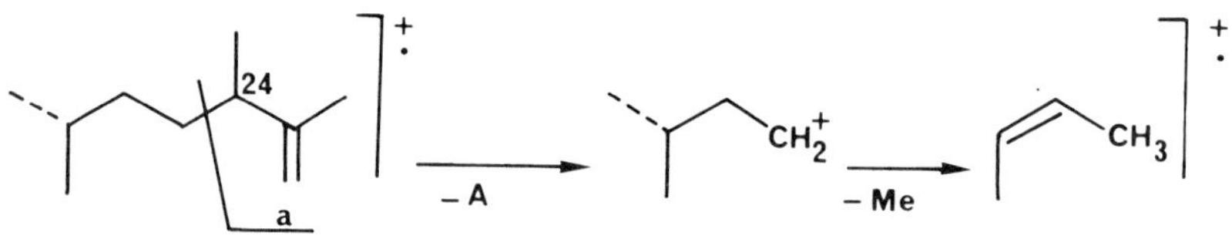

Figure 11 Fragmentation of $\Delta^{25(27)}$-sterols.

IV. INFLUENCE OF THE PRESENCE OF METHYLS AT THE C4 AND C14α POSITIONS ON THE RELATIVE INTENSITIES OF THE FRAGMENTATION PATTERN OF STEROLS

As shown in Table 18, 14α-methylsterols very easily lose the 14α-methyl group, leading to strong $|M\text{-}Me|^{+}$ and/or $|M\text{-}Me\text{-}ROH|^{+}$ fragments. In the case of Δ^{8}-14α-methyl-sterols, the fragment $|x\text{-}Me|^{+}$ is always stronger that the parent $|x|^{+}$ fragment.

The fragments that retain the C-4 and C-14 methyl group(s), $|M\text{-}SC|^{+}$, $|M\text{-}SC\text{-}2H|^{+}$ and so on, are useful to diagnose the presence or absence of methyls at these positions. Moreover, fragments that retain only the C-4 methyl groups—such as $|M\text{-}SC\text{-}42\text{-}ROH|^{+}$, which appears, for example, at *m/e* 227 for 14α-methyl

Table 18 Influence of the presence of methyls at the C-4 and C-14 positions on the fragmentation pattern of sterols

Sterols R	**6L** Ac	**11L** Ac	**12L** Ac	**13L** Ac	**10L** Ac	**14L** Ac	**15L** Ac	**16L** Ac
M^+	440(100)	454(30)	454(100)	468(34)	454(8)	468(6)	482(10)	440(45)
M^+-Me	425 —	439(100)	439 —	453(100)	439(6)	453(4)	467(23)	425(100)
M^+-ROH	380(64)	394(14)	394(25)	408(20)	394(100)	408(100)	422(100)	422(10)
M^+-ROH-Me	365 —	379(71)	379 —	393(96)	379(98)	393(81)	407(74)	407(40)
M^+-a	356(7)	370 —	370(3)	385 —	370 —	385 —	399(3)	399(8)
M^+-a-Me	341 —	355(16)	355 —	369(10)	355 —	369 —	384 —	384 —
M^+-SC	315(10)	329 —	329(2)	343 —	329(6)	343 —	357(6)	315 —
M^+-SC-2H	313(49)	327 —	327(35)	341–	327 —	341 —	355(6)	313 —
M^+-a-ROH	296(3)	310 —	310 —	324 —	310(10)	324(6)	339(10)	339 —
M^+-a-ROH-Me	281 —	295(25)	295 —	309(20)	295 —	309 —	324(3)	324(5)
M^+-SC-42	273(32)	287(17)	287(10)	301(11)	287 —	301 —	315(3)	273(10)
M^+-SC-ROH	255(31)	269 —	269(20)	283 —	269(60)	283(31)	297(35)	297 —
M^+-SC-ROH-Me	241 —	255(18)	255	269(25)	255 —	269 —	282(16)	282(10)
M^+-SC-2H-ROH	253(30)	267 —	267(15)	281 —	267(19)	281 —	295 —	295 —
M^+-SC-42-ROH	213(100)	227(31)	227(78)	241(29)	227(20)	241(15)	255(10)	255(10)
Other prominent fragments					300(11)	300(9)	300(14)	

Source: Data for **16L** from Patterson (1984).

$\Delta^{8,24(28)}$-ergostadienol **11L** whereas it appears at *m/e* 241 for the 4α-methyl derivative **13L** and at *m/e* 255 for the 4,4-dimethyl derivative **16L**—are of value in diagnosing the presence of methyls at this position.

V. CONCLUSION

This chapter shows the possibilities of identifying the numerous plant and fungi sterol structures by MS. Although MS is a powerful analytical method, which when combined with GC is of great use to identify most structures from a few micrograms of a complex sterol mixture, some limitations, such as the impossibility of differentiating the C-24 alkyl isomers or the C-20 isomers, exist. In addition, the precise discrimination between Δ^{8}-, $\Delta^{8(14)}$-, and $\Delta^{9(11)}$-sterols is difficult on the basis of MS fragmentations. Thus MS, especially GC/MS, provides a unique combination of selectivity and sensitivity, even more powerful when used in conjunction with complementary spectroscopic methods (e.g., NMR, UV, and IR) that permit the complete identification of certain isomeric sterols after complete purification.

REFERENCES

Akilusa, T., Schimizu, N., Tamura, T., and Matsumoto, T. (1986). Structures of three new 24,24-dimethyl-Δ^{7}-sterols from *Gynostemma pentaphyllum. Lipids* **21**, 515–517.

Aplin, R. T., and Hornby, J. (1966). Application of mass spectrometry to the structural investigation of 9,19-cyclosterols and triterpenes. *J. Chem. Soc. B* pp. 1078–1079.

Audier, H. E., Bengelmaus, R., and Das, B. C. (1966). Mass spectrometry of tetracyclic triterpenes. Part II. The lanostane group: Influence of the 9,19-cyclopropane ring. *Tetrahedron Lett.* **36**, 4341–4347.

Benveniste, P. (1986). Sterol biosynthesis. *Annu. Rev. Plant Physiol.* **37**, 275–308.

Blattler, W. A. (1978). Sterischer Verlauf der Bildung und Offnung des Cyclopropaninges in der Biosynthese von Phytosterinen. Dissertation ETH 6127.

Bouvier, P., Rohmer, M., Benveniste, P., and Ourisson, G. (1976). $\Delta^{8(14)}$-steroids in the Bacterium *Methylococcus capsulatus. Biochem. J.* **159**, 267–271.

Brooks, C. J. W., Horning, E. C., and Young, J. S. (1968). Characterization of sterols by gas chromatography—Mass spectroscopy of the trimethylsilyl ethers. *Lipids* **3**, 394–402.

Brooks, C. J. W., Knights, B. A., Sucrow, W., and Raduchel, B. (1972). The characterization of 24-ethylidene-sterols. *Steroids* **20**, 487–497.

Budzikiewicz, H., Djerassi, C., and Williams, D. H. (1964). "Structural Elucidation of Natural Products by Mass Spectroscopy," Vol. 2. Holden-Day, San Francisco, California.

Caarlson, R. M. K., Popov, S., Massey, I., Delseth, C., Ayanoglu, E., Varkony, T. H., and Djerassi, C. (1978). Minor and trace sterols in marine invertebrates. *Bioorg. Chem.* **7**, 453–479.

Campbell, C. E., and Kircher, H. W. (1980). *Senita cactus*: A plant with interrupted sterol biosynthetic pathways. *Phytochemistry* **19**, 2777–2779.

Djerassi, C. (1979). Recent advances in the mass spectrometry of steroids. *Pure Appl. Chem.* **50**, 171-184.

Djerassi, C. (1981). Recent studies in the marine sterol field. *Pure Appl. Chem.* **53**, 873–890.

Dumazer, M., Farines, M., and Soulier, J. (1986). Identification de sterols par spectrometrie de masse. *Rev. Fr. Corps Gras* **33**, 151–156.

Galli, G., and Maroni, S. (1967). Mass spectrometric investigations of some unsaturated sterols biosynthetically related to cholesterol. *Steroids* **10**, 189–197.

Garg, V. K., and Nes, W. R. (1984). Studies at the C-24 configurations of Δ^7-sterols in the seeds of *Cucurbita maxima*. *Phytochemistry* **23**, 2919–2923.

Gilpin, J. A., and McLafferty, F. W. (1957). Mass spectrometric analysis. Aliphatic aldehydes. *Anal. Chem.* **29**, 990–994.

Gupta, M. M., Lal, R. N., and Shukla, Y. N. (1981). 5α-stigmast-9(11)-en-3β-ol, a sterol from *Costus speciosus* roots. *Phytochemistry* **11**, 2557–2559.

Knights, B. A. (1967). Identification of plant sterols using combined GLC/mass spectrometry. *J. Gas Chromatogr.* **5**, 273–282.

Lenton, J. R., Goad, L. J., and Goodwin, T. W. (1973). Sterol of *Xanthoria parientina*: Evidence for two sterols' pools' and the identification of a novel C_{28} triene, ergosta-5,8,22-triene-3β-ol. *Phytochemistry* **12**, 1135–1140.

Li, L. N., Sjöstrand, U., and Djerassi, C. (1981). Minor and trace sterols in marine invertebrates. Isolation, structure, elucidation, and partial synthesis of 25-methylxestosterol. *J. Org. Chem.* **46**, 3867–3870.

Lin, Y. Y., and Smith, L. L. (1984). Chemical ionization mass spectrometry of steroids and other lipids. *Mass Spectrom. Rev.* **3**, 319–355.

Massey, I. J., and Djerassi, C. (1979). Structural and stereochemical applications of mass spectroscopy in the marine sterol field. Synthesis and electron impact induced mass spectral fragmentation of Δ^{24} and $\Delta^{24(28)}$-3β-hydroxy-Δ^5-sterols. *J. Org. Chem.* **44**, 2448–2456.

Matsumoto, T., Asano, S., and Itoh, T. (1983a). 24-methylene-25-methyl cholesterol, a sterol from the seeds of *Brassica juncea*. *Phytochemistry* **22**, 2619–2620.

Matsumoto, T., Osawa, Y., and Itoh, T. (1983b). A methyl-5α-cholest-8(14)-en-3β-ol from the seeds of *Capsicum annuum*. *Phytochemistry* **22**, 2621–2622.

Misso, N. L. A., and Goad, L. J. (1984). Investigations on the Δ^{23}, $\Delta^{24(28)}$ and Δ^{25}-sterols of Zea mays. *Phytochemistry* **23**, 73–82.

Nes, W. R. (1977). The biochemistry of plant sterols *Adv. Lipid Res.* **15**, 233–324.

Nes, W. R. (1985). A comparison of methods for the identification of sterols: Mass spectrometry. *In* "Methods in Enzymology" (J. H. Law and H. C. Rilling, eds.), Vol. III, pp. 27–29. Academic Press, Orlando, Florida.

Nes, W. R., Joseph, J. M., Landrey, J. R., Behzadons, S., and Conner, R. L. (1981). Steric Effects at C-20 and C-24 on the metabolism of sterols by *Tetrahymena pyriformis*. *J. Lipid Res.* **22**, 770–777.

Nes, W. O., Heupel, R. C., and Le, P. H. (1985). Biosynthesis of Ergosta-6(7),8(14),22(23)-trien-3β-ol by *Gibberella Fujikuroi*. Its importance to Ergosterols's metabolic Pathway. *J. Chem. Soc., Chem. Commun.* pp. 1431–1433.

Paterson, G. W. (1984). Chemical and physical methods in the analysis of plant sterols: Mass spectroscopy. *In* "Isopentenoids in Plants Biochemistry and Function" (W. D. Nes, ed.), pp. 307–312. Dekker, New York.

Paterson, G. W., Thompson, M. J., and Dutky, S. R. (1974). Two new sterols from *Cholerella ellipsoidea*. *Phytochemistry* **13**, 191–194.

Raederstorff, D. (1985). Renforcateurs membranaires de protozoaires. Thèse de doctorat, Université de Haute Alsace.

Schmitt, P., and Benveniste, P. (1979). Effect of AY-9944 on sterol biosynthesis in suspension cultures of Bramble cells. *Phytochemistry* **18**, 445-450.

Schmitt, P., Scheid, F., and Benveniste, P. (1980). Accumulation of $\Delta^{8,14}$-sterols in suspension cultures of bramble cells cultured with an azasterol antimycotic agent (A25822B). *Phytochemistry* **19**, 525–530.

Schmitt, P., Rahier, A., and Benveniste, P. (1982). Inhibition of sterol biosynthesis in suspension cultures of bramble cells. *Physiol. Veg.* **20**, 559–571.

Smith, A. G., Rubinstein, I., and Goad, L. J. (1973). The sterols of the *Echinoderm Asterias rubens*. *Biochem. J.* **135**, 443–455.

Taton, M., Benveniste, P., and Rahier, A. (1987). The use of rationally designed inhibitors to study sterol and triterpenoid biosynthesis. *Pure Appl. Chem.* **59**, 287–294.

Taylor, U. F., Kisic, A., Pascal, R. A., Izumi, A., Tsuda, M., and Schroepfer, G. J., Jr. (1981). Sterol synthesis: A simple method for the isolation of zymosterol from yeast and spectral properties of zymosterol. *J. Lipid Res.* **22**, 171–177.

Wyllie, S. G., and Djerassi, C. (1968). Mass spectrometry in structural and stereochemical problems. Mass spectrometric fragmentations typical of sterols with unsaturated side chains. *J. Org. Chem.* **33**, 305–313.

Zalkow, L. H.,. Cabat, G. A., Chetty, G. L., Ghosal, M., and Keen, G. (1968). Isolation of a novel sterol: Stigmasta-8(14),22-dien-3β-ol. *Tetrahedron Lett.* 5727–5729.

Zaretskii, Z. C. (1976). "Mass Spectrometry of Steroids." Wiley, New York.

Ziogas, B. N., Sisler, H. D., and Lusby, W. R. (1983). Sterol content and other characteristics of Pinaricin-resistant mutants of *Aspergillus nidulans*. *Pestic. Biochem. Physiol.* **24**, 320–329.

12

^{13}C-NMR Spectral Identification of Sterols

Toshihiro Akihisa (née Itoh)
College of Science and Technology, Nihon University
Chiyoda-ku, Tokyo, 101 Japan

I. INTRODUCTION

^{13}C nuclear magnetic resonance (NMR) spectra are considerably more useful than ^{1}H NMR spectra for structural analyses of complex molecules because of the great sensitivity of ^{13}C chemical shifts to structural changes and because each carbon atom in the molecule can usually be examined individually (Stothers, 1972). The ^{13}C chemical shifts of many steroids have been compiled and reviewed by Blunt and Stothers (1977) and Smith (1978). However, no systematic compilation of ^{13}C shift data of sterols has been published. This chapter compiles and reviews the ^{13}C chemical-shift data for a number of 4-demethylsterols with a hydroxyl group in the 3 position (including phytosterols) and their possible biosynthetic intermediates, that is, 4-monomethyl- and 4,4-dimethylsterols (Table 1). The discussion includes methods of signal assignments and ^{13}C chemical-shift compilations of sterols.

Table 1 Structural codes and names of sterols for which ^{13}C chemical shifts are compiled in the subsequent tables

Structural Code	Sterol Name
4-Demethylsterol	
(**1a**)	Cholestanol
(**2a**)	Epicholestanol
(**3a**)	Coprostanol
(**4a**)	Cholest-4-enol
(**5a**)	Cholesterol
(**5b**)	17(20)*E*-Dehydrocholesterol
(**5c**)	20(22)*Z*-Dehydrocholesterol
(**5d**)	20(22)*E*-Dehydrocholesterol
(**5e**)	22*E*-Dehydrocholesterol
(**5f**)	22*Z*-Dehydrocholesterol
(**5g**)	Desmosterol
(**5h**)	Campersterol
(**5i**)	22-Dihydrobrassicasterol
(**5j**)	22*E*-Dehydrocampesterol
(**5k**)	Brassicasterol
(**5l**)	24-Methylenecholesterol
(**5m**)	24-Methyldesmosterol
(**5n**)	Sitosterol
(**5o**)	Clionasterol
(**5p**)	Stigmasterol
(**5q**)	Poriferasterol
(**5r**)	Fucosterol
(**5s**)	Isofucosterol
(**5t**)	Clerosterol
(**5u**)	22*E*-Dehydroclerosterol
(**5v**)	24*E*-Propylidenecholesterol
(**6a**)	Lathosterol
(**7a**)	Cholest-8-enol
(**8a**)	Cholest-8(14)-enol
(**9k**)	Ergosterol
(**10a**)	Cholesta-7,14-dienol
(**11k**)	24β-Methylcholesta-7,9(11),22*E*-trienol
(**12a**)	Cholesta-8,14-dienol
(**13a**)	Cholesta-6,8,14-trienol
(**14a**)	Pollinastanol
(**15a**)	14α-Methylcholest-9(11)-enol
4-Monomethylsterol	
(**16a**)	4α-Methylcholestanol
(**17a**)	Lophenol
(**18a**)	4β-Methylcholestanol
(**19l**)	Cycloeucalenol
(**20l**)	Obtusifoliol
(**21a**)	31-Norlanost-9(11)-enol
4,4-Dimethylsterol	
(**22a**)	4,4-Dimethylcholestanol
(**23a**)	Lanostanol
(**24a**)	Cycloartanol
(**25a**)	24-Dihydrolanosterol
(**26a**)	24-Dihydroagnosterol

Sources for the ^{13}C-NMR data: (**11k**) (Abraham and Monasterios, 1974); (**5n**), (**5o**) (Akihisa *et al.*, 1986); (**5l**), (**5n**), (**5t**), (**5u**), (**17a**) (T. Akihisa, T. Tamura, and T. Matsumoto, unpublished results); (**5c**), (**5d**) (Anderson *et al.*, 1976); (**25a**) (Beierbeck *et al.*, 1977); (**3a**) (Blunt and Stothers, 1977); (**9k**) (Cushley and Filipenko, 1979); (**2a**) (Eggert *et al.*, 1976); (**15a**), (**21a**) (Goad *et al.*, 1985); (**16a**), (**18a**), (**22a**) (Iida *et al.*, 1982); (**201**) (Itoh *et al.*, 1981); (**14a**) (Khuong-Huu *et al.*, 1975); (**24a**) (Khuong-Huu *et al.*, 1975; Seo *et al.*, 1987); (**19l**) (Kikuchi *et al.*, 1986); (**23a**), (**26a**) (Knight, 1974); (**5b**) (Kobayashi *et al.*, 1979); (**5v**) (Kokke *et al.*, 1984): (**13a**) (Parish *et al.*, 1979); (**5r**), (**5s**) (Ricca and Nicotra, 1978); (**5l**), (**5n**)–(**5p**) (Seo *et al.*, 1983); (**1a**), (**4a**), (**5a**)–(**8a**), (**10a**), (**12a**) (Tsuda and Schroepfer), 1979b); (**5e**)–(**5k**), (**5p**), (**5q**) (Wright *et al.*, 1978).

II. METHODS FOR SIGNAL ASSIGNMENTS

The ^{13}C-NMR spectra of steroids and sterols are generally recorded in $CDCl_3$ with broadband proton decoupling. But, under these conditions, ^{13}C signals can be differentiated only on the basis of their relative intensity and chemical shifts, and the number of protons bonded to each carbon cannot be determined. Every signal in a broadband decoupled spectra can be assigned to a specific carbon by using one or a combination of several of the techniques described in the following sections.

A. Single-Frequency Off-Resonance Decoupled Technique and Others

The single-frequency off-resonance decoupled (SFORD) techniques, in which proton decoupling is done at the frequency of an "off-resonance" position (usually 1 or 2 kHz from the center of the proton spectrum), has the effect of removing the ^{13}C-^{1}H long-range couplings while retaining the direct couplings, although these are reduced from their true values ($J \sim$ 120–250 Hz) to small residual couplings ($J_r \sim$ 20–40 Hz). Thus, single peaks in a broadband decoupled spectrum become quartets, triplets, doublets, or remain singlets for methyl (CH_3), methylene (CH_2), methine (CH), and quarternary (C) carbons, respectively. However, in a congested spectral region, the overlap of multiplets and the residual line broadening often associated with the SFORD technique can make assignment of multiplicity very difficult.

Newly devised techniques, such as the attached proton test (APT), the insensitive nuclei enhanced by polarization transfer (INEPT), the distortionless enhancement by polarization transfer (DEPT), and the spin-echo Fourier transfer (SEFT), can be used to differentiate among methyl, methylene, methine, and quaternary carbons whenever strong overlap of partially decoupled multiplets in SFORD spectra makes the assignment difficult. Various two-dimensional NMR techniques, such as J-resolved ^{13}C, ^{13}C-^{13}C correlated, and ^{1}H-^{13}C correlated pulse techniques, have recently been introduced, which greatly increase the amount of information that can be extracted from complex spectra. The two-dimensional techniques offer unambiguous ^{13}C assignment, the establishment of C—C bonds from "carbon-carbon" connectivity plots, and great improvements of proton "resolution" from ^{1}H-^{13}C correlated spectra. These and other new NMR techniques are the subjects of recent reviews by Benn and Günther (1983), Morris (1986), and Shoolery (1984).

B. ^{13}C Chemical-Shift Range

The ^{13}C nuclei in steroids and sterols give signals in a wide range ($\sim$200 ppm), and each type of ^{13}C nucleus possesses a characteristic chemical-shift region that allows unambiguous assignment of some signals in the spectra simply on the basis of chemical-shift values. Thus, saturated carbons give ^{13}C signals at δ 10–60 ppm (from TMS), olefinic carbons at 120–170 ppm, carbinol carbons at 65–80 ppm, and carbonyl carbons at 170–220 ppm, with ketones at the low-field end and esters at the high-field end (Blunt and Stothers, 1977). Further assignments in this group cannot be made unambiguously on the basis of their chemical shifts alone, though it may be noted that the more highly substituted carbons resonate at the lower-field end of this range whereas the less substituted carbons, such as the methyl carbons, resonate at the high-field end.

C. Comparison of Spectra with Closely Related Compounds

One of the powerful features of ^{13}C spectra is the finding that within a family of compounds, a given substituent usually produces remarkably similar effects on the chemical shifts of the carbons at and near the site of substitution. In general, the substituent effects (the α-, β-, and γ-effects) are rapidly attenuated with increasing distance from the site of substitution. These substituent effects are consistent for steroids and sterols; hence, a useful approach to ^{13}C spectral assignments is to make comparisons with closely related compounds .

D. Chemical-Shift Rules

From a comparison of chemical-shift data of many ^{13}C-NMR spectra of steroids, various substituent effects have been deduced (Blunt and Stothers, 1977; Smith, 1978; Stothers, 1972). In general, the chemical shifts of carbons attached directly to various substituents reflect the electronegativity of the given substituents (the α-effect). In most cases the α-(allylic) effect produces deshielding. Carbons β (homallylic) to the point of substituent attachment are, with few exceptions, also deshielded (the β-effect). For carbons that are three bonds away from the carbon of interest, a more complex pattern of behavior is observed (the γ-effect). δ-Substituent effects are generally small. Smith (1978) has provided a simple set of guidelines for predicting ^{13}C chemical shifts of the skeletons and alkyl side chains of steroids; and Tsuda and Schroepfer (1979a) have presented several chemical-shift rules for allylic carbons, homoallylic carbons, and olefinic carbons of sterols. Using the ^{13}C prediction rules for saturated hydrocarbons presented by Lindeman and Adams (1971) and Grant and Paul (1964), one can calculate the ^{13}C chemical shifts of C_7-C_{11} saturated sterol side chains (Kelecom, 1980).

E. Derivatization

Information for signal assignment can be obtained by comparing the chemical shifts of the original compound with those of its derivatives. Acetylation has been successfully used, at least for the assignment of the hydroxyl-bearing carbon and adjacent carbons (Stothers, 1972). On acetylation, the 3β hydroxyl group of sterols produces a characteristic downfield shift of C-3 signals (~ 3 ppm), an upfield shift of the β-carbon (C-2 and C-4) signals (~ 4 ppm), and a smaller upfield shift of the γ-carbon (C-1 and C-5) signals (~ 0.3 ppm), whereas all other resonances are unchanged within 0.2 ppm (Abraham and Monasterios, 1974). For some sterols, differences in shift values between carbons of the free sterol and of its acetate are given in Table 2. A comparison of ^{13}C chemical-shift data of the free hydroxy compounds and their acetate, benzoate, 3-oxo, and 2α-brom-3-oxo derivatives has facilitated the assignment of the A-ring and C-4,4 dimethyl carbon signals of 4,4-dimethylsterols (Knight, 1974).

F. Lanthanide-Shift Reagent

The use of lanthanide-shift reagents (LSR) to simplify ^{13}C-NMR spectra is one of the most promising methods for structural analysis of molecules. Ytterbium-, europium-, and praseodymium-based reagents have been successfully used in the examination of

Table 2a ^{13}C Chemical shifts of some 4-demethylsterols

Carbons	(1a)	(2a)	(3a)	(4a)	(5a)	(6a)	(7a)	(8a)	(9k)	(10a)	(11k)	(12a)	(13a)	(14a)[e]	(15a)[e]
1	37.0	32.2	30.0	35.3	37.2	37.1	35.1	36.5	38.5	36.7	34.6	35.2	34.0	31.4[a]	35.3
		(0.7)		(−0.4)	(−0.3)	(−0.3	(−0.3)	(−0.3)	(−0.5)	(−0.2)	(−0.3)				
2	31.5	29.1	27.9	29.4	31.5	31.3	31.5	31.5	32.1	31.4	31.6	31.3	31.3	30.4[a]	27.2
		(−3.0)		(−4.4)	(−3.8)	(−3.9)	(−4.0)	(−4.0)	(−4.0)	(−3.9)	(−4.0)				
3	72.1	66.5	67.1	67.8	71.4	70.7	70.9	71.0	70.5	70.6	70.3	70.7	70.8	73.7	73.6
		(3.5)		(2.9)	(2.4)	(2.3)	(2.4)	(2.4)	(2.2)	(2.6)	(2.8)				
4	33.2	35.9[a]	33.6	123.1	42.2	37.8	38.2	38.2	40.9	37.8	37.7	37.9	35.9	38.5	34.3
		(−3.0)		(−4.4)	(−4.1)	(−4.0)	(−4.1)	(−4.2)	(−4.3)	(−4.1)	(−4.1)				
5	44.8	39.1	36.6	147.3	140.5	40.2	40.7	44.2	139.8	39.6	39.1	40.8	41.5	37.1	42.9
		(1.0)		(1.9)	(−1.1)	(−0.2)	(−0.2)	(−0.2)	(−1.5)	(−0.2)					
6	23.7	28.6	26.3	32.2	121.3	29.6	25.4	28.9	119.7	30.2	29.8	25.1	129.6	28.1[b]	28.5
					(1.1)										
7	32.1	32.0	26.7	33.0	31.8	117.2	27.1	29.6	116.4	119.9[a]	118.0[a]	26.4	124.0	27.8[b]	28.0
8	35.4[a]	35.5	35.7	35.9	31.8	139.3	128.0	126.1	141.3	134.2	135.7[b]	122.7	123.0	46.1	41.9
9	54.3	54.3	39.8	54.4	50.0	49.4	134.8	49.2	46.3	49.6	143.4[b]	140.4	142.2	23.5	145.9
10	35.5[a]	36.1	35.1	37.2	36.4	34.1	35.6	36.7	37.1	33.8	35.6	36.3	36.5	29.8	38.1
11	21.3	20.8	21.2	21.0	21.0	21.5	22.7	19.9	21.1	20.9	118.8[a]	21.7	22.0	24.6[c]	116.6
12	40.0	40.1	40.3	39.8	39.7	39.5	36.9	37.2	39.2	40.1	42.1	36.8	36.0	35.2	37.3
13	42.5	42.6	42.7	42.4	42.2	43.2	42.0	42.6	42.9	46.3	42.7	44.8	44.8	45.3	44.4
14	56.4	56.5	56.7	56.1	56.6	54.9	51.8	142.4	54.6	151.7	51.5	150.7	148.1	49.0	47.2
15	24.2	24.2	24.2	24.2	24.2	22.9	23.9	25.7	23.0	119.2[a]	23.1	117.1	117.9	32.9	34.0
16	28.2	28.2	28.3	28.2	28.2	27.9	28.7	27.0	28.3	35.1	28.8	35.7	35.9	27.1	27.6
17	56.2	56.2	56.4	56.1	56.1	56.1	54.8	56.8	55.9	58.6	56.0	57.0	57.1	52.3	51.1
18	12.1	12.1	12.1	12.0	11.8	11.8	11.2	18.2	12.1	16.4	11.4	15.6	15.5	17.5[d]	14.5
19	12.3	11.2	23.9	18.9	19.2	12.9	17.8	12.8	16.3	12.3	19.3	18.2	13.3	25.7[c]	19.2
20	35.7	35.8[a]	35.8	35.7	35.7	36.1	36.2	34.4	40.4	34.0	40.3	33.8	34.0	36.2	36.2
21	18.7	18.7	18.7	18.6	18.7	18.8	18.7	19.0	21.2	18.9	19.6	18.7	18.9	18.5[d]	18.4
22	36.1	36.2	36.2	36.1	36.1	36.1	36.1	35.9	135.6	36.0	135.0	35.9	36.0	36.5	36.6
23	23.8	23.9	23.9	23.8	23.8	23.9	23.7	23.7	132.1	23.7	131.5	23.6	23.7	24.2	24.2
24	39.5	39.5	39.5	39.4	39.4	39.4	39.4	39.5	42.9	39.4	42.7	39.3	39.4	39.6	39.6
25	28.0	28.0	28.0	27.9	27.9	27.9	27.9	27.9	33.1	27.9	32.9	27.8	27.9	28.1	28.0
26	22.5	22.5	22.5	22.5	22.5	22.5	22.4	22.5	22.0	22.5	20.6	22.4	22.5	22.9	22.6
27	22.8	22.8	22.8	22.8	22.7	22.7	22.7	22.7	19.7	22.7	19.8	22.6	22.7	22.9	22.8
28									17.6		17.6				
30															
31															
32														19.0[d]	18.4
$COCH_3$														170.0	170.6
$COCH_3$														21.5	21.4

Note: In ppm downfield from TMS (solvent $CDCl_3$). Figures in parentheses denote shifts from the alcohol values upon acetylation; positive value shows downfield shift and negative value indicates upfield shift.

[a–d] In some columns, the assignment of chemical shifts may be interchanged from certain sets of close-lying peaks; all elements of such a set have the same superscript (a, b, c, or d).

[e] Data for the acetyl derivatives.

Table 2b ^{13}C Chemical shifts of some 4-monomethyl- and 4,4-dimethylsterols

	4-Monomethylsterol						4,4-Dimethylsterol				
Carbons	(**16a**)	(**17a**)	(**18a**)	(**19l**)	(**20l**)	(**21a**)	(**22a**)	(**23a**)	(**24a**)	(**25a**)	(**26a**)
1	36.9	36.6	37.7	30.9	34.9	35.5	37.5	37.7	31.9	35.6	35.8
	(−0.4)		(−0.2)	(−0.4)	(−0.3)		(−0.4)		(−0.4)	(−0.3)	
2	31.2	27.1	26.4	34.9	31.1	31.3	27.7	27.7	30.3	27.7	28.2
	(−4.1)		(−3.5)	(−3.9)	(−4.0)		(−3.8)		(−3.6)	(−3.5)	
3	76.6	78.4	74.1	76.6	76.4	76.5	79.0	79.1	78.5	79.0	79.0
	(2.3)		(2.6)	(2.2)	(2.3)		(1.8)		(1.8)	(1.9)	
4	39.4	37.0	40.5	44.7	39.2	39.6	38.9	39.0	40.3	38.9	38.5
	(−3.2)		(−3.0)	(−3.1)	(−3.2)		(−1.0)		(−0.9)	(−1.0)	
5	51.1	46.7	48.6	43.4	47.0	49.5	55.0	55.1	47.0	50.4	49.2
6	24.2	26.6	27.2	24.7	20.7	24.2	20.7	18.3	21.0	19.1	23.0
7	32.2	117.1	32.8	25.2	28.2	28.1	33.0	29.0	26.0	26.5	120.1
8	36.1	139.1	36.0	46.9	133.5[a]	41.5	35.2	38.7	47.8	134.4	142.7
9	54.7	49.4	56.1	23.6	134.5[a]	146.6	56.7	48.8	20.0	134.4	145.9
10	34.9	34.7	35.8	29.7	36.3	38.8	36.6	37.2	26.0	37.0	37.4
11	21.1	21.3	20.7	27.1	21.7	116.4	21.4	20.1	26.5	21.0	116.3
12	40.2	39.5	40.0	33.0	25.5	37.5	40.1	21.7	32.8	31.0	37.9
13	42.6	43.3	42.6	45.5	44.5	44.4	42.6	45.3	45.1	44.5	43.8
14	56.6[a]	54.9	56.7	49.0	49.8	47.2	56.4	48.0	48.7	49.8	50.4
15	24.2	22.9	24.3	35.4	31.2	34.0	24.3	33.7	35.5	30.8	28.1
16	28.3	28.0	28.2	28.2	31.0	27.5	28.2	32.2	28.0	28.2	31.6
17	56.4[a]	56.1	56.4	52.3	50.3	51.2	56.4	51.1	52.2	50.5	51.1
18	12.0	11.9	12.1	17.8[a]	15.7	14.5	12.0	16.3	17.9	15.8	15.7
19	13.4	14.0	14.8	27.3	18.7[b]	20.6	14.4	13.9	29.8	18.3	22.8
20	35.8	36.2[a]	35.8	36.2	36.4	36.2	35.8	36.2	36.0	36.5	36.5
21	18.7	18.8	18.7	18.4	18.2[b]	18.5	18.7	18.7	18.3	18.7	18.6
22	36.2	36.1[a]	36.2	35.1	34.9	36.7	36.3	36.7	36.4	36.5	36.3
23	23.9	23.9	23.9	31.4	30.7	24.2	23.9	24.1	24.0	24.1	24.1
24	39.5	39.5	39.5	156.9	156.8	39.6	39.5	39.6	39.4	39.5	39.5
25	28.0	28.0	28.0	33.9	33.8	28.1	18.0	28.0	28.0	28.0	28.1
26	22.5	22.6	22.5	22.1[a]	21.8[c]	22.6	22.5	22.6	22.5	22.5	22.8
27	22.7	22.8	22.7	21.9[a]	22.0[c]	22.8	22.7	22.8	22.7	22.8	22.6
28				106.1	105.9						
30	15.1	15.1		14.5	15.0	15.3	28.2	28.3	25.4	27.9	27.9
31			8.8				15.5	15.6	14.0	15.4	15.8
			(0.8)				(1.1)		(1.1)	(1.2)	
32				19.2	24.4	18.5		14.4	19.3	24.3	25.6
$COCH_3$		170.8									
$COCH_3$		21.3									

Note: See footnotes for Table 2a.

steroid spectra, with a preference for the use of ytterbium for downfield shifts and praseodymium for upfield shifts because of the smaller contact shifts generated by these lanthanides (Blunt and Stothers, 1977; Smith, 1978). The usual approach is to determine the relative distances of each carbon from the lanthanide atom by measuring the incremental shifts of the chemical shift on successive additions of known quantities of the shift reagent to the substrate solution. As for 3-hydroxy steroids, the lanthanide-induced shifts (LIS) were largest at the carbinol carbon and

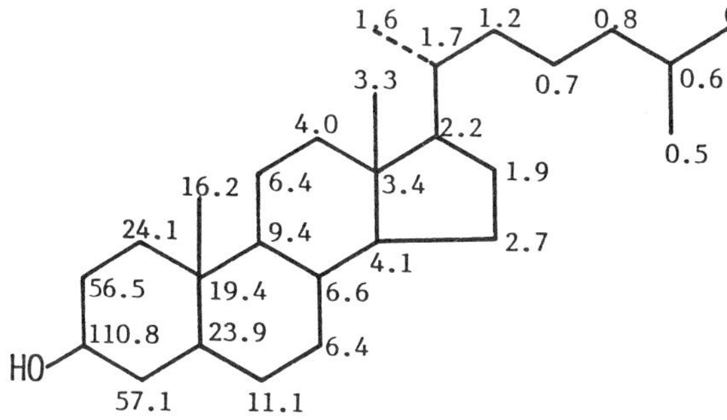

Figure 1 Yb(dpm)$_3$-induced ^{13}C-NMR shifts (ppm; substrate: LSR = 1:1 mol/mol) in cholestanol (**1a**).

are expected to decrease qualitatively in the following carbon order: $3 > 2 \sim 4 > 1 \sim 5 > 6 \sim 10 \sim 19 > 7 \sim 8 \sim 9 \sim 11 > 12 \sim 13 \sim 14 \sim 18 > 15 \sim 16 \sim 17$ (ApSimon *et al.*, 1973; Chadwick and Williams, 1974; Smith, 1978). The LIS of side chain ^{13}C signals are smaller than those of ring system signals. An example of the LIS values (ppm; substrate: LSR = 1:1 mol/mol) induced by Yb(dpm)$_3$ for the carbon signals of cholestanol (**1a**) is shown in Fig. 1 (Chadwick and Williams, 1974).

G. Spin-Lattice Relaxation Times

When signal assignments are difficult or impossible by the SFORD experiment, the use of spin-lattice relaxation time (T_1) data, which correlate with carbon type (CH_3, CH_2, CH, C) as well as structural location (e.g., rings or side chain), may be helpful (Blunt and Stothers, 1977; Smith, 1978; Stothers, 1972). As for sterols, the T_1 values for skeletal carbons depend on the number of attached hydrogens, with methylene carbons having T_1 values one-half of those found for methine carbons. Quaternary carbons have considerably larger T_1 values, and methyl carbons and carbons near the end of the sterol side chain also have T_1 values larger than those for the skeletal protonated carbons because of the extra degrees of freedom at motion associated with the former type of carbon. Thus, the comparison of the T_1 values can be useful for distinguishing various carbon types. The T_1 values of cholestanol (**1a**) determined using a 180°-τ-90° pulse sequence are shown in Fig. 2 (Chadwick and Williams, 1974).

H. Isotopic Labeling

Isotopic labeling has proved useful in making unequivocal assignments. The use of ^{13}C-labeled precursor compounds in biosynthetic studies of sterols not only enhances the signal intensity of a specifed carbon but also introduces ^{13}C-^{13}C coupling (Cushley and Filipenko, 1976; Nicotra *et al.*, 1985; Popjak *et al.*, 1977; Seo *et al.*, 1983). Specific deuteration is also an effective tool for identifying particular carbons. The signals for carbons α to carbonyl groups in several steroid ketones were identified in this way

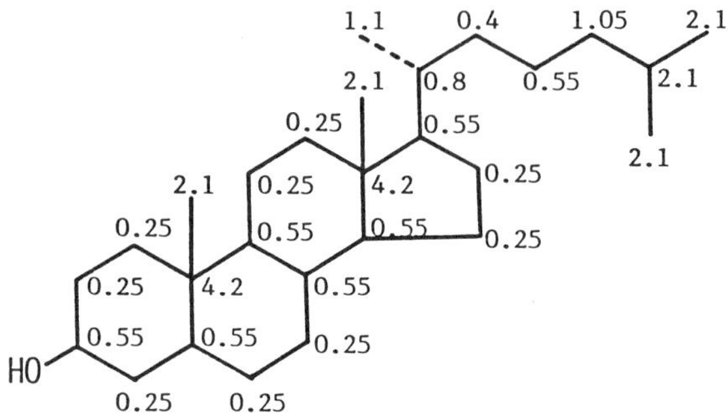

Figure 2 Relaxation times [T_1 (s)] of cholestanol (**1a**) obtained with 180°-τ-90° pulse sequence.

(Reich *et al.*, 1969). The signal for the deuterated carbon essentially disappears at the attainable signal-to-noise ratios (S/N) because of quadrupole broadening spin-spin splitting, and decreased Overhauser enhancement.

I. Solvent Effects

It may be useful to discuss the effects of the solvent on the ^{13}C chemical shift. Solvent effects are, in general, small for the ^{13}C-NMR shielding but are not negligible, especially for those carbons bearing polar substituents, such as hydroxyl, or polarizable groups such as double bonds (Blunt and Stothers, 1977). Solvent effects were investigated on ^{13}C-NMR spectra of cholesterol (**5a**) using the following solvents: benzene, pyridine, *p*-dioxane, $CHCl_3$, and CCl_4 (Mantsch and Smith, 1973). All carbon atoms were subject to solvent effects of varying sign and magnitude. The most solvent-sensitive carbons are the hydroxyl-bearing C-3 and the unsaturated C-6, both of which are shifted downfield by about 1 ppm in $CHCl_3$ and CCl_4 compared with benzene, pyridine, or *p*-dioxane. The chemical shifts in CCl_4 and $CHCl_3$ are nearly always identical (differences are less than 0.1 ppm) to those occurring in $CHCl_3$ at a slightly lower field.

III. ^{13}C CHEMICAL-SHIFT DATA OF STEROLS

Table 1 and Fig. 3 list the names (most of which are trivial names) and structures of the 47 sterols (4-demethyl-, 4-monomethyl-, and 4,4-dimethylsterols) for which ^{13}C shift data are compiled in Tables 2 and 3. All shift data in Tables 2 and 3 are determined in $CDCl_3$ and are given in ppm, as positive numbers representing downfield shifts from TMS. Most of the chemical-shift data have been published previously. For some sterols, the signal assignments were made in the author's laboratory using combinations of the techniques described in the previous section (T. Akihisa, T. Tamura, and T. Matsumoto, unpublished results). In some cases, the original assignments have been revised, either in the light of subsequent studies on the same sterols or to gain consistency with unambiguous assignments for closely related sterols.

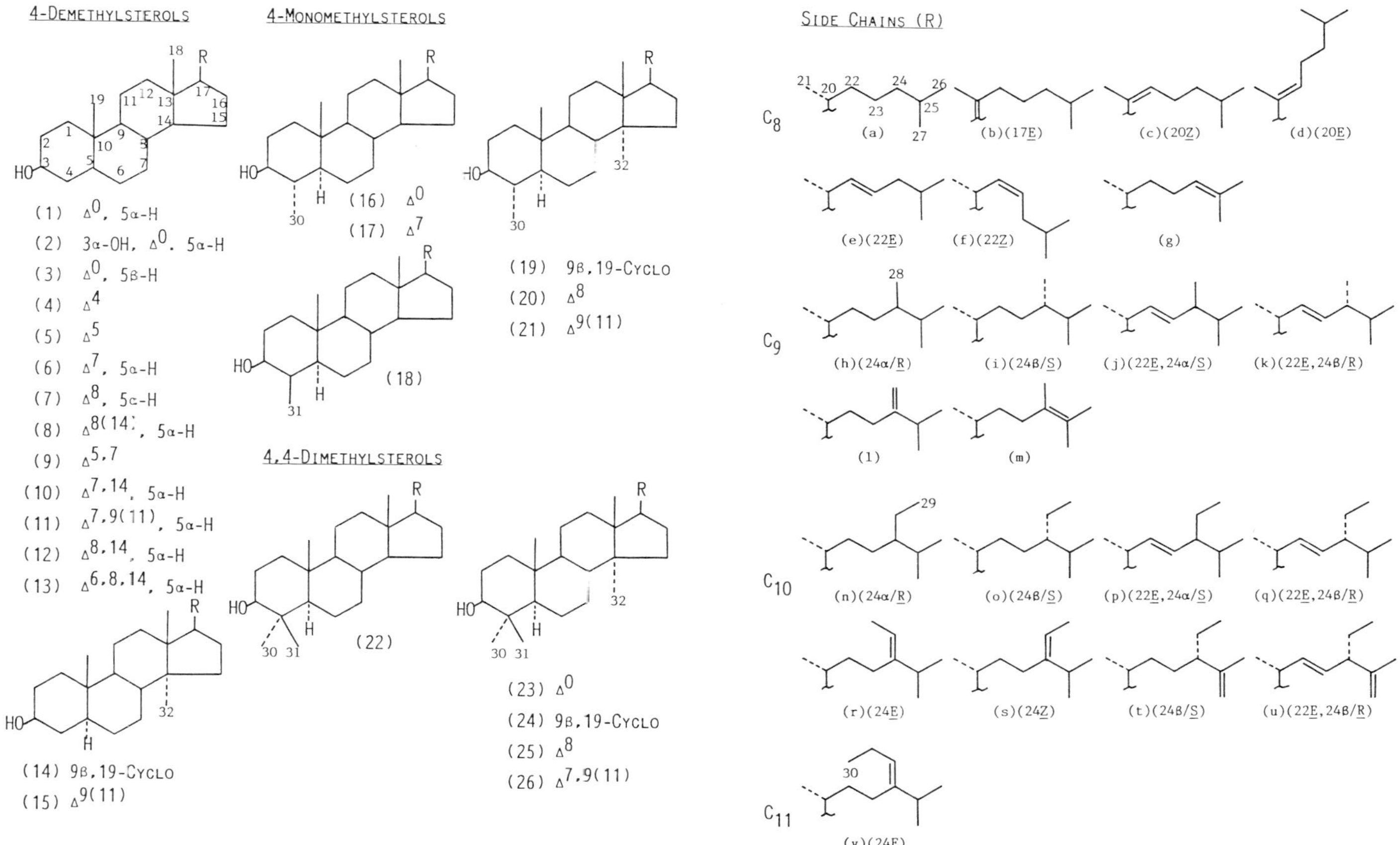

Figure 3 Structures of skeletons and side chains of sterols.

Table 3 ^{13}C Chemical shifts of C_8-C_{11} side chains and part of skeletons of some Δ^5-sterols

	C_8							C_9						C_{10}								C_{11}
Carbons	(**5a**)	(**5b**)[a]	(**5c**)	(**5d**)	(**5e**)	(**5f**)	(**5g**)	(**5h**)	(**5i**)	(**5j**)	(**5k**)	(**5l**)[a]	(**5m**)[a]	(**5n**)[a]	(**5o**)	(**5p**)	(**5q**)	(**5r**)	(**5s**)	(**5t**)[a]	(**5u**)[a]	(**5v**)
15	24.2	24.5	24.7	24.5	24.3	24.3	24.4	24.4	24.4	24.4	24.4	24.3	24.3	24.3	24.3	24.4	24.4	24.3	24.3	24.3	24.3	24.3
16	28.2	29.5	26.3	26.0	28.6	28.1	28.3	28.3	28.3	28.9	28.6	28.2	28.2	28.2	28.2	29.0	28.8	28.2	28.2	28.2	28.7	28.2
17	56.1	143.0	51.2	59.1	56.0	56.3	56.2	56.2	56.1	56.1	56.1	56.0	55.8	56.0	56.0	56.1	56.1	55.7	55.9	56.0	55.8	55.7
18	11.8	16.5	14.0	13.0	12.1	12.2	12.0	11.9	11.9	12.1	12.1	11.9	11.8	11.9	11.9	12.1	12.1	11.9	11.9	12.1	12.1	11.8
20	35.7	125.0	134.2	134.1	40.1	34.3	36.2	36.0	36.3	40.3	40.2	35.8	36.0	36.2	36.3	40.5	40.5	36.4	36.1	35.5	40.2	35.8
21	18.7	17.5	22.8	17.8	20.9	20.7	18.7	18.8	19.0	21.1	21.1	18.7	18.8	18.8	18.8	21.1	21.0	18.7	18.8	18.7	20.8	18.7
22	36.1	36.8	129.6	126.1	138.1	137.2	35.7	33.8	33.8	136.1	135.8	34.7	34.3	33.9	33.9	138.4	138.3	35.2	35.9	33.6	137.1	34.6
23	23.8	25.3	24.7	24.9	126.2	125.5	24.8	30.4	30.7	131.8	131.8	31.0	31.1	26.1	26.4	129.3	129.4	25.7	27.9	29.4	130.0	26.0
24	39.4	39.1	38.5	38.9	42.0	36.8	125.3	38.9	39.2	43.1	42.9	156.7	128.3	45.8	46.1	51.3	51.3	146.7	145.7	49.5	52.0	145.4
25	27.9	27.9	28.0	28.0	28.6	28.8	130.9	32.5	31.5	33.3	33.2	33.8	123.2	29.2	29.0	31.9	31.9	34.8	28.6	147.4	148.4	36.4
26	22.5	22.7	22.6	22.6	22.3	22.4	17.7	20.3	17.7	19.7	20.0	21.9	20.0	19.8	19.6	21.3	19.0	22.2	21.1	17.8	20.3	22.3
27	22.7	22.7	22.6	22.6	22.3	22.6	25.7	18.3	20.6	20.2	19.7	22.0	20.5	19.0	19.0	19.0	21.2	22.1	21.1	111.4	109.6	22.2
28								15.4	15.5	18.1	17.7	105.9	18.4	23.1	23.0	25.4	25.4	115.4	116.3	26.5	25.7	123.8
29														12.0	12.3	12.3	12.4	13.1	12.7	11.9	12.2	20.9
30																						14.8

Note: In ppm downfield from TMS (solvent $CDCl_3$). Most of the ^{13}C chemical shifts of skeletal carbon signals were omitted from this table because these shifts were almost consistent with those of cholesterol (**5a**) or its acetate.

[a] Data for the acetyl derivatives.

A. Skeletal Carbon Chemical Shifts

Table 2 shows the ^{13}C chemical shifts of 26 sterols, all of which are 3β-monohydroxy compounds except (**2a**), which is a 3α-hydroxy steroid. The sterols in Table 2 have 26 different skeletons: fifteen 4-demethylsterols [skeletons (**1**)–(**15**)], six 4-monomethylsterols [(**16**)–(**21**)], and five 4,4-dimethylsterols [(**22**)–(**26**)]. Whereas most shift data correspond to the free alcohols, some correspond to the acetyl derivatives. When shift data for free sterols and for their acetates are available, the characteristic shift data upon acetylation (which are defined as shifts from the alcohol values) are presented in parentheses. Positive values of the shifts denote downfield shifts whereas negative values indicate upfield shifts. The shift data in Table 2 are extremely useful for determining the skeletal structures of unknown sterols because substituents occurring in the side chain, such as alkylation at C-24, have little, if any, effect on the shielding of skeletal carbons unless the substituents occur in close proximity to the skeleton, such as the $\Delta^{20(22)}$ [(**c**), (**d**)] double bond (cf. Table 3).

B. Side-Chain Carbon Chemical Shifts

The chemical-shift data of side-chain carbons together with the D-ring (C-15, C-16, and C-17) and C-18 carbons of twenty-two Δ^5-sterols, which possess either of the twenty-two C_8-C_{11} side chains (**a**)–(**v**), are listed in Table 3. The ^{13}C shift data of side-chain carbons allow unambiguous differentiation between each of the double-bond isomers of $\Delta^{20(22)}$-[(**c**) and (**d**)], Δ^{22}-[(**e**) and (**f**)], and 24-ethylidene-[(**r**) and (**s**)] sterols. Various C-24 alkylated sterols occur as the major sterols in plants and microorganisms, and both C-24 diastereoisomers have been found to occur naturally (Nes and McKean, 1977). Although high-resolution ^{1}H-NMR spectroscopy (frequency $\gtrsim$220 MHz) has been used for the differentiation and identification of C-24 epimers of 24-alkylsterols (Akihisa *et al.*, 1986; Chiu and Patterson, 1981; Nes *et al.*, 1977; Rubinstein *et al.*, 1976), the ^{13}C shift data have proven more useful (Akihisa *et al.*, 1986; Koizumi *et al.*, 1979; Wright *et al.*, 1978). For the 24-methylsterols, (**5h**) and (**5i**), the C-28 carbon signal and other side-chain signals provide a basis for assigning the configuration at C-24. The C-24 diastereoisomers of the 24-ethylsterols, (**5n**) and (**5o**), are readily distinguishable on the basis of the shift data of the carbon signals of C-23–C-26 and C-29. The most useful ^{13}C signals for distinguishing the epimers of the 24-methyl-Δ^{22}-sterols, (**5j**) and (**5k**), are those of C-28 and C-16. These signals are more shielded in the 24β-epimer (0.4 and 0.3 ppm, respectively). Although the differences between the ^{13}C shift data of the epimers of the 24-ethyl-Δ^{22}-sterols, (**5p**) and (**5q**), were not so pronounced, the configuration at C-24 can be determined by the C-16 and C-29 resonances. 24-Alkylsterols occur often as diastereoisomeric mixtures in organisms (Nes and McKean, 1977), and ^{13}C-NMR spectroscopy has been used successfully for the determination of the compositions of epimeric mixtures (Akihisa *et al.*, 1986; Wright *et al.*, 1978).

The ^{13}C shift data of the side chain carbons in Table 3 provide the basis for the determination of the side-chain structures of sterols with various skeletal substitutions since many structural changes (especially in rings A, B, and C) of the sterol appear to have little or no effect on the chemical shift of the side-chain resonances.

C. Characteristic ^{13}C Chemical-Shift Ranges of Sterols

Table 4 summarizes the chemical-shift ranges for the resonances of the carbons of a number of the sterols compiled in this review. The characteristic chemical-shift range in each of the saturated, carbinol, and olefinic carbon resonance regions provides important information for the structural analysis of sterols. Note that the cyclopropane ring of 9β,19-cyclosterols causes a considerable upfield shift of the C-9 and C-10 quaternary carbons and that 4-demethyl-, 4-monomethyl-, and 4,4-dimethylsterols can be differentiated on the basis of the shift of the C-3 (carbinol) carbon. Many useful empirical rules for the shifts of the carbons of steroids and sterols have already been established (Blunt and Stothers, 1977; Smith, 1978; Tsuda and Schroepfer, 1979a). Further work using the data in Tables 2 and 3 might result in the formulation of additional rules.

Table 4 Characteristic ^{13}C chemical-shift range of sterols

Carbon Types		Approximate ^{13}C Chemical-shift range (δ, ppm)
$—CH_3$		9–29
$—CH_2—$		18–42
>CH—		28–59
>C<		34–50
	Cyclopropyl >C<	20–30
>CH—OH (C-3)	4-Demethylsterol	66–71
	4-Monomethylsterol	74–77
	4,4-Dimethylsterol	78–79
H_2C^*=C<		106–111
—HC*=C	—HC*=C<	115–130
	—HC*=CH—	126–138
>C*=C	>C*=C<	123–143
	>C*=CH—	131–152
	$>C^*=CH_2$	147–157
$O=C^*(CH_3)O—$		170–171

Note: Summarized using ^{13}C shift data of the sterols listed in Tables 2 and 3.

ACKNOWLEDGMENTS

The author is grateful to Dr. W. C. M. C. Kokke (Smith Kline and French Laboratories, Philadelphia) for his careful examination of the manuscript.

REFERENCES

Abraham, R. J., and Monasterios, J. R. (1974). ^{13}C Nuclear magnetic resonance spectra of some ergosta-dienes and -trienes. *J. Chem. Soc., Perkin Trans. 2* pp. 662–665.

Akihisa, T., Thakur, S., Rosenstein, F. U., and Matsumoto, T. (1986). Sterols of Cucurbitaceae: The configurations at C-24 of 24-alkyl-Δ^5-, Δ^7- and Δ^8-sterols. *Lipids* **21**, 39–47.

Anderson, W. G., Byon, C. Y., Gut, M., and Bissett, F. H. (1976). ^{13}C NMR studies of the four, 20,22-epoxycholesterols and the two 20(22)-dehydrocholesterols. *Tetrahedron Lett.*, pp. 2193–2196.

ApSimon, J. W., Beierbeck, H., and Saunders, J. K. (1973). Lanthanide shift reagents in ^{13}C nuclear magnetic resonance: Quantitative determination of pseudocontact shifts and assignment of ^{13}C chemical shifts of steroids. *Can. J. Chem.* **51**, 3874–3881.

Beierbeck, H., Saunders, J. K., and ApSimon, J. W. (1977). The semiempirical derivation of ^{13}C nuclear magnetic resonance chemical shifts. Hydrocarbons, alcohols, amines, ketones, and olefins. *Can. J. Chem.* **55**, 2813–2828.

Benn, R., and Günther, H. (1983). Modern pulse methods in high-resolution NMR spectroscopy. *Angew. Chem., Int. Ed. Engl.* **22**, 350–380.

Blunt, J. W., and Stothers, J. B. (1977). ^{13}C N.m.r. spectra of steroids—A survey and commentary. *Org. Magn. Reson.* **9**, 439–646.

Chadwick, D. J., and Williams, D. H. (1974). The full assignment of the carbon-13 nuclear magnetic resonance spectrum of 5α-cholsetan-3β-ol with the aid of the lanthanide shift reagent $Yb(dpm)_3$. *J. Chem. Soc., Perkin Trans. 2* pp. 1903–1908.

Chiu, P.-L., and Patterson, G. W. (1981). Quantitative estimation of C-24 epimeric sterol mixtures by 220 MHz nuclear magnetic resonance spectroscopy. *Lipids* **16**, 203–206.

Cushley, R. J., and Filipenko, J. D. (1976). ^{13}C Fourier transform n.m.r. XIII. Reassignment of the ^{13}C spectrum of ergosterol. *Org. Magn. Reson.* **8**, 308–309.

Eggert, H., VanAntwerp, C. L., Bhacca, N. S., and Djerassi, C. (1976). Carbon-13 nuclear magnetic resonance spectra of hydroxy steroids. *J. Org. Chem.* **41**, 71–78.

Goad, L. J., Garneau, F.-X., Simard, J. L., ApSimon, J W., and Girard, M. (1985). Isolation of $\Delta^{9(11)}$-sterols from sea cucumber *Psolus fabricci.* Implication for holothurin biosynthesis. *Tetrahedron Lett.* **26**, 3513–3516.

Grant, D. M., and Paul, E. G. (1964). Carbon-13 magnetic resonance. II. Chemical shift data for the alkanes. *J. Am. Chem. Soc.* **86**, 2984–2990.

Iida, T., Kikuchi, M., Ishikawa, T., Tamura, T., and Matsumoto, T. (1982). Carbon-13 NMR spectra of some C-4 methylated sterols and their derivatives. *Org. Magn. Reson.* **19**, 228–229.

Itoh, T., Kikuchi, Y., Shimizu, N., Tamura, T., and Matsumoto, T. (1981). 24β-Ethyl-31-norlanosta-8,25(27)-dien-3β-ol and 24β-ethyl-25(27)-dehydrolophenol in seeds of three Cucurbitaceae species. *Phytochemistry* **20**, 1929–1933.

Kelecom, A. (1980). Use of calculated carbon chemical shift tables of saturated C-7 and C-11 sterol side chains for structure elucidation. *Bull. Soc. Chim. Belg.* **89**, 343–352.

Kikuchi, T., Kadota, S., and Tsubomo, K. (1986). Studies on the constituents of orchidaceous plants. IV. Proton and carbon-13 signal assignment of cycloeucalenol-type triterpenes from *Nervilia purpurea* Schlechter by two-dimensional nuclear magnetic resonance spectroscopy. *Chem. Pharm. Bull.* **34**, 2479–2486.

Khuong-Huu, F., Sangare, M., Chari, V. M., Bekaert, A., Devys, M., Barbier, M., and Lukacs, G. (1975). Carbon-13 nuclear magnetic resonance spectral analysis of cycloartanol and related compounds. *Tetrahedron Lett.* pp. 1787–1790.

Knight, S. A. (1974). Carbon-13 NMR spectra of some tetra- and pentacyclic triterpenoids. *Org. Magn. Reson.* **6**, 603–611.

Kobayashi, M., Tomioka, A., and Mitsuhashi, H. (1979). Marine sterols. VIII. Isolation and structure of sacosterol, a new sterol with a $\Delta^{17(20)}$-double bond from the soft coral *Sarcophyton glaucum*. *Steroids* **34**, 273–284.

Koizumi, N., Fujimoto, Y., Takeshita, T., and Ikekawa, N. (1979). Carbon-13 nuclear magnetic resonance of 24-substituted steroids. *Chem. Pharm. Bull.* **27**, 38–42.

Kokke, W. C. M. C., Shoolery, J. N., Fenical, W., and Djerassi, C. (1984). Biosynthetic studies of marine lipids. 4. Mechanism of side chain alkylation in (*E*)-24-propylidenecholesterol by Crysophyte alga. *J. Org. Chem.* **49**, 3742–3752.

Lindeman, L. P., and Adams, J. Q. (1971). Carbon-13 nuclear magnetic resonance spectroscopy chemical shifts for the paraffins through C_9. *Anal. Chem.* **43**, 1245–1252.

Mantsch, H. H., and Smith. I. C. P. (1973). A study of solvent effect on the ^{13}C nuclear magnetic resonance spectra of cholesterol, pyridine, and uridine. *Can. J. Chem.* **51**, 1384–1391.

Morris, G. A. (1986). Modern NMR techniques for structure elucidation. *Magn. Reson. Chem.* **24**, 371–403.

Nes, W. R., and McKean, M. L. (1977). "Biochemistry of Steroids and Other Isopentenoids." University Park Press, Baltimore, Maryland.

Nes, W. R., Krevitz, K., Joseph, J., Nes, W. D., Harris, B., Gibbons, G. F., and Patterson, G. W. (1977). The phylogenetic distribution of sterols in Tracheophytes. *Lipids* **12**, 511–527.

Nicotra, F., Ronchetti, F., Russo, G., Toma, L., and Ranzi, B. M. (1985). Application of biosynthetic ^{13}C enrichment using [1,2-$^{13}C_2$]acetate as precursor for ^{13}C NMR spectral assignment of the isopropyl methyls of (24β)-ethylsterols. *Org. Magn. Reson.* **23**, 134–136.

Parish, E. J., Tsuda, M., and Schroepfer, G. J., Jr. (1979). Synthesis and spectral properties of 5α-cholesta-6,8,14-trien-3β-ol. *Chem. Phys. Lipids* **25**, 111–124.

Popjak, G., Edmond, J., Anet, F. A. L., and Easton, N. R., Jr. (1977). Carbon-13 NMR studies on cholesterol biosynthesis from [^{13}C]mevalonates. *J. Am. Chem. Soc.* **99**, 931–935.

Reich, H. J., Jautelat, M., Messe, M. T., Weigert, F. J., and Roberts, J. D. (1969). Nuclear magnetic resonance spectroscopy. Carbon-13 spectra of steroids. *J. Am. Chem. Soc.* **91**, 7445–7454.

Ricca, G. S., and Nicotra, F. (1978). Carbon-13 nuclear magnetic resonance spectra of some phytosterols. *Gazz. Chim. Ital.* **108**, 713–715.

Rubinstein, I., Goad, L. J., Clague, A. D. H., and Mulheirn, L. J. (1976). The 220 MHz NMR spectra of phytosterols. *Phytochemistry* **15**, 195–200.

Seo, S., Uomori, A., Yoshimura, Y., and Takeda, K. (1983). Stereospecificity in the biosynthesis of phytosterol side chains: ^{13}C nmr signal assignments of C-26 and C-27. *J. Am. Chem. Soc.* **105**, 6343–6344.

Seo, S., Uomori, A., Yoshimura, Y., Sankawa, U., Ebizuka, Y., Seto, H., and Takeda, K. (1987). Stereospecificity in the side-chain formation of 24β-ethylsterols in tissue cultures of *Trichosanthes kirilowii*. *J. Chem. Soc., Chem. Commun.* pp. 1876–1878.

Shoolery, J. N. (1984). Recent developments in ^{13}C- and proton-NMR. *J. Nat. Prod.* **47**, 226–259.

Smith, W. B. (1978). Carbon-13 NMR spectroscopy of steroids. *Annu. Rep. NMR Spectrosc.* **8**, 199–226.

Stothers, J. B. (1972). "Carbon-13 NMR Spectroscopy." Academic Press, New York.

Tsuda, M., and Schroepfer, G. J., Jr. (1979a). Nuclear magnetic resonance spectroscopy of sterols. ^{13}C Olefinic carbon shieldings in sterols and related cyclic compounds. *Chem. Phys. Lipids* **25**, 46–68.

Tsuda, M., and Schroepfer, G. J., Jr. (1979b). Carbon-13 nulcear magnetic resonance studies of C_{27} sterol precursors of cholesterol. *J. Org. Chem.* **44**, 1290–1293.

Wright, J. L. C., McInnes, A. G., Shimizu, S., Smith, D. G., Walter, J. A., Idler, D., and Khalil, W. (1978). Identification of C-24 alkyl epimers of marine sterols by ^{13}C nuclear magnetic resonance spectroscopy. *Can. J. Chem.* **56**, 1898–1903.

13

Identification of Sterols and Biologically Significant Steroids by Ultraviolet and Infrared Spectroscopy

Patricia Acuña-Johnson
Escuela de Química y Farmacía
Universidad de Valparaiso
Valparaiso, Chile

A. C. Oehlschlager
Department of Chemistry
Simon Fraser University
Burnaby, British Columbia, Canada

I. INTRODUCTION

Ultraviolet (UV) and infrared (IR) absorption spectroscopies are used as ancillary tools in the assignment of structure. Both methods are excellent for the confirmation of the presence and relative locations of absorbing functional groups. Several books and reviews are available (Dence, 1980; Dobriner *et al.*, 1953; Dorfman, 1953; Dyer, 1965; Morton, 1975; Nakanishi and Solomon, 1977; Rao, 1964, 1967; Roberts *et al.*, 1958; Scott, 1964). Theoretical and biochemical aspects of the analysis of steroids by absorption spectroscopy are covered elsewhere (Bellamy, 1975; Brand and Eglinton, 1965; Brande, 1962; Caspi and Scrimshaw, 1967; Cole, 1956; Fieser and Fieser, 1959; Gillam and Stern, 1970; Gore, 1962; Görög, 1982; Nes and McKean, 1977; Silverstein *et al.*, 1981).

We have selected examples in which absorptions in these radiation ranges are useful in assignment of position or stereochemistry of UV and IR active functional groups. We have not covered the use of chiroptical techniques.

Analysis of Sterols and Other Biologically Significant Steroids

UV absorption spectroscopy yields information about the presence and relative positions of unsaturated functional groups, and IR spectroscopy yields similar information concerning both unsaturated and saturated functional groups. Since many steroids exhibit similar UV spectra, IR has been widely used as a complementary tool in structure elucidation. IR absorption has the advantage that it yields spectra that are unique to the molecule. Overlapping of absorptions occurs in both UV and IR spectra, which reduces their diagnostic value.

II. ULTRAVIOLET ABSORPTION SPECTROSCOPY

Compounds containing single chromatographic groups absorb strongly in the far-UV and very weakly in the near-UV regions. The effective spectral range of conventional UV spectrophotometers is 200–400 nm. Most naturally occurring steroids possess chromophores that absorb in this region.

Absorptions in the UV region are usually associated with $\pi \rightarrow \pi^*$ or $n \rightarrow \pi^*$ transitions. Both the position and intensity of UV absorption bands provide structural information. The intensity of absorption at a given wavelength is conventionally expressed as the molar extinction coefficient or the molar absorptivity (ε) or as its logarithm to base 10 (log ε). If A is the optical density or absorbance, c the concentration of the solution (in mol·liter^{-1}), and d the thickness of the cell that contains the solution (in cm), then for a given absorption, ε is calculated by the expression.

$$\varepsilon = \frac{A}{c \cdot d}$$

and has the units liter·mol^{-1}·cm^{-1}. Plots of absorption intensity (log ε) versus wavelength (λ) are presented semilogarithmically. Because the resulting spectrum often includes more than one band, each corresponding to a different excited electronic state of the molecule, tabular representation is preferred. For solutions of unknown composition the intensity of absorption can be expressed in terms of

$$E^{1\%}_{1\,\text{cm}} = \frac{A}{c \cdot d}$$

where c is the concentration in grams per 100 milliliters and d the pathlength through the sample in centimeters.

A. Simple Chromophores

1. Unconjugated Olefins

Sterols containing isolated double bonds absorb in the range 190–210 nm, and their absorption maxima are attributed to $\pi \rightarrow p^*$ transitions. Characterization of monounsaturated steroids by examination of their UV spectra is difficult because few clear relationships between location of unsaturation and position of absorption exist.

Bladon *et al.* (1952) have reported the UV spectra of many monosubstituted steroids. Increasing substitution, as in the change from I to II, shifts the absoption maximum to longer wavelength and increases the intensity.

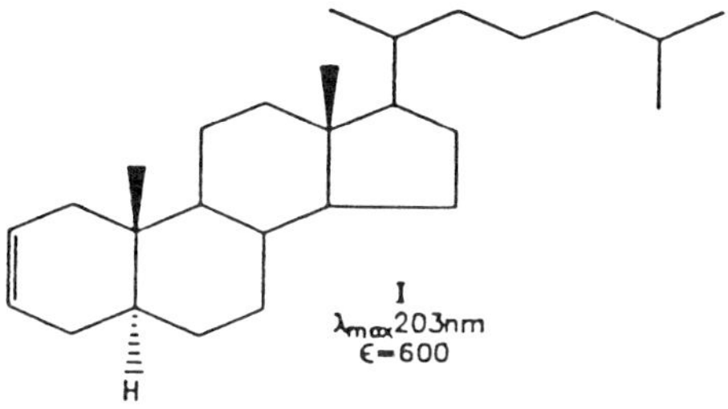

I
λ_{max} 203nm
ϵ=600

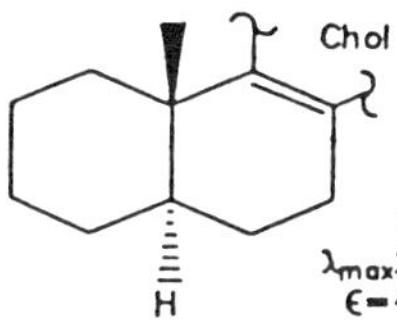

II
λ_{max} 207nm
ϵ=4,600

2. Conjugated Olefins

Conjugated polyenes exhibit intense UV absorption due to $\pi \rightarrow \pi^*$ transitions. This absorption occurs in the 215–285 nm region for dienes. Acyclic conjugated dienes prefer the s-trans to the s-cis conformation. The s-trans conformers exhibit more intense absorptions ($\varepsilon = 12{,}000$–$18{,}000$) at lower wavelength than the s-cis conformers ($\varepsilon = 5{,}000$–$15{,}000$). The position and intensity of absorption of dienes increase with the degree of alkyl substitution.

Sterols containing s-trans diene systems such as III, recently isolated from a soft coral (Gebreyesus *et al.*, 1985), as well as those containing annular s-trans diene systems (IV and V), absorb strongly in the range 225–239 nm.

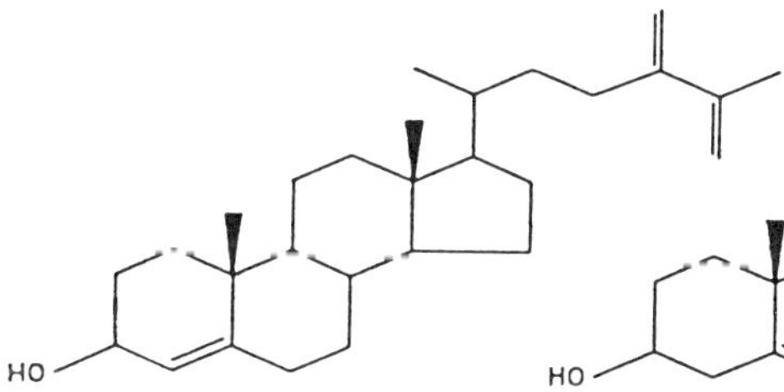

III
λ_{max} 227nm

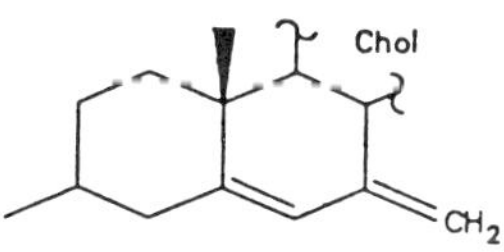

IV
λ_{max} 239nm

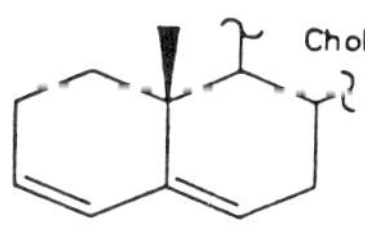

V
λ_{max} 235nm

The diene moieties of homoannular unsaturated sterols, cholesta-2,4-diene (VI) and ergosterol (VII) are constrained to the s-cis conformation and exhibit absorption maxima in the 275–285 nm region.

The $\Delta^{5,7}$-system of VII occurs in major fungal sterols and in minor sterol metabolites of higher plants and animals. Such diene chromophores can be readily identified on the basis of their multipeaked UV absorption spectra. If s-trans and s-cis dienes are present in a sterol (as in VIII), both can be readily detected by UV spectroscopy (Breivik *et al.*, 1954).

Extending the conjugation increases the intensity and wavelength of the absorption maxima. Steroids containing conjugated trienes are usually encountered as

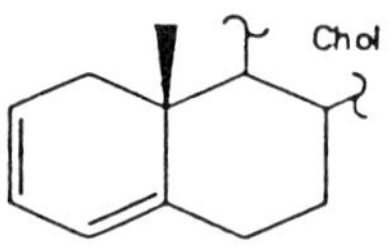

VI
λ_{max} 275nm
ϵ=10,000

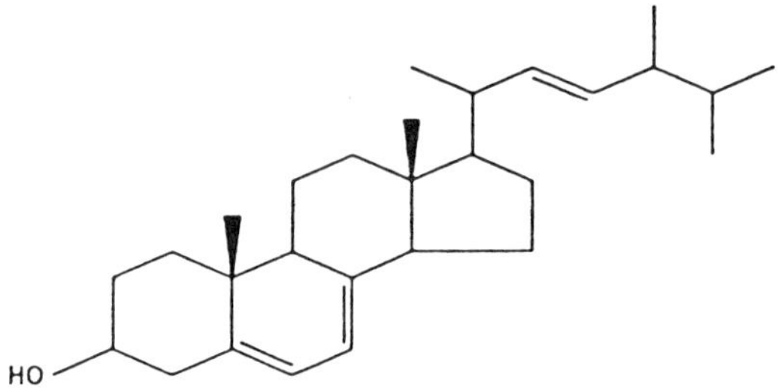

VII
λ_{max} 282nm
ϵ=11,900

products of UV irradiation of $\Delta^{5,7}$-sterols. UV spectroscopy has been particularly useful in the identification of B-ring cleaved sterols generated during these processes. Two of the most important of these seco-derivatives, previtamin D (IX) and calciferol (X), show intense absorption maxima at longer wavelength than their $\Delta^{5,7}$-dienic precursor. Absorption of IX is less intense than that of X, presumably due to lower π planarity in the former.

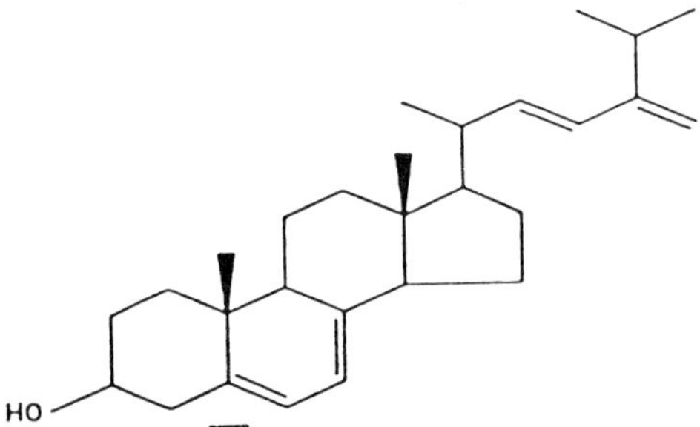

VIII
λ_{max} 293nm, ϵ=6,900
λ_{max} 281.5nm, ϵ=12,800
λ_{max} 271nm, ϵ=12,200
λ_{max} 230nm, ϵ=21,400

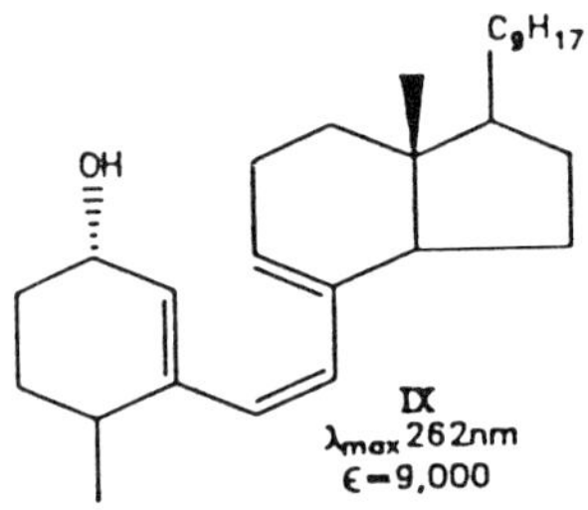

IX
λ_{max} 262nm
ϵ=9,000

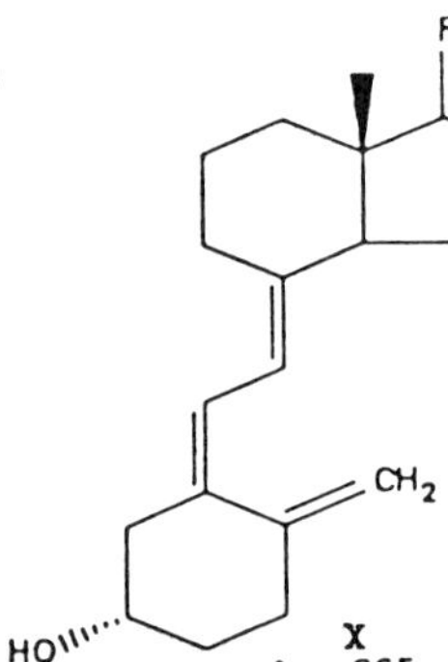

X
λ_{max} 265nm
ϵ=18,300

Empirical correlations of the position of the UV absorption maximum for steroidal 1,3-dienes have been formulated by Booker *et al.* (1940) and by Woodward (1942a). These correlations have been useful in the prediction of the positions of absorption maxima of conjugated steroidal polyenes (Fieser and Fieser, 1959). The success of the rules depend upon taking into account the planarity of the π system. Accurate predictions of planarity are available from molecular mechanics calculations (Ulrich and Allinger, 1982). In general, these rules are applied reasonably well for conjugated systems containing four double bonds or less.

3. Ketones

Saturated ketones show a broad band and low-absorption maxima ($\varepsilon \sim 30$–370) around 270–300 nm due to an $n \rightarrow \pi^*$ forbidden transition. A band of medium intensity near 190 nm that results from an $n \rightarrow \sigma^*$ transition is also characteristic of this group. Although the $n \rightarrow \pi^*$ absorption of ketones is weak, it is characteristic and therefore valuable for confirming the presence of this group. Presence of an α-halogen or other polar substituent (e.g., α-acetoxyl) increases the intensity of the $n \rightarrow \pi^*$ absorption and changes the position of the absorption maximum. The magnitude and direction of the latter change is determined by the angular relationship between the polar α substituent and the carbonyl σ C—O bond. For cyclohexyl systems in chair conformations, hypsochromic shifts on the order of 5–10 nm are seen when the group is equatorial (XI $\rightarrow$ XII, dihedral angles $\sim 4^\circ$), whereas bathochromic shifts ranging between 10 and 30 nm occur when the substituent is axial (XI $\rightarrow$ XIII, dihedral angles $\sim 110^\circ$) (Cookson, 1954; Cookson and Dandegaonker, 1955).

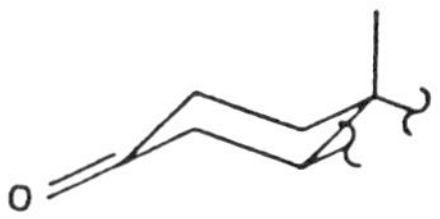

XI
λ_{max} 286nm
ϵ=23

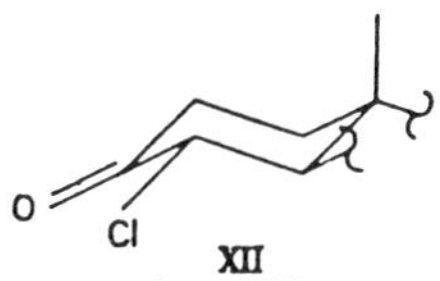

XII
λ_{max} 279nm
ϵ=40

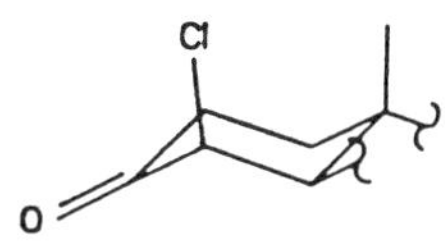

XIII
λ_{max} 299.5nm
ϵ=34

4. α-Diketones

Acyclic α-diketones, such as diacetyl, show two characteristic absorption bands of low intensity: one near 280 nm due to an $n \rightarrow \pi^*$ transition and the other near 450 nm due to interactions between the two carbonyl groups. The absorption occurring in the visible region corresponds to the s-trans conformation. This band shifts into the ultraviolet region when the carbonyl groups are forced to adopt noncoplanar relationships, as found in cyclic α-diketones.

Cyclic α-diketones containing α-hydrogens exist in the more stable enolic form. Thus, the absorption of cyclic α-diketones is similar to that of α,β-unsaturated ketones, and the Woodward rules are applicable to these systems (Woodward, 1941, 1942b). The absorption maxima of cyclic α-diketones and their enol derivatives (e.g., enol esters and ethers) are displaced relative to α,β-unsaturated ketones due to the presence of the polar enol group. For instance, the 3α-hydroxy-11,12-diketocholanic acid (XIV) shows a weak band corresponding to a $n \rightarrow \pi^*$ transition at 281 nm ($\varepsilon = 7{,}000$), close to the calculated wavelength for the enolic form (XV, $\lambda_{max} = 279$ nm). The enol acetate (XVI) exhibits its maximum at 243 nm (calc. 250 nm). In strong alkaline solution the absorption maxima of α-diketones shift to longer wavelengths (281–330 nm) due to formation of the enolate (XVII) (Brand and Eglinton, 1965).

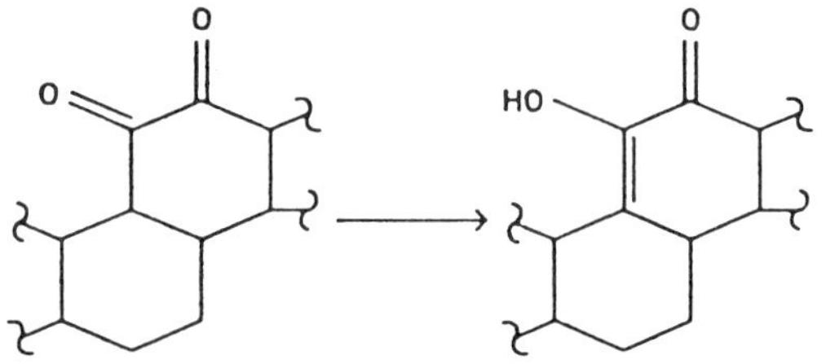

XIV XV

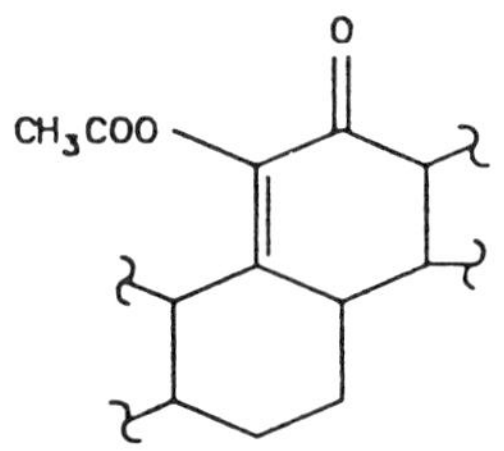

XVI

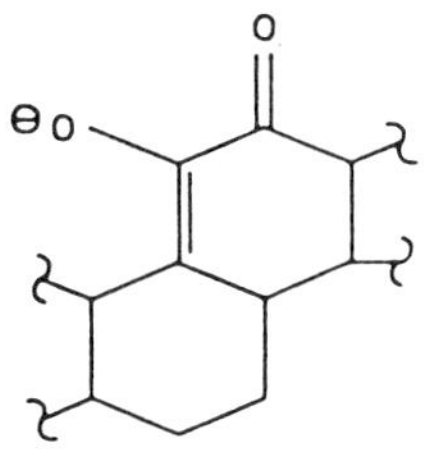

XVII

5. *Unsaturated Ketones*

Steroids containing α,β-unsaturated ketones show intense absorptions in the 225–250 nm region (ε ~ 10,000–20,000) due to $\pi \rightarrow \pi^*$ transitions. In addition, low-intensity absorptions due to $n \rightarrow \pi^*$ transitions at 310–330 nm (ε ~ 60–100) are also observable. The absorption spectra of many steroidal unsaturated ketones are available for comparison (Morton, 1975). Because of the polar nature of the carbonyl group, the positions of the absorption maxima are dependent on the polarity of the solvent. Increasing solvent polarity generates a hypsochromic shift for the low-intensity $n \rightarrow \pi^*$ band whereas the strong $\pi \rightarrow \pi^*$ band undergoes a bathochromic displacement. Calculations of the position of absorption maxima of enones are conducted using rules similar to those described for dienes (Fieser and Fieser, 1959). The exact wavelength of an absorption maximum depends, once again, on the degree of substitution. Likewise, extinction coefficients of s-cis enones are usually less than 10,000 whereas those of s-trans enones are greater than 10,000.

The Woodward-Fieser rules have been widely used for predicting the position of the $\pi \rightarrow \pi^*$ band for α,β-unsaturated steroidal ketones. It has been suggested that reliability of these rules is due to a fortuitous cancellation of effects (Liljefors and Allinger, 1978). The original rules did not take into account differences in the electronic character of s-trans and s-cis conformations of the conjugated systems. Moreover, precise calculations of the position of $\pi \rightarrow \pi^*$ absorption for cyclic enones that possess ring strain were not available.

Reevaluation of the Woodward-Fieser rules with special attention to the torsion angle bewteen the carbonyl and the olefin components has yielded a new and simpler set of rules. The new rules are applicable to planar or moderately twisted systems, whether cyclic or acyclic, and use a parent value of 209 nm for s-trans and 215 nm for s-cis systems. The shifts resulting from alkyl substitution are predicted as usual, that is, + 10 nm for α- and + 12 nm for β-substitution. A ring closure correction of + 17 nm is added if the double bond is endocyclic in a 6-membered ring. These rules apply only if ethanol is used as a solvent; with other solvents, corrections must be made according to Fieser and Fieser (1959). A more detailed calculation of the ultraviolet spectrum for α,β-unsaturated enones involves the torsion angle between the carbonyl and olefin and permits prediction of the absorption maxima for both the lowest energy (~225–250 nm) and the higher energy (~200–220 nm) band, which is forbidden for near-planar enones but is pronounced in twisted systems (Liljefors and Allinger, 1978).

Conjugated enones and dienones are common in several classes of physiologically important steroids. The hormones such as Δ^4-androstendione (XVIII), testosterone (XIX), and progesterone (XX) possess α,β-unsaturated ketone groups that are clearly identified by the appearance of absorptions at 241 nm (ε = 16,000–17,000). The insect moulting hormones, the ecdysteroids (XXI), contain Δ^7-6-keto groups that exhibit strong ultraviolet absorptions characteristic for α,β-unsaturated ketones. The 5-membered α,β-unsaturated lactone rings (butenolides) of cardiac glycosides (XXII) (e.g., digoxin, α-methyldigoxin, and ouabain) show intense absorption near 215 nm (ε ~ 15,000). Absorption intensities of bufadienolides (XXIII) are much lower and are displaced to longer wavelengths (λ_{max} ~ 300 nm; ε = 6000) due to the presence of additional unsaturation in the lactone ring.

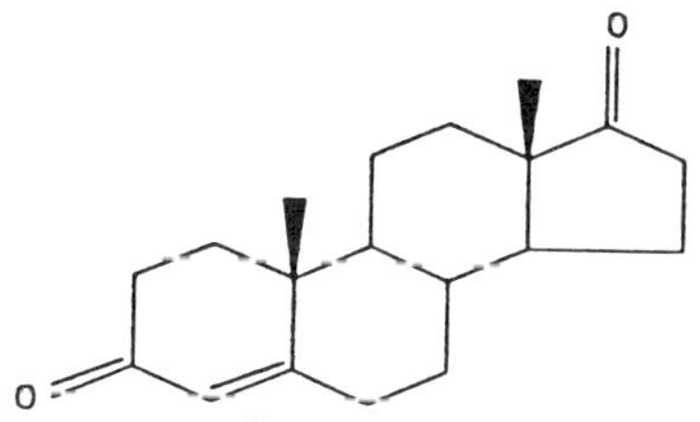

XVIII

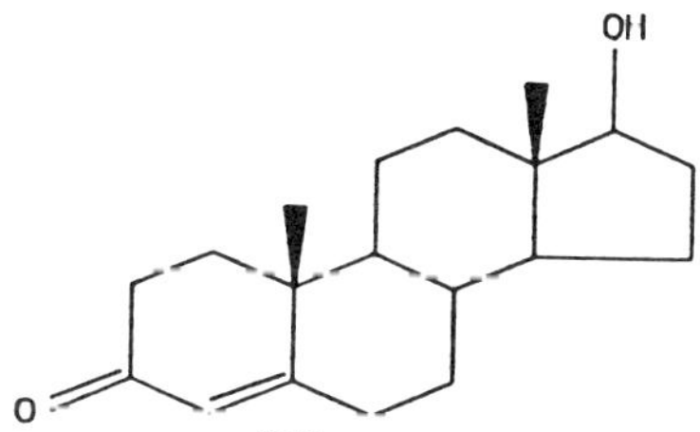

XIX

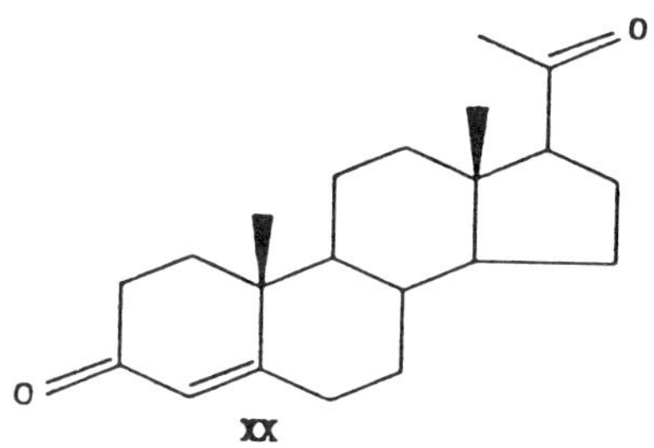

XX

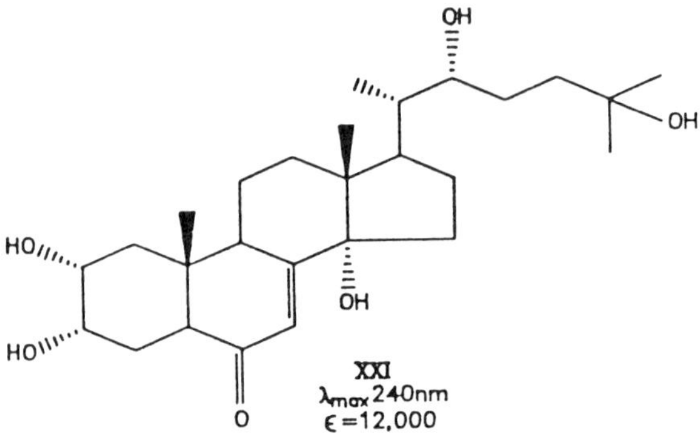

XXI
λ_{max} 240nm
ϵ=12,000

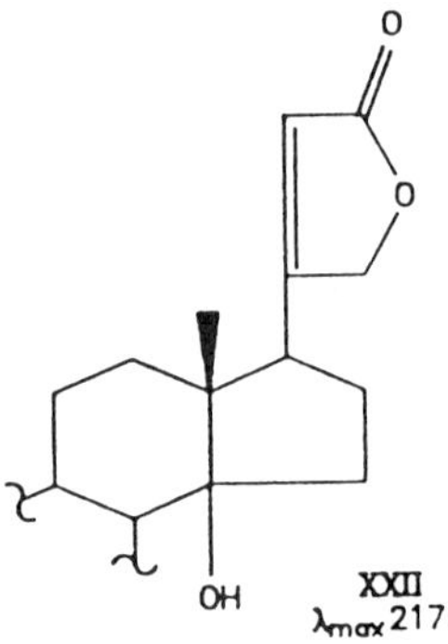

XXII
λ_{max} 217nm

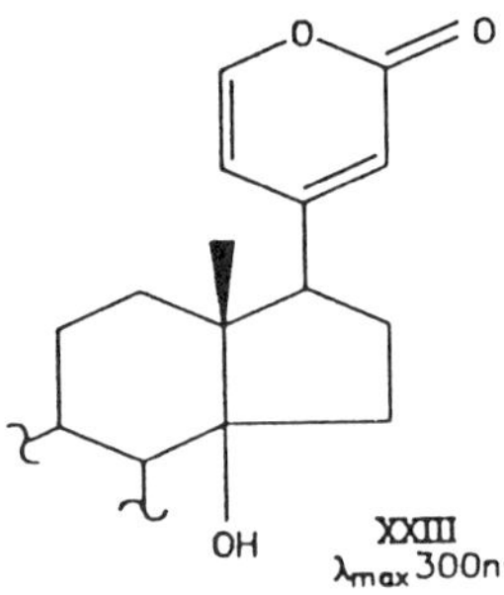

XXIII
λ_{max} 300nm

6. *Dienones*

Additional unsaturation, conjugated with enones, can be located adjacent to the olefin (extended conjugation) or adjacent to the carbonyl (cross conjugation). Either arrangement of a second double bond produces bathochromic shifts and increased absorption intensities of the $\pi \rightarrow \pi^*$ band. The effect of additional conjugation on the wavelength of this absorption is much larger for dienones possessing extended conjugation (e.g., XXIV → XXV) than for those with cross conjugation (XXIV → XXVI) (Brand and Eglinton, 1965).

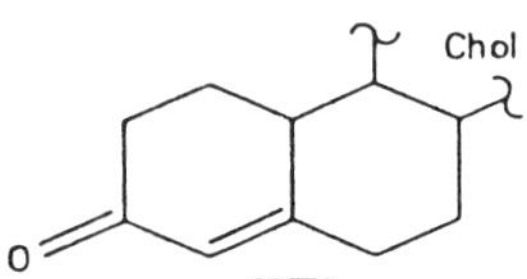

XXIV
λ_{max} 241nm
ϵ=16,600

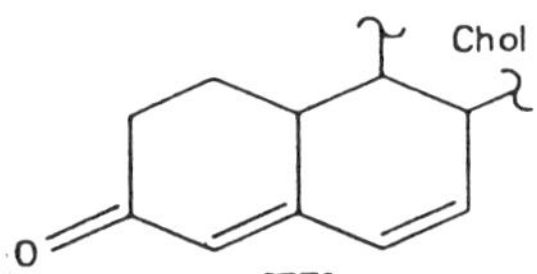

XXV
λ_{max} 284nm
ϵ=28,000

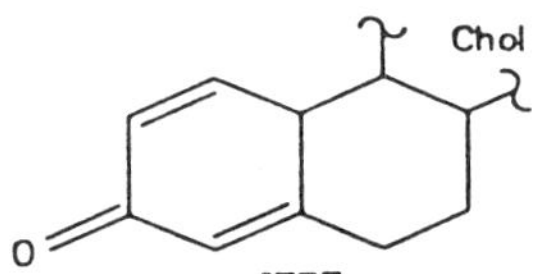

XXVI
λ_{max} 244nm
ϵ=15,000

7. *Enediones*

Enediones that possess s-trans conformations absorb more intensely and at longer wavelengths than those possessing the s-cis conformations. This is seen by comparing the absorption spectrum of the s-trans enedione, diketoeuphorbenyl acetate (XXVII), with that of the s-cis endione, ergost-8-ene-7,15-dione (XXVIII) (Brand and Eglinton, 1965).

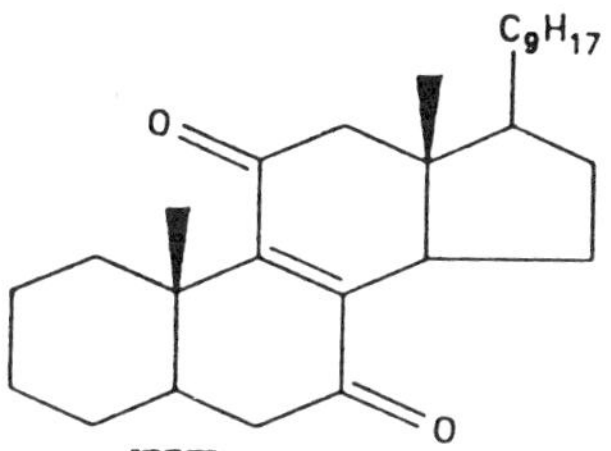

XXVII
λ_{max} 270nm
ε = 7,400

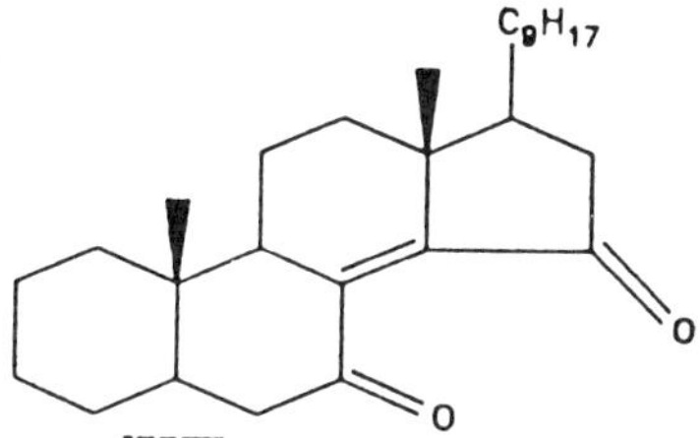

XXVIII
λ_{max} 259nm
ε = 11,300

B. Aromatic Chromophores

Single aromatic rings display three bands that correspond to $\pi \rightarrow \pi^*$ transitions: 184 nm ($\varepsilon \sim 60{,}000$), 204 nm ($\varepsilon \sim 7900$), and 256 nm ($\varepsilon \sim 200$). The intense bands observed at the shortest wavelength result from allowed transitions and are difficult to observe. The other bands result from forbidden transitions and are usually used in diagnosing structure.

Attachment of alkyl and alkenyl substituents produce bathochromic shifts, the magnitude of which is different for each transition. These shifts are attributed to hyperconjugation. Addition of a second alkyl group in a para position is most effective in producing a bathochromic change. Aromatic chromophores found in sterols related to ergosterol, such as neoergosterol (XXIX), exhibit UV spectra similar to those of tetraalkylbenzenes (Fieser and Fieser, 1959).

The absorption spectra of naturally occurring steroids that contain a 3 hydroxy aromatic ring such as estrone (XXX) resemble those of dialkylphenols. Although characteristic, the intensities are quite weak (λ_{max} 280 nm, $\varepsilon = 2000$). In general, steroids that contain a phenolic A-ring exhibit extinction coefficients in the range 2000–7000 for the band at 280 nm. The high absorptivity can be used to distinguish aromatic A-ring steroids from those with the aromatic B-ring ($\varepsilon \sim 400$–700).

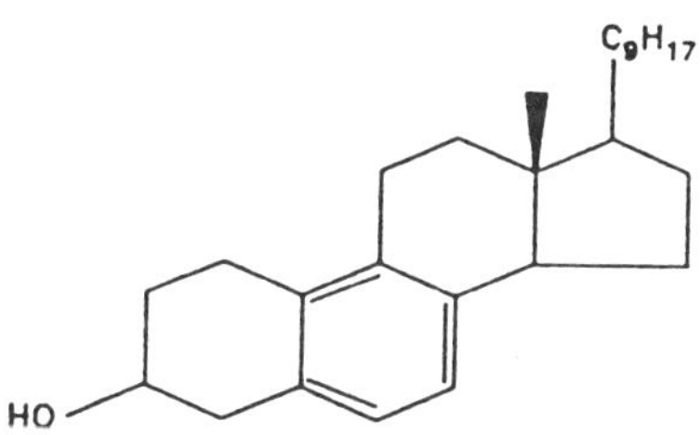

XXIX
λ_{max} 268nm
ε = 500

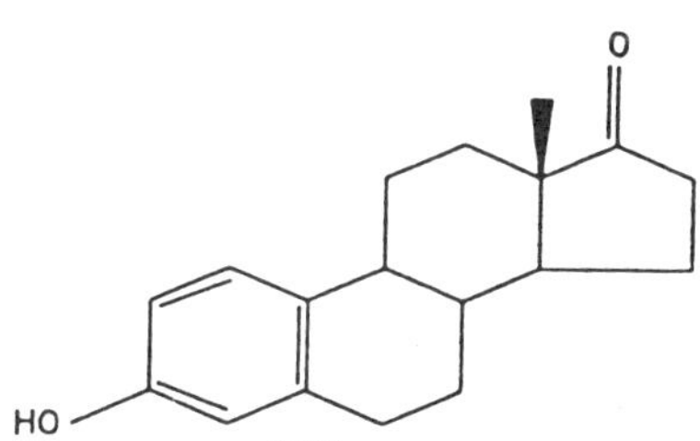

XXX
λ_{max} 280nm
ε = 2,300

The absorption bands of an aromatic ring undergo a bathochromic shift when the ring is fused to another that is unsaturated, as in the case of naphthalene. This bathochromic shift is different for each of the three bands, and the spectrum that results usually contains additional bands. For instance, 15-dehydroequilin-17-one (XXXI) absorbs at 230, 270, and 321 nm (ε = 77,600, 6800, and 660, respectively). In XXXI the intensity and position of the naphthalene absorptions mask the absorption corresponding to the α,β-unsaturated chromophore.

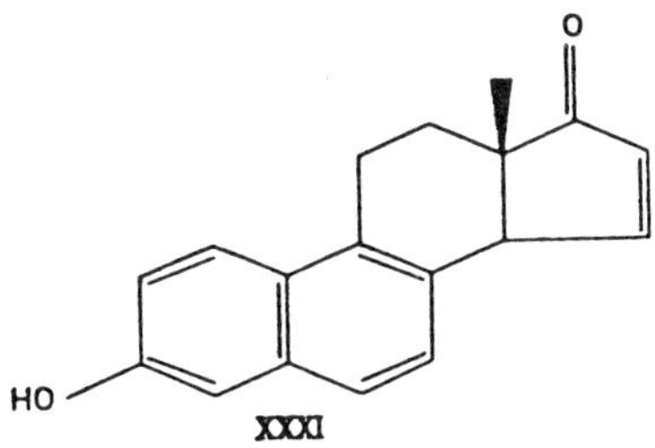

XXXI

III. INFRARED ABSORPTION SPECTROSCOPY

The usefulness of IR spectroscopy for the identification and analysis of steroids is limited to the determination of the presence of absorbing functional groups and their stereochemical relationships. The functional groups that are easily identified by IR are those that contain polar bonds absorbing in the region between 1600 and 400 cm^{-1}. Infrared absorption occurs when absorbing bonds undergo an increase in their amplitude of vibration. The two types of vibrational motion that commonly occur during the absorption of infrared light are stretching and bending. The wave number of absorption (ν, cm^{-1}) is directly proportional to the absorbed energy ($E = h\nu$). The approximate value of the atoms M_1 and M_2 (in grams), the velocity of light (c), and the stretching constant of the bond (k, in dyn/cm) according to the expression

$$\nu = \frac{1}{2\pi c}\left(\frac{k}{(M_1M_2/M_1 + M_2)}\right)^{1/2}$$

The magnitude of the extinction coefficient in infrared spectroscopy varies from nil to around 2000 and is proportional to the square of the change in the dipole moment of the bond undergoing absorption. Absorptions due to stretching motions are usually the most intense bands in the spectrum.

A. Carbonyl Stretching

1. Saturated Ketones

The carbonyl stretching frequency (in solution) observed for steroids containing saturated ketones at all positions in rings A–C (C-1–C-12) and the side chain is in the range 1704–1722 cm^{-1} with the average absorption being 1708 cm^{-1}. Only when keto groups are located in the 5-membered D-ring do they give rise to distinctive infrared absorptions. D-ring keto-sterols such as XXX are characterized by C=O absorption frequencies in the range 1738–1749 cm^{-1}. The higher frequency of absorption of 5-membered versus 6-membered ketones is due to the ring strain imposed on the carbonyl of the smaller 5-membered ring. This differential (1708 versus 1741 cm^{-1}) is suffficient to allow both 5- and 6-membered ring ketones to be identified in a steroid.

The position and intensity of the C═O stretching frequency of ketones are also altered by the presence of adjacent polar groups. For instance, the intensity and wavelength of the C═O absorption of the 20-keto group of progesterone (XX) increase considerably upon acylation at either α position (e.g., XX → XXXII and XXXII → XXXIII) (Holley *et al.,* 1980). The frequency shift is dependent on the electronic nature of the ester group, with the highest shift observed in 21-trichloroacetoxy and 21-phenoxyacetoxy derivatives (Egyed *et al.,* 1983). Such α-substituent–induced frequency shifts are attributed to inductive effects whereas intensity shifts are considered to be due to mesomeric effects (Brownlee *et al.,* 1975; Brownlee and Topsom, 1975; Deady *et al.,* 1975).

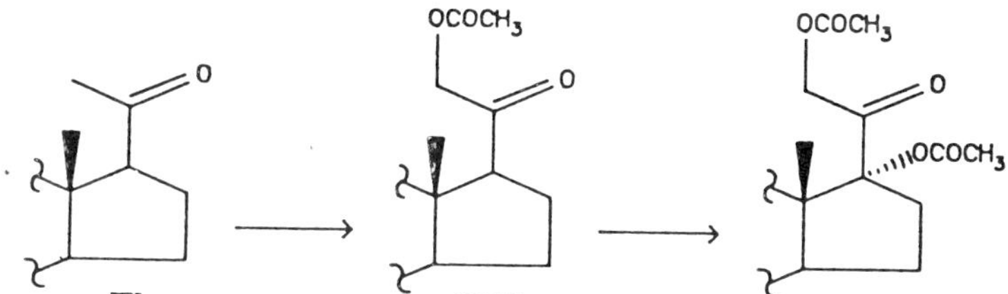

XX 1707cm^{-1} XXXII 1725cm^{-1} XXXIII 1732cm^{-1}

Positional isomers of D-ring monoketones can be differentiated by the absorptions in the range 1410–1438 cm^{-1}, which are due to scissoring of adjacent methylenes (—CO—CH_2—) (Bridgman *et al.,* 1970). The IR spectra of several keto-steroids have provided correlations between the location of the carbonyl and the intensity of these methylene absorptions (Boul *et al.,* 1971). For instance, the C—O frequencies of 17- and 15-keto steroids (XXX and XXXIV, respectively) are very close. However, the intensities of adjacent methylene absorptions are sufficiently different to distinguish between the two isomers. Likewise, the IR spectra of 16-keto-sterols (XXXV) show bands twice as intense as those of similarly substituted 15- and 17-ketones (Boul *et al.,* 1971).

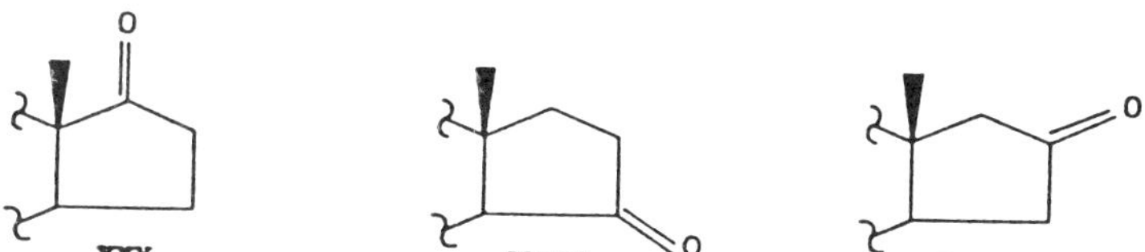

XXX 1738cm^{-1} XXXIV 1749cm^{-1} XXXV 1741cm^{-1}

When two ketones are present in a steroid, each can influence the absorption position of the other, even when they are well separated. The frequency shift observed in such cases is in the range 0–+13 cm^{-1} (Boul *et al.,* 1971).

2. α,β-Unsaturated Ketones

Conjugation of a carbonyl with a double bond lowers the frequency of the C=O stretching band and increases its intensity. The IR absorption due to carbonyl stretching of conjugated acyclic and 6-membered ring ketones is in the 1660–1685 cm^{-1} range. Ketones such as XIX show this absorption at 1677–1681 cm^{-1}. D-ring α,β-unsaturated ketones (e.g., XXXI) absorb at correspondingly higher frequencies (~1716 cm^{-1}). The presence of a second double bond, extending the conjugation, produces a bathochromic frequency shift in the range 12–15 cm^{-1}.

Characteristic C=C stretching bands around 1600 cm^{-1} are also present in the IR spectra of α,β-unsaturated ketones. Overlapping C=O and C=C absorption in the stretching region often makes IR spectra of α,β-unsaturated keto steroids difficult to interpret. This problem can be solved by measuring the individual intensities of overlapping bands, provided that the characteristic intensities of various C=O groups in a steroid are known (Jones *et al.*, 1952a).

3. Esters: Carboxylic Acid Esters and Lactones

Carbonyl stretching absorptions of carboylic acid esters and acetates appear at 1737–1742 cm^{-1} and 1733–1739 cm^{-1}, respectively. These functional groups are best recognized by the presence of an additional strong, sharp C=O stretching absorption at 1135–1155 cm^{-1} for carboxylic acid esters and at 1200–1250 cm^{-1} for acetates. Equatorial acetates yield a single band and axial acetates yield doublet or triplet bands in this region.

The positions and intensities of the C=O stretching absorptions of esters are affected by their conformations and neighboring unsaturation. Introduction of unsaturation, as in enol acetates and phenolic acetates, shifts the C=O stretching frequency to 1748——1762 cm^{-1}. The C=O bands of primary, secondary, and tertiary acetoxy groups display characteristically different intensities (Aruldhas *et al.*, 1980; Holly *et al.*, 1980;). IR spectra of cardinolides (XXII) such as digitoxigenin, gitoxigenin, and digoxigenin exhibit C=O stretching of the lactone ring at 1739 cm^{-1} and C=O stretching at 1621–1618 cm^{-1} (Yamaguchi, 1970). The α-pyrone moiety of bufadienolides (XXIII) is characterized by peaks at 1538 and 830 cm^{-1}.

4. Amides

Absorption due to CO—N stretching is in the 1630–1680 cm^{-1} region. However, α-hydroxyl groups, when present in steroidal alkaloid structures such as tomatine (XXXVI), shift the amide C=O band from its usually observed frequency (1640 cm^{-1}) to ~1730 cm^{-1}, which is more characteristic of esters than amides (Kastelic-Suhadolc, 1983). This effect is not observed in non-steroidal α-hydroxy amides (XXXVII).

B. Absorptions of Methylene Groups

1. C=C and C=CH Stretching

Absorptions corresponding to C=C stretching of isolated ethylene groups are observed in the region 1620–1650 cm^{-1}. They are moderately weak in most

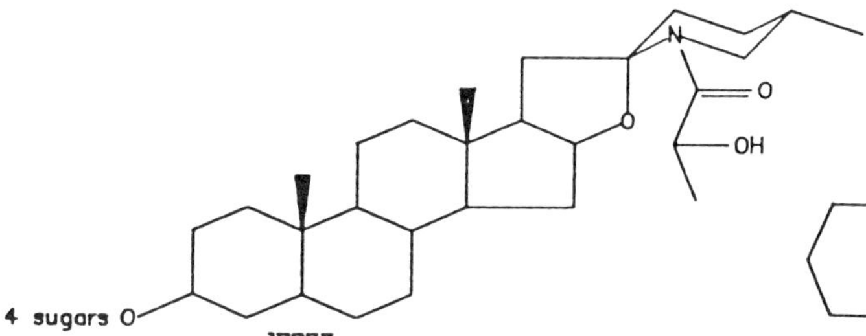

XXXVI
1733cm^{-1}

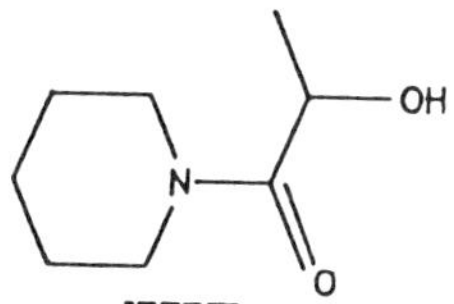

XXXVII
1640cm^{-1}

monounsaturated compounds and have not been widely used to elucidate steroid structures. Conjugation of ethylenic groups displaces these absorptions to 1575–1630 cm^{-1}. The C=C stretching absorption is most useful in confirming the presence of an α,β-unsaturated carbonyl (see Section III. A.2).

Absorptions due to stretching of olefinic and aromatic C=C—H stretching occur in the region 3300–3100 cm^{-1}. The C—H stretching absorptions of saturated CH, CH_2, and CH_3 are near 2850–2950 cm^{-1}. These absorptions can be useful if IR spectra are obtained at high resolution (Smith and Eddy, 1959).

2. C—H Bending

Bending absorptions due to methylene groups adjacent to carbonyl groups can provide guidance in the determination of structures of α,β-unsaturated ketones. These C—H absorptions are in the range 1415–1438 cm^{-1}. For instance, steroids bearing a C=O at C-3 give IR absorptions around 1420 cm^{-1} due to methylenes at C-2 and C-4. In the case of cholestan-7-one, this absorption ($C6H_2$) appears at 1433 cm^{-1}. Deuterium exchange at these methylene groups causes these bands to disappear.

When the methylene is adjacent to a C=O in the 5-membered D-ring, the absorption due to methylene bending appears at 1404–1411 cm^{-1}. 16-Ketosteroids (XXXV) that possess an adjacent methylene group exhibit a peak at 1410 cm^{-1}. The position of this methylene band is useful to differentiate this type of carbonyl from those corresponding to esters and acetates.

Most naturally occurring plant and fungal sterols (e.g., VII and VIII) possess a trans olefin between C-22 and C-23. The absorption due to vinyl C—H bending of this unsaturation is very strong and occurs at around 967 cm^{-1}. In general, those bands that appear in the region 1000–660 cm^{-1} are associated with the C—H out-of-plane bending of the C=C—H group. This particular absorption is characteristic of trans 1,2-disubstituted olefins.

When comparing the IR spectra of steroids that contain unsaturation in the side chain with those of steroids that contain saturated side chains in the same position, the band that corresponds to the C—H bonding vibration is the only difference. Absorptions due to bending of vinyl C—H associated with trisubstituted olefins appear in the range 790–850 cm^{-1}. These are much weaker and usually overlap with other absorptions occurring in this frequency range. Sterols containing $\Delta^{5,7}$-diene systems such as ergosterol (VII) exhibit a characteristic doublet of medium intensity near 805 cm^{-1} and 840 cm^{-1} (the stronger) (Nes and McKean, 1977). Monounsaturated Δ^5- and Δ^7-steroids exhibit triplets in the same region. For instance, Δ^5-steroids show two peaks of equal intensity at 802 and 845 cm^{-1} and a weaker third peak at 830 cm^{-1}.

C. Hydroxyl Absorptions

Absorptions corresponding to O—H stretching appear in the region 3200–3650 cm^{-1}. The position of this absorption is dependent on solvent and the presence of sterochemically accessible neighboring groups that possess nonbonding electrons, which are available for intramolecular hydrogen bonding. In dilute solutions non-hydrogen-bonding hydroxyls show sharp peaks at 3590–3650 cm^{-1}. Primary alcohols exhibit this absorption at 3640 cm^{-1} whereas the corresponding absorptions for secondary and tertiary alcohols are at 3630 and 3620 cm^{-1}, respectively.

Intramolecularly hydrogen-bonded hydroxyls exhibit sharp bands at 3450–3600 cm^{-1} that are not affected by dilution. Investigations of the OH absorption of a great number of steroids (in CS_2) have shown complex OH bands, which have been interpreted in terms of intramolecular OH···H interactions (Winman, 1967). Intramolecular hydrogen bonding in steroidal diols and hydroxy-ketones has been extensively studied by IR (Dalton *et al.*, 1963; Davey *et al.*, 1968; Joris and von R. Schleyer, 1968; Oki *et al.*, 1968; Tichy, 1965). IR continues to be useful in the establishment of the relative stereochemistry of steroidal hydroxyls and other functional groups with which they can hydrogen bond (Boul *et al.*, 1971; Higa *et al.*, 1981). For example, equatorial hydroxy-ketone, XXXVIII, which can easily form an OH···O bond exhibits a single band at 3485 cm^{-1}. The corresponding axial compound (XXXIX) exhibits two bands, one near 3615–3620 cm^{-1} due to an unassociated OH and the other near 3600–3610 cm^{-1} due to a π associated OH. When competition occurs between OH···O and OH···π bonding as in XL, only bands due to the OH···O are observed (Suga *et al.*, 1972).

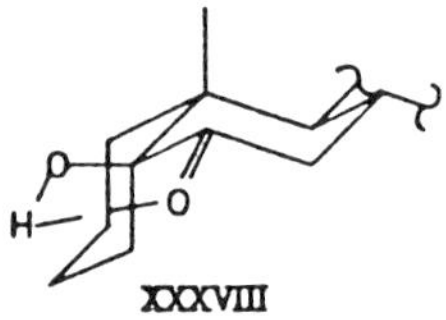

XXXVIII

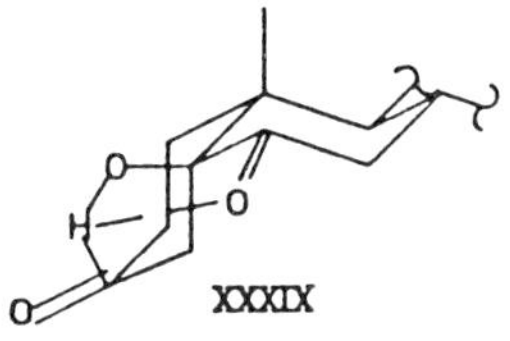

XXXIX

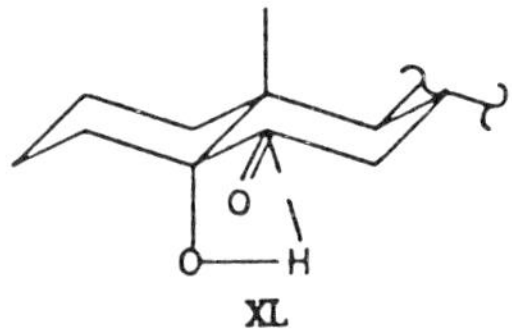

XL

The presence of various hydroxyl rotamers in 17-hydroxy steroids (in CCl_4) has recently been established by IR (Visser and van der Maas, 1983), as has the intermolecular association of 5α-cholestan-3α- and 3β-ols in solution (Kinst *et al.*, 1979).

D. Solvent Effects

Hydrogen bonding with solvent broadens O—H and usually lowers the frequency of these absorptions. Thus, an intermolecularly hydrogen-bonded hydroxyl gives a broad band at 3200–3550 cm^{-1} that disappears upon dilution.

The oxygens of carbonyl groups are sites capable of electron donation and are able to form hydrogen-bonded complexes with proton-donating solvents (Bellamy and Williams, 1959). The degree of this interaction in steroidal systems depends on the steric environment of the carbonyl. The influence of solvent on the absorption due to C=O stretching of C-3 and C-17 steroid esters has been extensively investigated (Jones and Herling, 1954; Jones *et al.*, 1948, 1950, 1952b). The effect of solvents on the IR spectra of carboxylic esters of androstan-17β-ol derivatives has also been studied (James and Noyce, 1971). Solute–solvent interactions are responsible for the shifts in the carbonyl stretching frequency and correlate with the length of the ester chain and with the hydrogen-bonding strength of the solvent. Since carbonyls assume increasing single-bond character when conjugated with double bonds, the strength of this type of interaction can be expected to increase with unsaturation (James and Ramgoolam, 1978).

REFERENCES

Aruldhas, G., Jalsovszky, G., and Holly, S. (1980). Infrared absorption intensities of steroids. *Acta Chim. Acad. Sci. Hung.* **104**, 117–122.

Bellamy, L. J. (1975). "The Infrared Spectra of Complex Molecules," 3rd ed. Chapman & Hall, London.

Bellamy, L. J., and Williams, R. L. (1959). Infra-red spectra and solvent effects. Part 2. Carbonyl absorptions. *Trans. Faraday Soc.* **55**, 14–18.

Blandon, P., Henbest, H. B., and Wood, G. W. (1952). Studies in the sterol group. Part LV. Ultraviolet absorption spectra of ethylenic centres. *J. Chem. Soc.* pp. 2737–2744.

Booker, H., Evans, L. K., and Gillam, A. E. (1940). Effect of Molecular environment on the absorption spectra of organic compounds in solution. I. Conjugated dienes. *J. Chem. Soc.* pp. 1453–1463.

Boul, A. D., Blunt, J. W., Browne, J. W., Kumar, V., Meakins, G. D., Pinhey, J. T., and Thomas, V. E. M. (1971). Microbiological hydroxylation of steroids. Part II. Structural information and infrared spectrometry. Carbonyl, preturbed methylene and hydroxy-vibrations of steroidal ketones and alcohols. *J. Chem. Soc. C* pp. 1130–1136.

Brand, J. C. D., and Eglinton, G. (1965). "Application of Spectroscopy to Organic Chemistry." Oldbourne Press, London.

Brande, E. A. (1962). *In* "Determination of Organic Structures by Physical Methods" (E. A. Brade and F. C. Nachod, eds.), 3rd ed. Academic Press, London.

Breivik, O. N., Owades, K. L., and Light, R. F. (1954). A new tetraethenoid sterol of yeast. *J. Org. Chem.* **19**, 1734–1740.

Bridgman, J. E., Cherry, P. C., Clegg, A. S., Evans, J. M., Jones, E. R. H., Kasal, A., Kumar, V., Meakins, G. D., Morisawa, Y., Richards, E. E., and Woodgate, P. D. (1970). Microbiological hydroxylation of steroids. Part I, Proton magnetic resonance spectra of ketones, alcohols and acetates in the androstane, pregnane and oestrane series. *J. Chem. Soc. C* pp. 250–257.

Brownlee, R. T. C., and Topsom, R. D. (1975). Correlations between i.r. frequencies and substituent constants. I. General considerations and aliphatic compounds. *Spectrochim. Acta, Part A* **31A**, 1677–1683.

Brownlee, R. T. C., di Stefano, J., and Topsom, R. D. (1975). Correlations between i.r. frequencies and substituent constants. 2. Substituted benzenes. *Spectrochim. Acta, Part A* **31A**, 1685–1693.

Caspi, E., and Scrimshaw, G. F. (1967). *In* "Steroid Hormone Analysis" (H. Carstensen, ed.), Vol. 1. Dekker, New York.

Cole, A. R. H. (1956). Infrared spectra of natural products. *Fortschr. Chem. Org. Naturst.* **13**, 27–60.

Cookson, R. C. (1954). Absorption spectra of ketones. Part I. α-halogeno-ketones. *J. Chem. Soc.* pp. 282–286.

Cookson, R. C., and Dandegaonker, (1955). Absorption spectra of ketones. Part II. The configuration of some bromo-derivatives of 6-oxocholestanyl acetate. Absorption spectra of α-ketols. *J. Chem. Soc.* pp. 352–355.

Dalton, F., McDougall, J. I., and Meakins, G. D. (1963). Hydroxy-steroids. Part II. The conformations and infrared spectra of steroid 3,5-diols and related compounds. *J. Chem. Soc.* pp. 4068–4075.

Davey, C. W., McGinnis, E. L., McKeown, J. M., Meakins, G. D., Pemberton, M. W., and Young, R. N. (1968). Hydroxy-steroids. Part XI. The preparation and infrared spectra of vicinal cholestanediols. *J. Chem. Soc. C* pp. 2674–2684.

Deady, L. W., Harrison, P. M., and Topsom, R. D. (1975). Frequency and intensity measurement of the carbonyl stretching vibration in substituted methyl benzoates and pyridine carboxylates. *Spectrochim. Acta, Part A* **31A**, 1671–1676.

Dence, J. B. (1980). "Steroids and Peptide." Wiley (Interscience), New York.

Dobriner, K., Katzenellenbogen, E., and Jones, R. N. (1953). "Infrared Absorption Spectra of Steroids—An Atlas." Wiley (Interscience), New York.

Dorfman, L. (1953). Ultraviolet absorption of steroids. *Chem. Rev.* **53**, 47–144.

Dyer, J. R. (1965). "Application of Infrared Absorption Spectroscopy of Organic Compounds." Prentice-Hall, Englewood Cliffs, New Jersey.

Egyed, O., Jalsovszky, G., and Holly, S. (1983). Infrared intensities of pregn-1,4-diene-3,20-dione derivatives. *J. Mol. Struct.* **99**, 133–136.

Fieser, L. F., and Fieser, M. (1959). "Steroids." Reinhold, New York.

Gebreyesus, T., Stoilov, I., Lou, F.-T., and Djerassi, C. (1985). Minor and trace sterols in marine invertebrates 55. The isolation, structure elucidation and synthesis of ergosta-5,24(28),25-trien-3β-ol. *Steroids* **45**, 447–452.

Gillam, A. E., and Stern, E. S. (1970). *In* "Electronic Absorption Spectroscopy in Organic Chemistry" (E. S. Stern and E. J. Timmons, eds.), 3rd ed. Arnold, London.

Gore, R. C. (1962). *In* "Determination of Organic Structures by Physical Methods" (E. A. Brande and F. C. Nachod, eds.), 3rd ed. Academic Press, London.

Görög, S., (1982). "Advances Steroid Analysis." Akadémiai Kiadó, Budapest.

Higa, T., Tanaka, J., Tsukitani, Y., and Kikuchi, H. (1981). Hippuristanols, cytotoxic polyoxygenated steroids from the Gorgonian *Isis hippuris*. *Chem. Lett.* pp. 1647–1650.

Holly, S., Jalsovszky, G., and Egyed, O. (1980). Infrared intensities of pregn-4-ene-3,20-dione derivatives. *J. Mol. Struct.* **60**, 139–142.

James, K. C., and Noyce, P. R. (1971). An infrared study of solvent effects on the carbonyl stretching bands of some androgen esters. *J. Chem. Soc. B* pp. 2045–2048.

James, K. C., and Ramgoolam, M. (1978). Solvent effects on carbonyl and ethylenic stretching frequencies in 3-keto unsaturated steroids. *Spectrochim. Acta, Part A* **34A**, 1145–1149.

Jones, R. N., and Herling, F. (1954). Characteristic group frequencies in the infrared spectra of steroids. *J. Org. Chem.* **19**, 1252–1268.

Jones, R. N., Williams, V. Z., Whalen, M. J., and Dobriner, K. (1948). Steroid metabolism. IV. Characterization of carbonyl and other functional groups in steroids by infrared spectrometry. *J. Am. Chem. Soc.* **70**, 2024–2034.

Jones, R. N., Humphries, P., and Dobriner, K. (1950). Steroid metabolism. IX. Further observations on the infrared absorption spectra of ketosteroids and steroidal esters. *J. Am. Chem. Soc.* **72**, 956–961.

Jones, R. N., Ramsey, D. A., Keir, D. S., and Dobriner, K. (1952a). The intensities of carbonyl bands in the infrared spectra of steroids. *J. Am. Chem. Soc.* **74**, 80–88.

Jones, R. N., Humphries, P., Herling, F., and Dobriner, K. (1952b). Steroid metabolism. XII. Determination of the structure of the side chains of C-21 steroids by infrared spectrometry. *J. Am. Chem. Soc.* **74**, 2820–2828.

Joris, L., and von R. Schleyer, P. (1968). Intramolecular hydrogen bonding in aliphatic hydroxy ketones. *J. Am. Chem. Soc.* **90**, 4599–4611.

Kastelic-Suhadolc, T. (1983). IR-spectra of amides of steroidal alkaloids with lactic acid. *Experientia* **39**, 259–260.

Kinst, M., van Duijn, D., and Bordewijk, P. (1979). Hydrogen bonding of 5α-cholestanol in carbon tetrachloride. *Recl. Trav. Chim. Pays-Bas* **98**, 262–267.

Liljefors, T., and Allinger, N. L. (1978). Conformational analysis. 128. The Woodward-Fieser rules and α,β-unsaturated ketones. *J. Am. Chem. Soc.* **100**, 1068–1073.

Morton, R. A. (1975). "Biochemical Spectroscopy," Vols. 1 and 2. Wiley, New York.

Nakanishi, K., and Solomon, P. H. (1977). "I.R. Absorption Spectroscopy," 2nd ed. Holden-Day, New York.

Nes, W. R., and McKean, M. L. (1977). "Biochemistry of Steroids and Other Isopentenoids." University Park Press, Baltimore, Maryland.

Oki, M., Iwamura, H., Aihara, J., and Iida, H. (1968). Intramolecular interaction between hydroxyl group and carbonyl moiety in keto-alcohols. *Bull. Chem. Soc. Jpn.* **41**, 176–182.

Rao, C. N. R. (1964). "Chemical Applications of Infrared Spectroscopy." Academic Press, New York.

Rao, C. N. R. (1967). "Ultraviolet and Visible Spectroscopy, Chemical Applications," 2nd ed. Butterworth, London.

Roberts, G., Gallagher, B., and Jones, R. N. (1958). "Infrared Absorption Spectra of Steroids—An Atlas," Vol. 2. Wiley (Interscience), New York.

Scott, A. I. (1964). "Interpretation of Ultraviolet Spectra of Natural Products." Pergamon, Oxford.

Silverstein, R. M., Bassler, G. C., and Morrill, T. C. (1981). "Spectrometric Identification of Organic Compounds," 4th ed. Wiley, New York.

Smith, A. M., and Eddy, C. R. (1959). High resolution infrared spectra of steroids in the carbon-hydrogen stretching region. *Anal. Chem.* **31**, 1539–1542.

Suga, T., Shishibori, T., and Matsuura, T. (1972). Intramolecular hydrogen bonding in hydroxy-keto steroids. *J. Chem. Soc., Perkin Trans. I* pp. 171–173.

Tichy, M. (1965). *Adv. Org. Chem.* **5**.

Ulrich, B., and Allinger, N. L. (1982). "Molecular Mechanics." *Am. Chem. Soc.*, Washington, D.C.

Visser, T., and van der Maas, J. H. (1983). Structural information from OH-stretching vibrations. XII. The orientation of the hydroxyl in 17-ethynyl-17-hydroxy- and 17-methyl-17-hydroxy steroids. *Spectrochim. Acta, Part A* **39A**, 921–924.

Winman, J. (1967). Vibration de valence ν(OH) libre des hydroxyles stérödiques: fréquences intensité et forme de la bande. *Bull. Soc. Chim. Fr.* pp. 4259–4270.

Woodward, R. B. (1941). Structure and absorption spectra of α,β-unsaturated ketones. *J. Am. Chem. Soc.* **63**, 1123–1126.

Woodward, R. B. (1942a). Structure and absorption spectra. III. Normal conjugated dienes. *J. Am. Chem. Soc.* **64**, 72–75.

Woodward, R. B. (1942b). Further observations on α,β-unsaturated ketones. *J. Am. Chem. Soc.* **64**, 76–77.

Yamaguchi, K. (1970). "Spectral Data of Natural Products." Elsevier, Amsterdam.

14

Raman Spectra of Steroids

Ian S. Butler and Monique Doyon
Department of Chemistry, McGill University
Montreal, Quebec, Canada

I. INTRODUCTION

The first detailed examination of the scattering of monochromatic light by a vibrating molecule was reported in 1928 by C. V. Raman, an Indian physicist (Raman, 1928; Raman and Krishnan, 1928a,b,c). He verified experimentally the 1923 predictions of Smekal. Raman's dramatic discovery quickly led to the Nobel Prize in Physics in 1930, a knighthood, and ultimately to his name being given to the new spectroscopic technique. The method was widely exploited during the 1930s in establishing the structures of many simple molecules. It fell into disfavor, however, during the 1940s because of its limitations with colored compounds, the very long exposure times necessary to detect the effect with photographic plates, and the development during World War II of routine infrared (IR) spectrometers for the rapid identification of synthetic rubbers. However, the discovery of continuous-wave (CW) visible lasers in the 1960s and the first experiments using lasers to excite Raman spectra have renewed interest in the technique. Laser Raman spectrometers now are fairly widespread, though still much more expensive than their IR counterparts and not as simple to operate.

Both IR and Raman spectroscopy provide information about molecular vibrations, but the selection rules are different. For a molecular vibration to be IR active, there must be a change in dipole moment derivative $(\partial\mu/\partial Q)_0 \neq 0$, where μ is the dipole moment and Q the normal coordinate that describes the relative motions of the atoms in the molecule during the vibration. For Raman activity, on the other hand, there must be a change in the molecular polarizability derivative $(\partial\alpha/\partial Q)_0 \neq 0$ during the vibration. An important consequence of these selection rules in the case of centrosymmetric systems is the rule of mutual exclusion, which states that molecular vibrations that are Raman active are IR inactive and *vice versa*. The non-coincidence of

Analysis of Sterols and Other Biologically Significant Steroids

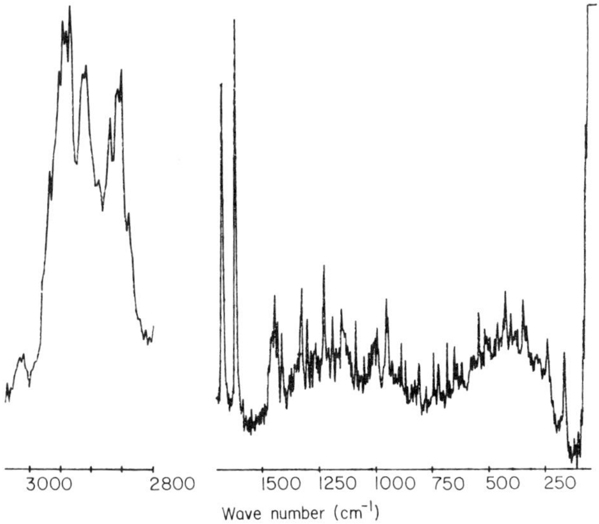

Figure 1 Raman spectrum of solid Δ^4-cholesten-3-one. Conditions: excitation, 514.5-nm Ar^+-ion laser (~ 40 mW at sample); slit widths, 300 μm; microRaman mode (4X magnification); baseline corrected below 1700 cm^{-1}.

IR and Raman peaks in the spectra of a compound is thus good evidence for the presence of a center of symmetry. This situation does not apply in the case of a steroid, however, because these molecules have no symmetry at all, except for the identity; and so all molecular vibrations are both IR and Raman active. Moreover, since steroids are relatively large organic molecules, containing 30 or more atoms, there should be at least 80 peaks in each spectrum because of the $3n - 6$ rule for the number of vibrational modes, where n is the number of atoms. Figure 1 shows the numerous peaks that appear in the Raman spectrum of a typical steroid, Δ^4-cholesten-3-one.

A convenient way to illustrate qualitatively the principles of laser Raman spectroscopy is shown in Fig. 2. This figure is a schematic representation of the possible interactions of a monochromatic beam of light of frequency ν_0 from a laser source with a vibrating, diatomic molecule (e.g., N_2) of vibrational frequency ν_1. The light can be scattered either elastically (no energy exchange) or inelastically (energy exchange). Elastic scattering implies scattering with the same frequency as the incident beam; this is referred to as Rayleigh scattering. (In fact, Rayleigh scattering is the reason why our sky appears blue: Most of the radiation being scattered by the water molecules in the upper atmosphere lies in the blue region of the electromagnetic spectrum.) On the other hand, for inelastic scattering, energy exchange occurs, leading to the Raman effect [Stokes, $h(\nu_0 - \nu_1)$; anti-Stokes, $h(\nu_0 + \nu_1)$]. In both cases, the energy difference between the Rayleigh line and the Raman peak corresponds to the vibrational energy ν_1 of the diatomic molecule.

From the Boltzmann distribution it can be shown that at normal temperature most of the diatomic molecules are located in the ground-state level ($v = 0$), and so the peak

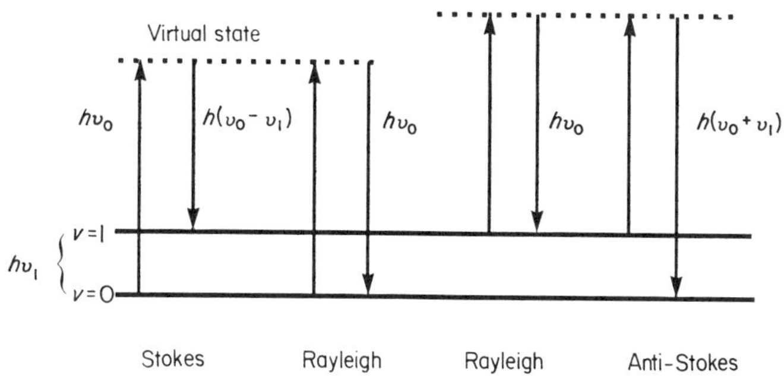

Figure 2 Qualitative description of the vibrational Raman effect for a diatomic molecule with a vibrational frequency ν_1.

on the Stokes side of the Rayleigh line will be significantly more intense than that on the anti-Stokes side, which derives from the first vibrational level ($v = 1$). For this reason, Raman spectra are usually scanned in the direction of decreasing absolute wavenumber.

Carbon tetrachloride is an excellent scatterer and is usually the compound chosen by the instrument manufacturers to illustrate the Raman effect and the performance of their spectrometers (Fig. 3). The 459 cm^{-1} peak is due to ν(C—Cl), the in-phase C—Cl stretching mode; and under high-resolution conditions ($\sim$ 1 cm^{-1}) this peak is split into several components due to the presence, in natural abundance, of the isotopic species $C^{35}Cl_4$, $C^{35}Cl_3{}^{37}Cl$, and so on.

The layout of a Raman spectrometer is illustrated in Fig. 4. Usually, the scattered radiation is analyzed at 90° to the incident laser beam. The Raman effect is about 10^4

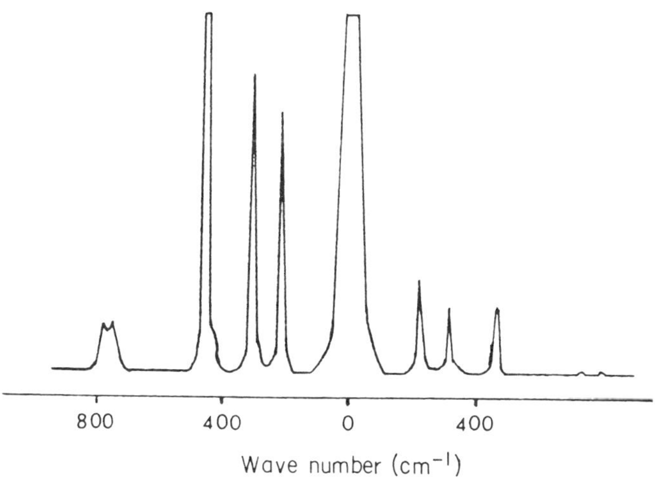

Figure 3 Raman spectrum of liquid CCl_4 showing the Rayleigh line (center) and the Stokes and anti-Stokes bands.

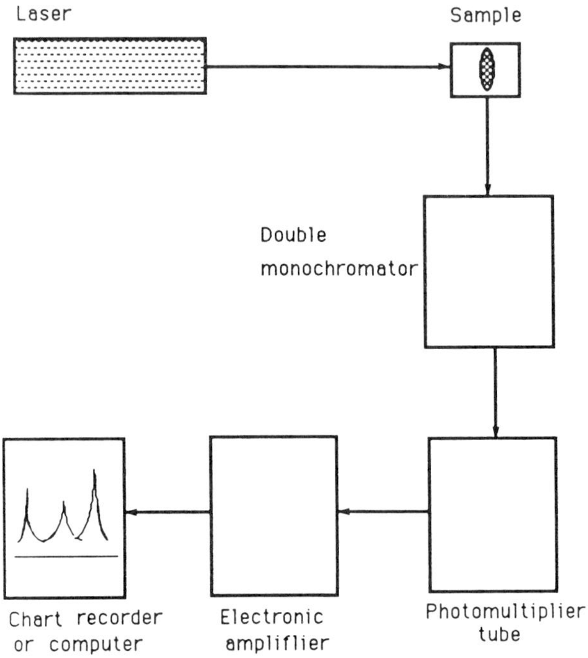

Figure 4 Block diagram showing the principal components of a modern Raman spectrometer.

times weaker than Rayleigh scattering; so it is necessary to have an efficient double monochromator with a low stray-light level to detect the weak Raman signals, especially at energies close to the very strong Rayleigh line due to the exciting laser line. Today, the detection systems are almost always based on photon counting, and excellent signal-to-noise ratios can be obtained because the instruments are interfaced to on-line minicomputers so that many scans can be co-added. The peak positions can be located easily and accurately by the software packages supplied with the computers.

Raman spectroscopy requires only small amounts of sample because the exciting laser line can be focused to a fraction of a millimeter. Some instruments are equipped with microscopes so that particles with cross sections of about 25 μm^2 can be examined without too much difficulty using 100 × magnification. The spectrum shown in Fig. 1 was recorded for a small cluster of crystals on a microscope slide on a microRaman spectrometer using 4 × magnification. In both normal and microRaman spectroscopy, gases, liquids, and solids can be studied, either in the free state or in glass vessels (e.g., melting point capillaries) since glass is a poor Raman scatterer. Large solid particles usually scatter better than small ones. Aqueous solutions can also be easily investigated because water is a weak scatterer; this affords a distinct advantage of the Raman technique over IR, particularly in biological work. Other advantageous features of Raman spectroscopy are the ready accessibility to low-energy vibrations that are sensitive to conformational changes and the ability to detect homonuclear vibrations that are only weakly (if at all) IR-active (e.g., S—S and N—N). Multiple bonds (e.g., C≡C and C═N) lead to particularly intense Raman peaks because they involve large changes in the molecular polarizability derivatives and because the Raman peak intensities are proportional to $(\partial\alpha/\partial Q)_0^2$.

There are, of course, disadvantages to Raman spectroscopy. For example, some compounds fluoresce markedly, which raises the background, making the detection of the Raman signal more difficult. However, computer software routines (e.g., baseline subtraction) are now available that help overcome this difficulty. Sample recrystallization often helps to reduce fluorescence backgrounds, especially for organic compounds such as steroids. Although Raman measurements do not take so long as they used to, it usually requires at least an hour to record a complete good-quality spectrum unless multichannel detection is employed. Detailed comparisons of the advantages and disadvantages of Raman and IR spectroscopy are given in Tobias (1967a,b) and Schrader and Steigner (1973).

Following this brief introduction to the Raman technique, we now turn to the Raman investigations on steroids that have been reported over the past 15 years. Owing to solubility limitations, almost all the work has been on crystalline solids or powders, and the main objective of the work has been to discover spectra–structure correlations of practical use to the synthetic steroid chemist. In 1973, Schrader and Steigner, who did much of the pioneering work in this field, published an excellent review of the earlier applications of Raman spectroscopy of steroids. Most of these earlier studies, therefore, will not be considered in the present survey. The range of compounds that has been investigated by Raman spectroscopy is indicated by the compilation given later in Table 2.

II. STRUCTURAL CORRELATION CHARTS

Considerable effort has been made to analyze systematically the Raman spectra of steroids and to correlate specific bands with molecular structure. In 1973, Schrader and Steigner published the results of an exhaustive study of the spectra of about 80 commercially available, crystalline steroids chiefly related to sexual and adrenal hormones. The spectra were recorded using both Hg-arc and Ar^+-ion laser excitation.

They examined five major spectral regions: (a) 4000–2800, (b) 2800–1350, (c) 1350–800, (d) 800–200, and (e) 200–20 cm^{-1}. In the 4000–2800 cm^{-1} range, they found that O—H stretching modes had low Raman intensity as do the C—H stretching modes of acetylenic groups. The N—H, C—H (aliphatic), and C—H (olefinic) stretching modes all exhibit medium-intense bands. The C≡C and C═C stretching motions appear in the 2800–1350 cm^{-1} region as strong bands. At around 1600 cm^{-1}, the C═O stretching modes are weaker than ν(C═C). The C—H bending modes at ~ 1450 cm^{-1} are of medium intensity. This region is particularly useful in indicating the type of steroid skeleton concerned. The stretching vibrations of the steroid skeleton and the wagging, twisting, and rocking deformations of the C—H bonds appear in the 1350–800 cm^{-1} region with varying intensities. The 800–200 cm^{-1} region displays deformation peaks characteristic of the steroid

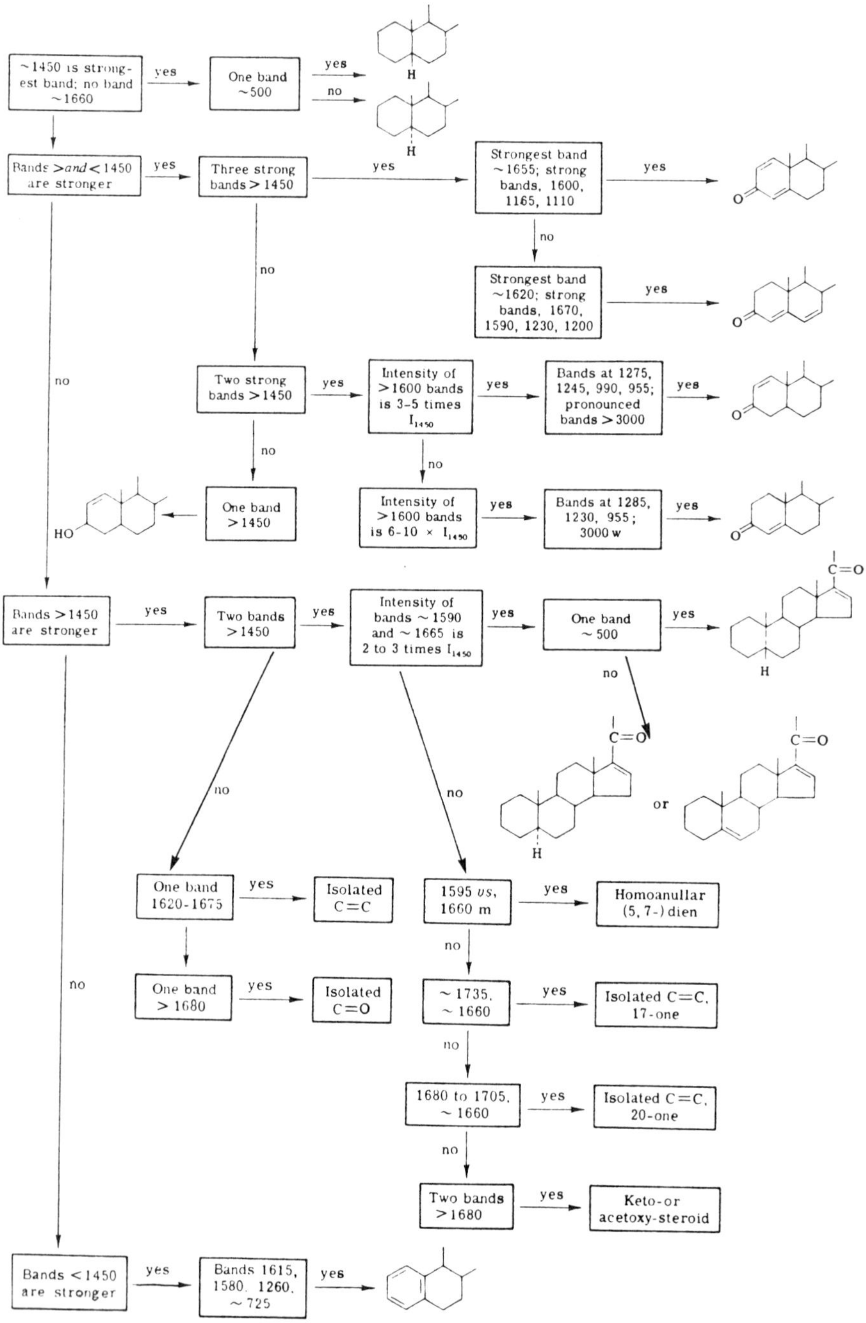

Figure 5 Correlation scheme for the elucidation of steroid skeletons on the basis of Raman spectral data. Reproduced from Schrader and Steigner (1973).

skeleton. A band near 725 cm^{-1} suggests the presence of an aromatic steroid, and a peak at 500 ± 5 cm^{-1}, with about half the intensity of the peak near 1450 cm^{-1}, is considered to be indicative of a 5-saturated steroid. The 500 cm^{-1} band is weak or absent for 5-steroids. The very low energy region (200-20 cm^{-1}) is where the translational and rotational modes of the rigid skeleton are expected. Finally, the peaks are particularly intense in the spectra when there are distinctly different electron polarizabilities along the chief axes of inertia. Moreover, a convenient intensity order is observed: aromatic ring >—C=C—C=C— (conjugated) >—C=C— (unconjugated) > saturated steroids.

Schrader and Steigner (1973) subjected their accumulated spectral data (peak positions and intensities) to computer analysis in an attempt to locate bands specific to certain steroidal structures, and they proposed the extensive structural correlation scheme shown in Fig. 5 in their review article. The indicated intensities are relative to an internal standard: the strongest band in the 1460–1440 cm^{-1} region due to the deformations of the CH_2 and CH_3 groups that every steroid exhibits. This correlation scheme affords an extremely rapid and convenient means of steroidal skeleton identification. Some typical Raman spectra in the 1700–1500 cm^{-1} region of the six main types of steroids investigated by Schrader and Steigner are shown in Fig. 6.

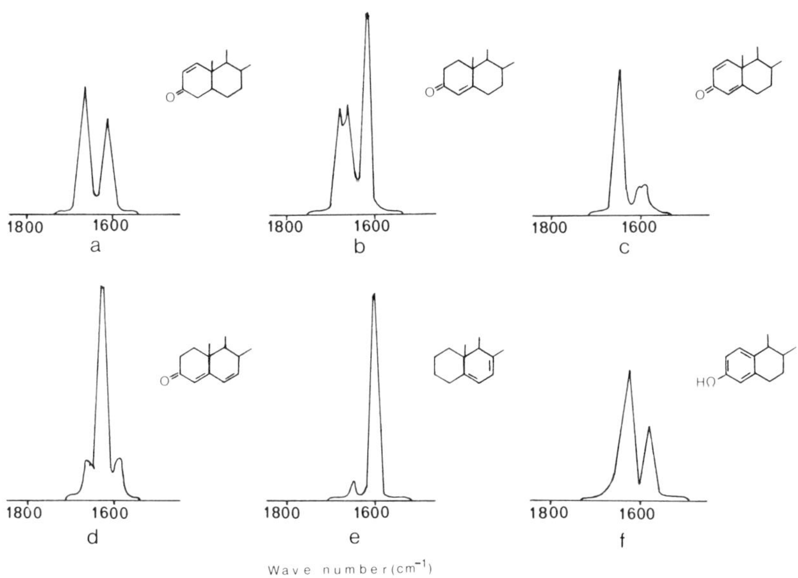

Figure 6 Raman spectra in the 1700–1500 cm^{-1} region of typical examples of the six main types of solid steroids investigated by Schrader and Steigner in the 1700–1500 cm^{-1} region (adapted from Schrader and Steigner, 1973):
(a) 17β-hydroxy-5α-androst-1-en-3-one, (b) 17β-hydroxy-4-androsten-3-one,
(c) 17β-hydroxyl,4-androstadiene-3-one, (d) 17β-hydroxy-4,6-androstadien-3-one,
(e) 3α-acetoxy-5,7-cholesta-diene, and (f) 1,3,5(10)-estratriene-3,17α-diol.

About ten years after Schrader and Steigner's comprehensive study, Pouskouleli *et al.* (1983) recorded the Raman spectra of 17 solid hormonal steroids representative of conjugated dieno-keto, conjugated keto, and saturated steroids, and steroids with isolated double bonds (C=C), using Ar^+-ion laser excitation (514.5 nm, ~180 mW at the samples). There was no visible evidence of thermal decomposition at this laser power. The vibrational data provided support for Schrader and Steigner's structural correlation scheme, though it was emphasized that the scheme must be used with caution when there are substituents present that contain ketonic groups. Since the spectra recorded in this work (and in that by Schrader and Steigner) were for the solids, reliance upon numbers of peaks is unwise because peak splitting, due to solid-state effects (site or factor group splitting) or polymorphism, is a distinct possibility. Nevertheless, taking into account all the possible intensity variations, it is possible to use the correlation chart with considerable success.

One of the steroids investigated by Pouskouleli *et al.* (1983) was the catatoxic drug 3β-hydroxy-20-oxo-5-pregnene-16α-carbonitrile (pregnenolone-16α-carbonitrile, PCN; see structure). A more thorough study of this compound has also been reported by Kourounakis and Theophanides (1981) and Theophanides (1978). The keto and cyano groups are clearly evident in the Raman spectra of the solid and of a $CHCl_3$ solution (Fig. 7). Two keto peaks are observed for C-20 in both cases (for solid:

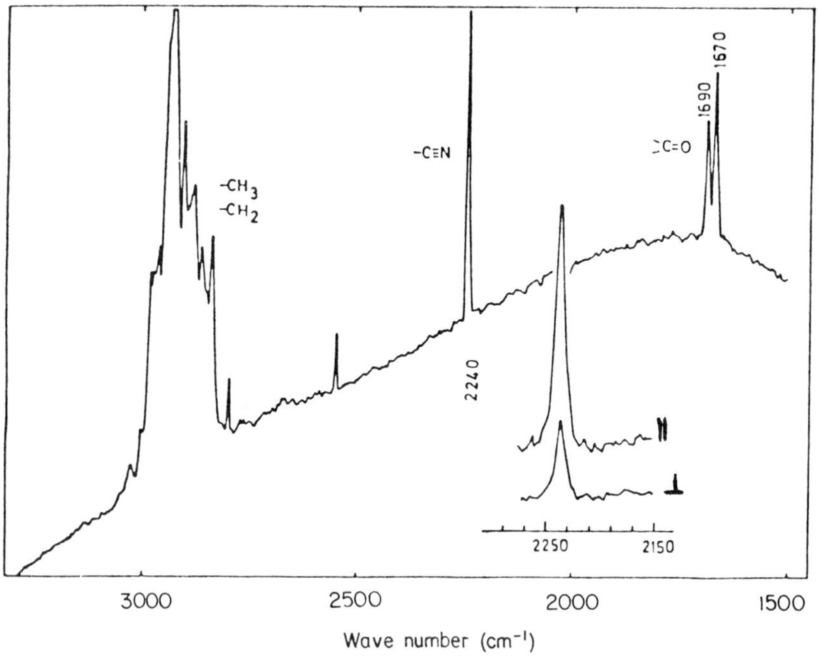

Figure 7 Partial Raman spectrum of solid PCN (inset: polarization data for $CHCl_3$ solution). Adapted from Kourounakis and Theophanides (1981) and Theophanides (1978).

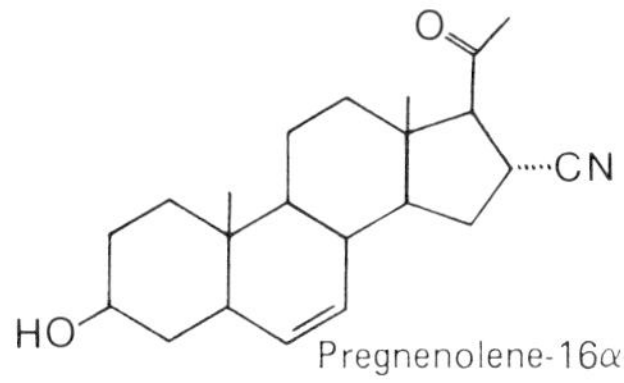

Pregnenolene-16α-carbonitrile (PCN)

1690, 1670 cm^{-1}; for solution, 1705, 1670 cm^{-1}), possibly due to the presence of two conformational rotamers resulting from rotation about the C-17/C-20 bond. The ν(CN) peak appears close to 2240 cm^{-1} for both the solid and $CHCl_3$ solution and is almost completely polarized in the solution spectrum. The polarization data were interpreted by Kourounakis and Theophanides to mean that the CN group lies principally in the mean, pseudoplane formed by the four carbon atoms C-16, C-17, C-14, and C-15′ but that there is a small percentage of the molecules with the CN group located out of the plane. The polarization results are not too surprising because X-ray diffraction analysis had shown that the CN group lies above the pseudoplane.

III. FLUOCORTOLONE DERIVATIVES

In the mid-1970s, Fleury and his co-workers demonstrated that it is possible to use Raman spectroscopy to identify steroids in picogram amounts from high-performance liquid chromatography (HPLC) fractions (Gamiot *et al.*, 1977). They compared the Raman spectra in the 4000–150 cm^{-1} region of polycrystalline fluocortolone caproate (CAF) (see structure), a corticosteroidal hormone, with the spectra of two related steroids, fluocortolone base, and its trimethylacetate (TMAF). There are several spectral regions in which the structures can be distinguished. In the

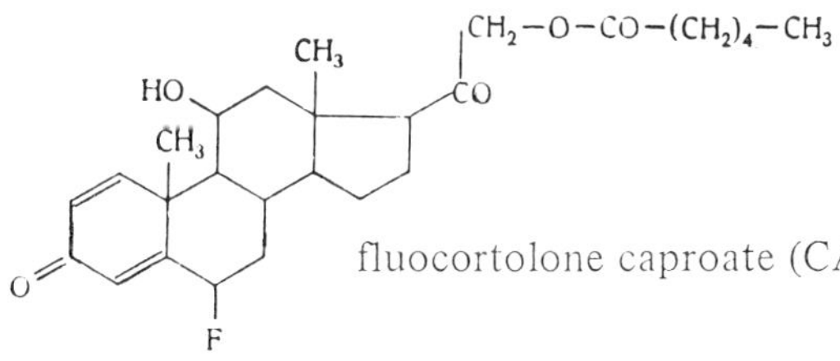

fluocortolone caproate (CAF)

1580–1690 cm^{-1} region are some intense bands that are specific to conjugated $\Delta^{1(4)}$-3-ones (Fig. 8). The 1690–1750 cm^{-1} range indicates not only a ketone group on the lateral chain but also the presence of an ester function: One (TMAF, 1728 cm^{-1}) or two peaks (CAF, 1723, 1745 cm^{-1}) are observed. The fluocortolone base displays a unique peak at 1635 cm^{-1}. Other spectral regions of interest that are representative of ester groups in the lateral chain are fixed on C-21, trimethylacetate chain (340–360, 570–610, 750–810 cm^{-1}). CAF can be distinguished from TMAF by the absence of the 796 cm^{-1} peak. The caproate chain exhibits a characteristic set of peaks at 1350–1310 cm^{-1}.

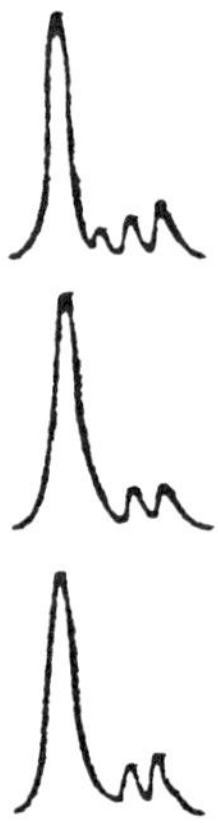

		$\nu \cdot cm^{-1}$	
Base	1606	1625	1666
Trimethylacetate	1608	1629	1662
Caproate	1604	1623	1660

Figure 8 Comparison of the Raman spectra of solid fluocortolones in the 1690–1580 cm^{-1} region. Adapted from Gamiot *et al.*, 1985.

Fleury's research group has also reported an analysis of the low-frequency Raman spectra of polycrystalline CAF as a function of temperature (Gamiot *et al.*, 1985). Fifteen bands were observed in the region below 200 cm^{-1} at 123 K, but only six at 423 K. These bands were assigned to rotational and translational lattice, internal, and overall modes of vibrations. For example, the authors assigned the bands at 191.4, 181.3, 147, 132.5, and 75.8 cm^{-1} to internal vibrational modes (torsions or vibrations

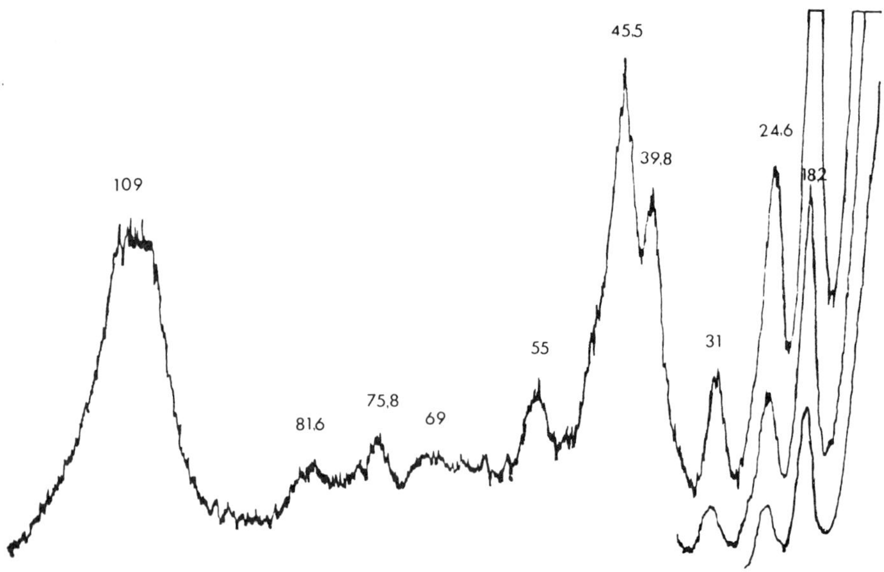

Figure 9 Raman spectrum of CAF at 123 K (Ar^+-ion laser excitation, 488.0 nm; slit widths ~ 2 cm^{-1}). Adapted from Gamiot *et al.* (1985).

of the molecule as a whole). The bands appearing at 55, 39.8 and 31 cm^{-1} were attributed chiefly to rotational lattice modes. A typical spectrum of CAF recorded at 123 K is shown in Fig. 9.

IV. NONCONJUGATED OLEFINIC STEROIDS

In 1976, Davies and co-workers published Raman data for 27 steroids containing nonconjugated olefinic bonds in a range of positions. The spectra were recorded for the solids and $CHCl_3$ solutions and, in some cases, for CCl_4 solutions. Particular attention was paid to two regions: 3100–3000 cm^{-1} (olefinic C—H stretching) and 1700–1600 cm^{-1} (olefinic double bond stretching). All the nuclear disubstituted olefins exhibit a band in the 3028–3013 cm^{-1} region. Several of the trisubstituted olefins give a band between 3040–3035 cm^{-1}, but the others, like the tetrasubstituted olefins, display strong bands between 1676 and 1632 cm^{-1}. The authors concluded that the frequency ranges for the various double-bond positions often overlap, but the ranges for Δ^{8}-, $\Delta^{9(11)}$-, and Δ^{11}-olefins are different from those of other tetra-, tri-, and disubstituted C═C double bonds, respectively. A comparison of the IR and Raman-active ν(C═C) peaks for typical di-, tri-, and tetrasubstituted steroids is shown in Fig. 10, which illustrates the intensity differences observed. Table 1 presents a useful correlation of the wavenumber ranges for ν(C═C) for the solids and in solution for various types of olefins. These Raman peaks agree quite well with the IR data for the same types of complexes, but the Raman spectra are much easier to obtain. The frequencies of tetrasubstituted double-bond vibrations are not available from IR spectroscopy.

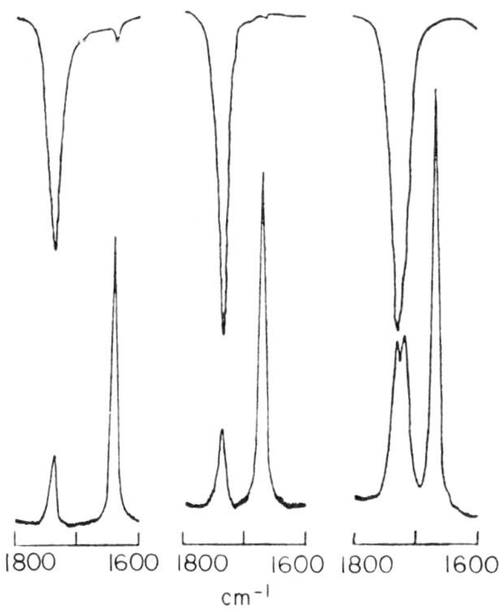

Figure 10 Infrared (upper trace) and Raman (lower trace) spectra of typical di-, tri-, and tetrasubstituted olefinic steroids: left, solid 5α-cholest-6-en-3β-yl acetate; middle, cholest-5-en-3β-yl acetate in CCl_4 solution; right, 3β,17α-diacetoxy-6-methylpregn-5-en-20-one in $CHCl_3$ solution. Adapted from Davies *et al.* (1976).

Table 1 Wavenumber ranges for ν(C=C) for the different types of olefinic steroids studied in Davies *et al.* (1976).

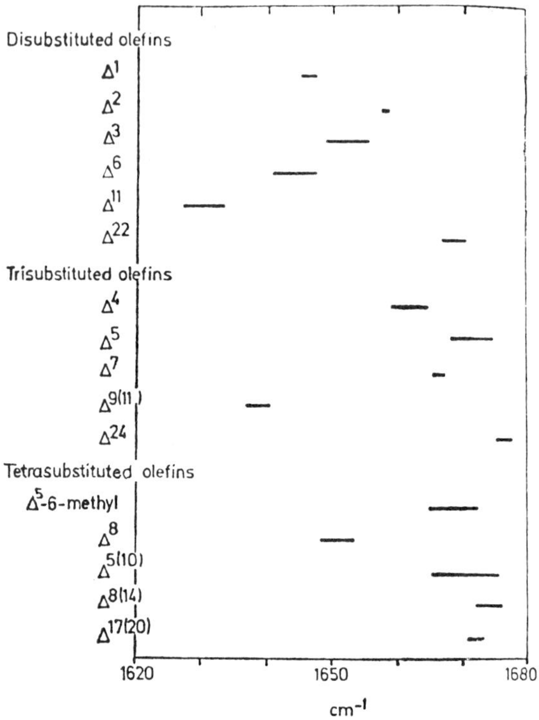

V. CHOLESTEROLS

In another attempt to obtain empirical correlations between Raman data and steroid structure, Faiman (1977) has investigated the Raman spectra of a number of chloresterols and their derivatives in the crystalline state. Although the data are extremely complex, three spectral regions were shown to be useful for distinguishing chain packing in each form: < 300 cm^{-1}, giving information on inter- and intramolecular vibrations in the chloresterol moiety; the methylene rocking/deformation region (1400–1500 cm^{-1}), giving information on packing in the crystalline state; and the C—H stretching region (3100–2700 cm^{-1}), which suggests a correlation between branching in the side chains of the cholesterols, polarity of the substituent groups in the various derivatives studied, and relative chain order in the packing arrangements in the crystalline state. A study of two branched-chain aerosol derivatives, bis(2-octyl)sodium sulpho-succinate and its isomer bis(di-2-ethylhexyl-sodium sulpho-succinate, indicated that branched-chain amphiphiles are good Raman spectroscopic models for the cholesterols, in accord with earlier Raman work that showed straight-chain amphiphiles to be good models for more complex phospholipids.

The effects of anesthetic and nonanesthetic steroids on dipalmitoyl phosphatidylcholine liposomes were studied by O'Leary *et al.* (1984) by making use of high-sensitivity scanning calorimetry and Raman spectroscopy. Calorimetric measurements indicated that both anesthetic and nonanesthetic steroids depressed and broadened the gel to liquid-crystalline phase transition. There was no correlation between the perturbations by the steroids on the primary gel to liquid-crystalline phase transition temperature and anesthetic potency. The magnitudes of the steroid-induced transition broadening and lowering of the pretransition temperature, however, correlated well with anesthetic potency. This effect appeared to arise from the projection from the plane of the D-ring of substituents at the C-17 position of the steroid nucleus. Raman spectroscopic measurements demonstrated that the steroid molecule is localized in the acyl region of the bilayer and that effects of the steroid do not extend to either the head-group or interface regions of the lamellae. The data are consistent with unitary hypotheses relating general anesthesia to lipid perturbations. For model systems, perturbations to the subtle structural and dynamical properties of the bilayer pretransition may provide a more sensitive marker than the main-phase transition in assessing the significance of lipid mediation in inducing anesthetic action.

VI. SAPOGENINS

Hunter *et al.* (1981) have used Raman spectroscopy, in conjunction with HPLC analysis, to identify six common isomeric steroidal sapogenin acetates in the solid state that were obtained from the degradation of plant materials. The sapogenins in question are diosgenin, yamogenin, togogenin, neotigogenin, smilagenin, and sarsasapogenin. Since these molecules contain almost 80 atoms, the spectra are extremely complex. All six compounds exhibit a series of bands near 1450 cm^{-1} due to the CH_2 scissoring mode of comparable relative intensity to the bands in the corresponding IR spectra. The ester ν(C=O) mode in the Raman at about 1730 cm^{-1} is 1/10 to 1/4 the relative intensity of the band in the IR (normalized against the 1450 cm^{-1} bands). These data are the first ever published for steroidal sapogenins.

VII. CONCLUSIONS

Raman spectroscopy continues to be a useful probe of steroid structure. The time required to obtained a complete spectrum is still rather long, but only small regions of the spectra need be scanned when using the spectra–structure correlations described in this chapter. If only the 1600–1400 cm^{-1} region is being examined, it is possible to scan the region in a matter of seconds using a multichannel Raman spectrometer. The microRaman technique should prove particularly useful for steroid analysis in the future because a single microcrystal is sufficient to obtain a good spectrum. This is an area that is worthwhile exploring. It will not be necessary to build up a large databank specifically for microRaman spectra of steroids because these spectra closely resemble those of the bulk materials. There is still a need for a complete catalog of Raman spectra of steroids (see Table 2).

Table 2 Examples of steroids that have been studied by raman spectroscopy

Steroid	Reference
6α-Fluoro-11β,17α-21-trihydroxy-16α-methyl-1,4-pregnadiene-3,20-dione, 21-acetate (paramethasone acetate)	5
17α,21-Dihydroxy-1,4-pregnadiene-3,11,20-trione, 21-acetate (prednisone acetate)	5
11β,17α,21-Trihydroxy-6α-methyl-1,4-pregnadiene-3,20-dione (medrol)	5
9α-Fluoro-11β,17α,21-trihydroxy-16α-methyl-1,4-pregnadiene-3,20-dione, 21-acetate (dexamethasone acetate)	5
11β,16α,17α,21-Tetrahydroxy-1,4-pregnadiene-3,20-dione (triamcinolone)	5
9α-Fluoro-11β,17α,21-trihydroxy-16β-methyl-1,4-pregnadiene-3,20-dione, 21-acetate (betamethasone acetate)	5
11β,17α,21-Trihydroxy-1,4-pregnadiene-3,20-dione, 21-acetate (prednisolone acetate)	5
17β-Hydroxy-1,4-androstadien-3-one	4,5
17α,21-Dihydroxy-4-pregnene-3,11-dione, 21-acetate (cortisone acetate)	5
11β,17α,21-Trihydroxy-4-pregnene-3,20-dione, 21-acetate (hydrocortisone acetate)	5
7α-Sulfhydryl-17-hydroxy-3-oxo-4-androstene-17α-propionic acid, γ-lactone	5
17α-Methyl-17-hydroxyl-1α, 7α-dithioacetyl-4-androsten-3-one (emdabol)	5
17-Hydroxy-7α-thioacetyl-3-oxo-4-androstene-17α-proionic acid, γ-lactone (spironolactone)	5
17-Hydroxy-7α-thioethyl-3-oxo-4-androstene-17α-propionic acid, γ-lactone	5
3β-Hydroxy-6β-thioacetyl-20-oxo-5α-pregnane-16α-carbonitrile (pregnasone)	5
3β-Hydroxy-6β-thioacetyl-5α-cholestane (cholethiate)	5
3β-Hydroxy-20-oxo-5-pregnene-16α-carbonitrile	5,6
17β-Hydroxy-19-nor-4-pregnen-20-in-3-one	4
4-Androstene-3,17-dione	4
17β-Hydroxy-4-androsten-3-one	4
17β-Hydroxy-4,6-androstadien-3-one	4
3β-Acetoxy-5,7-cholestadiene 1,3,5(10)-estradiene-3, 17-diol	4
3β-Acetoxy-5β-pregn-16-en-20-one	4
3β-Hydroxy-5α-androstan-17-one	4
3-Methoxy-19-nor-1,3,5(10)-pregnatrien-20-en 17β-ol	4
17β-Hydroxy-5α-androst-1-en-3-one	4
5α-Androst-1-en-3β-ol	9
5α-Cholest-1-en-3β-ol	9
5α-Cholest-2-ene	9
5α-Cholest-2-en-6-one	9
5α-Pregn-2-en-20-one	9
5α-Cholest-3-one	9
Methyl 5β-chol-3-enoate	9
5α-Cholest-6-en-3β-yl acetate	9
3α-Hydroxy-5β-chol-11-enoic acid	9
(25R)-5α-Spirost-11-en-3β-yl acetate	9
Cholest-4-ene	9
Cholest-4-en-3β-yl acetate	9
Cholest-5-ene	9
Cholest-5-en-3-one	9
Cholest-5-en-3β-yl acetate	9

3β-Chlorocholest-5-ene	9
20-Methylpregna-5,17(20)-dien-3β-yl acetate	9
Stigmasta-5,22-dien-3β-yl acetate	9
5α-Cholest-7-en-3β-ol	9
5α-Androst-9(11)-ene-3β, 17β-diol	9
3β-Acetoxy-5α-androst-9(11)-en-17-one	9
(25R)-6-Methylspirost-5-en-3β-yl acetate	9
3β,17α-Diacetoxy-6-methylpregn-5-en-20-one	9
17α-Ethynyl-17β-hydroxyestr-5(10)-en-3-one	9
5α-Lanost-8-en-3β-ol	9
5α-Lanosta-8,24-dien-3β-ol	9
5α-Cholest-8(14)-en-3β-ol	9
Anhydrus cholesterol	10
Cholesterol monohydrate	10
Cholesterol sodium sulphate	10
Cholesterol dihydrogen monophosphate	10
Cholesterol iodide	10
Cholesterol acetate	10
Cholesterol linolenate	10
Bis(di-2-octyl)sodium sulphosuccinate	10
Bis(di-2-ethylhexyl)sodium sulphosuccinate	10
Fluocortolone caproate	7,8
Fluocortolone base	7,8
Fliocortolone trimethylacetate	7,8
Diosgenin acetate	12
Yamogenin acetate	12
Tigogenin acetate	12
Neotigogenin acetate	12
Smilagenin acetate	12
Sarsasapogenin acetate	12

REFERENCES

Davies, J. E. D., Hodge, P., and Khan, M. N. (1976). *J. Chem. Soc., Perkin Trans.* II, 841.

Faiman, F. (1977). *Chem. Phys. Lipids* **18**, 84.

Gamiot, A. P., Cuingnet, E., Vergoten, G., and Fleury, G. (1977). *Bulg. J. Phys. 4*, **6**, 679.

Gamiot, A. P., Vergoten, A. G., Saudemon, M., and Fleury, G. (1985). *Talanta* **32**, 373.

Hunter, I. R., Walden, M. K., Bailey, G. F., and Heftmann, E. (1981). *J. Nat. Prod.* **44**, 245–251.

Kourounakis, P., and Theophanides, T. (1981). *Pharmazie* **36**, 613–614.

O'Leary, T. J., Ross, P. D., and Levin, I. W. (1984). *Biochemistry* **23**, 4636.

Pouskouleli, G., Butler, I. S., and Kourounakis, P. (1983). *J. Mol. Struct.* **102**, 93–101.

Raman, C. V. (1928). *Indian J. Phys.* **2**, 387.

Raman, C. V., and Krishnan, K. S. (1928a). *Nature (London)* **121**, 501.

Raman, C. V., and Krishnan, K. S. (1928b). *Proc. R. Soc. London, Ser. A* **122**, 23.

Raman, C. V., and Krishnan, K. S. (1928c). *Indian J. Phys.* **2**, 399.

Schrader, B., and Steigner, E. (1973). *In* "Modern Methods of Steroid Analysis" (E. Heftmann, ed.), Chapter 9, pp. 231-243. Academic Press, New York.

Smekal, A. (1923). *Naturwiss enschaffen* **11**, 873.
Theophanides, T. (1978). *In* "Raman Spectroscopy" (E. D. Schmid, R. R. Krishnan, and W. Kiefer, eds.), Chapter 6, pp. 115–130. Heyden Press, London.
Tobias, R. S. (1967a). *J. Chem. Educ.* **44**, 2.
Tobias, R. S. (1967b). *J. Chem. Educ.* **44**, 70.

15

Physicochemical Determinations of Sterols by Deuterium and Carbon-13 Nuclear Magnetic Resonance

Ian C. P. Smith
Division of Biological Sciences
National Research Council of Canada
Ottawa, Canada K1A OR6

Erick J. Dufourc
Centre de Recherche Paul Pascal, CNRS
Domaine Universitaire
33405 Talence Cedex, France

I. INTRODUCTION

Chapter 12 has shown that nuclear magnetic resonance (NMR) spectroscopy is one of the more important methods of elucidating the structures of biological molecules. In this chapter, we shall describe how the dynamics of biologically important molecules, such as sterols, can be determined with deuterium (^2H) and carbon-13 (^{13}C) NMR. Sterol motional behavior will be described in its natural environment, the biomembrane.

II. PRINCIPLES OF THE METHODS

A. Magnetic Interactions

To measure a nuclear magnetic resonance one needs a nucleus with nonzero spin. The total energy of such a nucleus in a static magnetic field can be decomposed into a sum of several terms, each corresponding to a given interaction (or coupling) between a nuclear property and the surroundings. This can be explicitly written as

$$H = \underset{10^8}{H_Z} + \underset{10^6}{H_Q} + \underset{10^4\text{–}10^3}{H_{CSA}} + \underset{10^4\text{–}10^3}{H_D} + \underset{10}{H_J} \tag{1}$$

where H denotes the total nuclear Hamiltonian, i.e., the quantum mechanical description of the total nuclear magnetic energy of interactions; H_Z the interaction of the nuclear magnetic moment μ with the external magnetic field B_0; H_Q arises from an electronic interaction of the nuclear quadrupole moment of the nucleus with electric field gradients surrounding the nucleus; H_{CSA} denotes the interaction relative to the anisotropy of the chemical shift (sensitive to chemical structure and phase symmetry); H_D the dipolar interaction (coupling through space with neighboring spins); and H_J the scalar interaction (coupling through chemical bonds to neighboring spins).

It can be seen that any modification in the structure or dynamics of the surroundings of the nucleus under study is reported by a variation of a given term in the interaction energy. The numbers below each term of the total Hamiltonian in Eq. 1 represent the orders of magnitude of the static interaction (in hertz). Certain terms of the total Hamiltonian are more sensitive to structural variations, and others report on dynamics.

In liquids, where isotropic fast motions occur, H_Q, H_D, and the anisotropic part of H_{CSA} are averaged to zero. Spectra report only on scalar and (isotropic) chemical-shift interactions. Information on quadrupolar, dipolar, and chemical-shift anisotropy coupling can nonetheless be obtained from relaxation phenomena (*vide infra*).

Biological membranes are, by definition, liquid crystals; in other words, they are anisotropic fluid media. The amphipathic molecules that comprise such membranes (phospholipids, sterols, proteins, etc.) do not orient randomly in water; instead they usually align locally in one direction: the normal to the bimolecular leaflet. A well-known picture of a biomembrane is the fluid-mosaic model proposed by Singer and Nicolson (1972). Although well organized, the membrane components are highly dynamic. Under such conditions, the quadrupolar, dipolar, and chemical-shift anisotropy interactions no longer cancel, though their magnitudes may be reduced by the anisotropic molecular motions, if the motions have the appropriate frequency relative to that of the interaction energy.

In the case of ^{2}H-NMR (deuterium, spin $I = 1$, having been incorporated in the biological molecule of interest by chemical synthesis), the total Hamiltonian can be approximated by

$$H \simeq H_Z + H_Q \tag{2}$$

The other terms of Eq. (1) do not contribute significantly to the total magnetic interaction energy and can be neglected.

In the case of ^{13}C-NMR (natural abundance or synthetic incorporation of a single ^{13}C nucleus), the Hamiltonian becomes

$$H \simeq H_Z + H_{CSA} + H_D \tag{3}$$

H_Q does not exist for nuclei with spin $I = 1/2$ (such as ^{13}C), and H_J is omitted in Eq. (3). H_D, which represents the proton-carbon dipolar interaction, may be suppressed by proton decoupling.

One can simplify the analysis by selecting the interaction of interest and monitor how a specific coupling is modified by the structure or the dynamics of the system. Calculation of energy levels and absorption lines has been detailed elsewhere (Seelig, 1977; Mehring, 1983); we shall only quote the results.

$$\text{Deuterium:} \quad \Delta\nu(\beta) = \frac{3}{2} A_Q S_{C\text{-}^2H} \left(\frac{3\cos^2\beta - 1}{2} \right) \tag{4}$$

$$\text{Carbon-13:} \quad \sigma(\beta) = \sigma_{iso} + \frac{2\Delta\sigma}{3} \left(\frac{3\cos^2\beta - 1}{2} \right) \tag{5}$$

Note in Eq. (4) that the frequency separation between the two absorption lines, called the quadrupolar splitting $\Delta\nu(\beta)$, is a function of the static quadrupolar coupling constant A_Q(A_Q = 170 kHz for methylene C-^{2}H bonds), the orientational order parameter $S_{C\text{-}^2H}$ and the angle β. In Eq. (5), the position of the absorption line, called the chemical shift $\sigma(\beta)$, is dependent on the isotropic chemical shift σ_{iso}, the residual chemical-shift anisotropy $\Delta\sigma$, and on β. In the usual analysis of fluid-phase spectra of both ^{2}H and ^{13}C, it is assumed that the system is axially symmetric and that the axis of symmetry is the bilayer normal n. The angle β represents the orientation of that axis relative to the direction of the external magnetic field B_0.

A typical variation of the resonance lines [Eqs. (4) and (5)] as a function of β is shown in Fig. 1.

The orientational order parameter $S_{C\text{-}^2H}$ gives a direct measure of the time-dependent angular excursions of a given C-^{2}H bond with respect to the principal axis of motion, usually taken to be the bilayer normal. In principle, $\Delta\sigma$ leads to the same information, but the order parameter cannot be extracted straightforwardly from measurement of the residual chemical-shift anisotropy.

Biological membranes do not usually orient themselves in the magnetic field. In other words, in a typical dispersion of biomembranes in water, one has a random

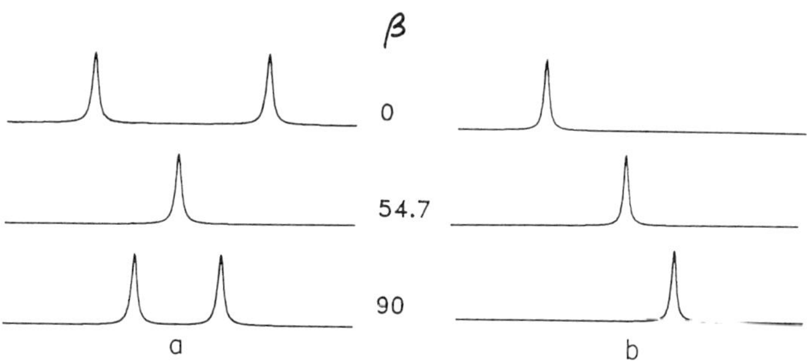

Figure 1 Variation of spectral frequencies as a function of β for nuclei subject to (a) quadrupolar and (b) chemical-shift anisotropy interactions. The angle β is defined in the text.

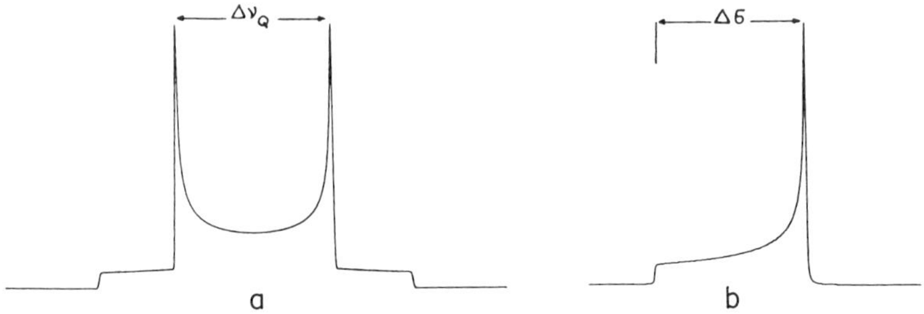

Figure 2 Axially symmetric powder patterns for nuclei subject to (a) quadrupolar and (b) chemical-shift anisotropy interactions.

distribution of local bilayer normals with respect to B_0, i.e., the angle β varies from 0° to 90°, and spectra are composed of a superposition of all resonances originating from all orientations of the motional averaging (symmetry) axis with respect to B_0. This random distribution can be described as if the axes were distributed around the surface of a sphere. The probability of having a normal that is oriented at β with respect to B_0 is described by a sin β function. With these considerations in mind, one obtains typical nonoriented spectra, as shown in Fig. 2, for nuclei subject to quadrupolar and chemical-shift anisotropy interactions. Such composite spectra are called *powder patterns* and may appear rather complex. However, one can still measure the quadrupolar splitting for $\beta = 90°$, called $\Delta\nu_Q$, and thus obtained $S_{C\text{-}^2H}$. The chemical-shift anisotropy $\Delta\sigma$ is measured directly from the chemical shifts due to $\beta = 0°$ and $\beta = 90°$ orientations.

As described above, the amplitude of molecular motions (angular excursions) is obtained from spectra. The rates of these motions can be estimated by measurement of relaxation times (see Sections II.B and IV).

B. Detection of Nuclear Magnetic Resonance Signals

Spectra such as those of Fig. 1 are usually obtained by Fourier transformation of the time evolution of the nuclear magnetic resonance (NMR) signal. Detection of this time-dependent signal relies on classical magnetic induction methods.

When a sample containing resonant spins resides in a magnetic field, the total magnetic interaction, described previously, promotes a separation of the magnetic energy levels. At equilibrium, the nuclear spins populate the energy levels according to Boltzmann statistics. The net effect is a resultant macroscopic magnetization M_0 along the external magnetic field direction z. Application of a strong impulse of radiofrequency (rf) field B_1, in a direction perpendicular to B_0 and hence to M_0, has the effect of rotating the resultant magnetization around B_1. The rotation angle depends on the energy of the pulse (in practice, the angle is determined by the length of the pulse, which is $\sim 10^{-5}$ s). Usually one uses rf pulses such that M_0 is projected onto the plane perpendicular to B_0, the x-y plane. Once B_1 is removed, the system starts relaxing back to its original equilibrium position.

Two relaxation processes then occur simultaneously: (1) The magnetization in the x-y plane M_{xy} diminishes due to the loss of phase coherence of the spins (spin-spin exchange, inhomogeneities in the external field, etc.), and (2) the equilibrium magnetization M_0 is gradually restored in the direction of the external field (the excited spins give up their energy to their surroundings, generally referred to as the lattice). These processes are assumed to follow exponential laws. The time constant of process (1) is the *transverse relaxation time* T_2 and that of process (2) the *longitudinal relaxation time* T_{1z}. It is clear that if one places a receiver coil in the x-y plane, the variation in time of M_{xy} will induce a time-decaying electric signal in the coil (the free induction decay, FID). This constitutes a means of detection.

Analysis of relaxation times can lead to detailed information on order parameters and rates of motions in dynamic systems (see Section IV).

The magnitudes of the various interactions [Eq. (1)] indicate that we are dealing in principle with very wide spectra, which can lead to technical problems in detection when using conventional pulse sequences (e.g., one-pulse acquisition). Fortunately, this drawback can be removed by the use of echo sequences such as the quadrupolar echo sequence for ^2H (Davis, 1979) and the Hahn echo sequence for ^{13}C (Rance and Byrd, 1983).

When dealing with complex powder patterns, spectral simplifications are sometimes needed. It will be shown below that one may have to perform spectral deconvolutions ("de-Pake-ing"; Bloom *et al.*, 1981) on powder spectra to obtain oriented-sample-like spectra (similar to those of Fig. 1).

III. ORDER PARAMETERS

A. Theoretical Aspects

The high degree of organization found in the lipids of biological membranes has been alluded to in Section II. In characterizing the states of membranes, one must find a means to define this organization more precisely. The problem was addressed some years ago for liquid crystals. (An excellent summary of contemporary thinking is given in the book edited by Emsley, 1985.) We shall present only a simplified version of the approach because the complex methods cannot be used for biological membranes. The ordering of a molecule may be thought of as a measure of the amplitude of rapid motion (on the time scale of the magnetic interaction used).

All membrane systems examined to date have the property of axial symmetry within the plane of the membrane (if the z-direction is perpendicular to the plane of the membrane, properties are identical in the x and y directions). This symmetry most likely arises due to rapid molecular motions that average axially asymmetric properties. The axis about which the system is symmetric is known as the *director*, and the ordering properties of the molecular segments are ultimately defined with respect to this director.

The description of ordering in axially symmetric systems is usually given in terms of the angle made by a direction, say a C-^{2}H bond vector, and an axis about which a rapid axially symmetric motion occurs. In this sense, the motional behavior of cholesterol in a membrane can be defined by a fast axial rotation and a fast wobbling of the molecule. In mathematical terms, the ordering can be written as

$$S_{\text{C-}^2\text{H}} = S_\alpha S_\gamma = \left(\frac{3\,\overline{\cos^2 \alpha} - 1}{2}\right)\left(\frac{3\,\overline{\cos^2 \gamma} - 1}{2}\right) \tag{6}$$

where $S_{\text{C-}^2\text{H}}$ is the orientational order parameter for the particular segment of the molecules, S_γ the order parameter for the C-^{2}H segment with respect to the rotation axis of cholesterol, and S_α (often called S_{mol}) the order parameter for that axis with respect to the director (i.e., the bilayer normal). In a rigid molecule such as cholesterol, the term S_γ merely accounts for the different angles γ made by the various carbon-deuterium bonds with the axis about which rapid rotation of the entire cholesterol molecule takes place. The term S_α measures the ordering of the entire cholesterol fused-ring system with respect to the director, thus providing an estimate of the amplitude of motion promoted by the wobbling of the cholesterol molecule; hence S_α can be called the molecular order parameter. In flexible molecules, such as the fatty acyl chains of membranes, the term S_α is dominated by gauche-trans interconversions of CH_2 groups, and therefore it has been called the segmental order parameter.

If several motions, say N motions, are present in a system, the observed partially averaged magnetic interaction is the result of the averages produced by each motion. In ^{2}H-NMR, the orientational order parameter $S_{\text{C-}^2\text{H}}$ may be considered as the product of the order parameters of motions having correlation times in the appropriate time scale (i.e., less than 10^{-6} s) (Dufourc and Smith, 1986).

$$S_{\text{C-}^2\text{H}} = \prod_i^N S_i \tag{7}$$

where S_i represents the ith motion of a hierarchy in time of N motions. If the motions are axially symmetric (which is usually assumed), $S_i = (3\,\overline{\cos^2 \beta_i} - 1)/2$, where β_i is the angle between the principal axis of the coordinate system attached to motion i and the principal axis of the coordinate system attached to motion $i - 1$. Note that Eq. (7) is the generalization of Eq. (6) to the case of N motions. These order parameters are an easy way to characterize membrane states. A state in which there are no fluctuations of angles β_i is called totally ordered and characterized by $S_i = 1$. Conversely, a totally disordered state (i.e., random fluctuations of angles β_i) has $S_i = 0$. Unfortunately, the decomposition according to Eq. (7) is not always possible, and one often reports only the variation of $S_{\text{C-}^2\text{H}}$ under certain constraints. In this situation, $S_{\text{C-}^2\text{H}} = (3\,\overline{\cos^2 \theta_{\text{C-}^2\text{H}}} - 1)/2$ is a measure of the fluctuations, promoted by all effective motions, of the angle $\theta_{\text{C-}^2\text{H}}$ between the C-^{2}H bond and the bilayer normal. Although less detailed, this information is nonetheless of first importance.

B. Experimental

In practical spectroscopic terms, the time- and ensemble-averaged quadrupole splitting observed for a C-^{2}H segment is given by

$$\Delta\nu_Q = \tfrac{3}{4}A_Q S_{\text{C-}^2\text{H}}$$
$$= \tfrac{3}{4}A_Q S_\alpha S_\gamma \qquad (8)$$

where A_Q is the quadrupolar coupling constant, which varies slightly with the chemical nature of the labeled site (Mantsch *et al.*, 1977). Note that for all positions of the fused-ring system of cholesterol, S_α (the molecular order parameter) is constant and $\Delta\nu_Q$ is thus sensitive to S_γ, providing a means to measure the location of the motional averaging axis within the cholesterol molecule (Taylor *et al.*, 1981; Dufourc *et al.*, 1984b).

In cholesteryl palmitate, where the 3β-hydroxyl group is esterified to palmitic acid, the axis of motional averaging has a much different location in the cholesterol framework (Chana *et al.*, 1985). The result of such calculations can be represented using computer-assisted spatial drawing routines such as PLUTO 78; the location of the axis of motional averaging for the fused-ring system of cholesterol and cholesteryl palmitate, in dipalmitoyl phosphatidylcholine (DPPC), is represented in Fig. 3, which shows the average orientations of both fused-ring systems undergoing fast reorientations around

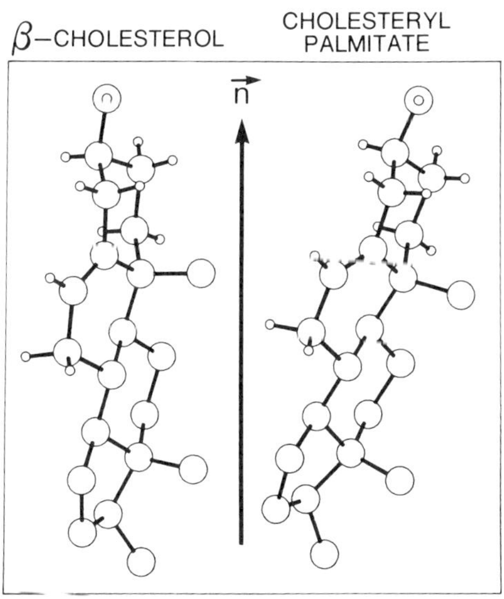

Figure 3 PLUTO 78 spatial representation of the fused-ring system of β-cholesterol and cholesteryl palmitate. The arrow indicates the direction of the rotation axis **n**, which for S_α (or S_{mol}) = 1, corresponds to the director (bilayer normal) and lies in the plane of the page. The symbol ◎ is the oxygen attached at C-3. From Chana *et al.* (1985).

their principal axis of rotational diffusion, **n**. This representation does not account for the angular fluctuations (wobbling) of the steroid moiety and can be considered as a "snapshot" of molecules when $S_\alpha = 1$. One sees clearly that the steroid skeleton of cholesteryl palmitate is markedly tilted away from the position of that of cholesterol. This reflects the presence of the palmitoyl chain attached to the oxygen at C-3. The palmitoyl chain is indeed known to fold back into the membrane (Gorrissen *et al.*, 1981) and therefore "pulls" the rigid cholesteryl skeleton away from the average orientation found for cholesterol.

Once the axis about which fast rotation occurs has been located, the molecular order parameter S_α (or S_{mol}), can be determined from Eq. (8). At 25°C, $S_\alpha = 0.80 \pm 0.03$ in dimyristoyl phosphatidylcholine (DMPC) (cholesterol:DMPC molar ratio of 3:7). This finding correlates well with that obtained by Taylor *et al.* (1981), ($S_\alpha \simeq 0.87$), for a higher concentration of cholesterol in the membrane (cholesterol was in 1:1 molar ratio with egg phosphatidylcholine). These authors found a higher value of S_α, which reflects the property that the order parameter increases when the concentration of cholesterol increases in the bilayer fluid phase (Oldfield *et al.*, 1978; Taylor *et al.*, 1981). The molecular order parameter of cholesterol is thus very high in most systems studied so far. A value of $S_\alpha = 0.76$ has also been determined for cholesterol in erythrocyte ghosts (Kelusky *et al.*, 1983). Even the apparently flexible tail of cholesterol has a relatively high order (Dufourc *et al.*, 1984b).

Figure 4 shows that the temperature dependence of the ordering of the fused-ring system in DMPC, S_{mol}^{chol}, is rather weak. The segmental order parameter as monitored at approximately the same bilayer depth of C-4′ of the acyl chains in the presence of cholesterol, $S_{mol,chol}^{4'}$, changes rather drastically over the same temperature range. It is interesting to note that below T_c ($T_c = 23$°C is the temperature of the gel-to-fluid phase transition of the pure lipid), the amplitudes of the motions of the C-^{2}H segments at C-4′ are almost the same as those of the cholesterol rigid body. It should be recalled that below T_c the lipid chains would not show any C-^{2}H angular excursions at all if β-cholesterol were not present. One can therefore interpret this "fluidizing" effect as a disordering effect: β-Cholesterol through its virtually temperature-independent angular fluctuations forces the lipid chains to fluctuate even below 23°C. Since between 10° and 35°C, S_α is almost the same for both the lipid at C-4′ and the steroid skeleton, it appears therefore that, in this temperature range, cholesterol controls the motions of the entire system through its own motions. In other words, the sterol increases the amplitude of acyl chain motions below T_c and decreases them above T_c (compared with systems lacking cholesterol); that is, it forces the ordering of the systems to its own level of ordering. It is interesting to note that at high temperatures, S_{mol}^{chol} is markedly greater than $S_{mol,chol}^{4'}$. The system is thus characterized by two kinds of angular fluctuations, those of the phospholipid and those of β-cholesterol. This point is rather important and emphasizes that measuring the segmental order parameter of β-cholesterol at 65°C would not give information about the amplitude of motions of the lipid chains. One would be measuring the property of the probe rather than that of the system.

The unnatural α-isomer of cholesterol, epicholesterol, which has the hydroxyl group essentially perpendicular to the plane of the A-ring, has been studied by the

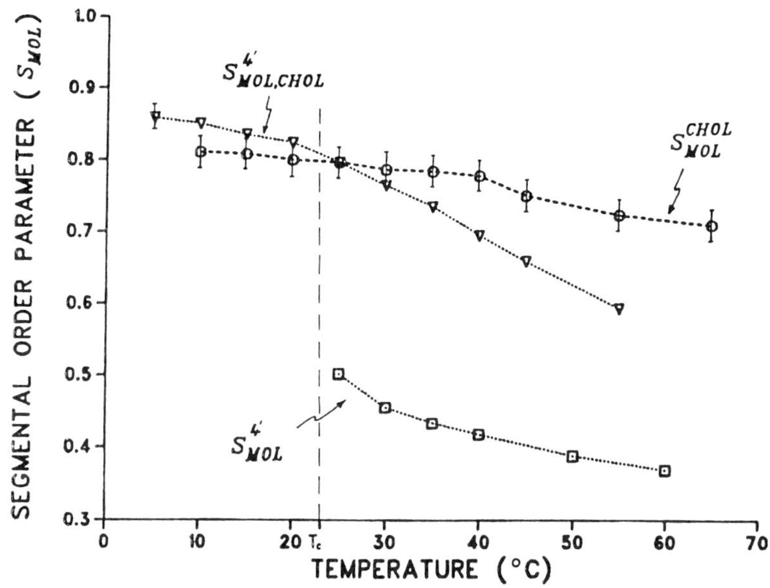

Figure 4 Temperature variation of the order parameter S_α of the β-cholesterol-DMPC (3:7) system. The $S^{4'}_{\text{mol,chol}}$ is the S_α of DMPC at C-4′, $S^{4'}_{\text{mol}}$, but in the presence of the sterol, and the $S^{\text{chol}}_{\text{mol}}$ is the S_α of the four rings of cholesterol in DMPC. From Dufourc *et al.* (1984b).

^{2}H-NMR method (Dufourc *et al.*, 1984b; Murari *et al.*, 1986). By comparison with the β-isomer, it was found to have a different location within the molecular framework for the axis of motional averaging, a higher order-parameter, a weaker effect on the acyl chains of surrounding lipids, and a steeper dependence of its order parameter on temperature. The different location for the axis of motional averaging of epicholesterol within the molecule indicates that this latter is markedly tilted with respect to the average orientation of β-cholesterol within the bilayer. This leads to a decrease in efficiency of regulation of acyl chain motions and can be proposed as a reason for its absence in natural systems.

Although the chemical-shift anisotropy of ^{13}C could, in principle, be used to measure order in membranes, it is usually not employed because of an insufficient number of observables and some uncertainty as to the directions of the CSA tensor within the molecular framework. An example of such spectra and their analysis is the paper by Blume *et al.* (1982).

IV. MOTIONAL RATES VIA RELAXATION TIMES

The preceding has shown that one can obtain information on the degree of order (the amplitude of molecular fluctuations) by measuring the partially averaged quadrupolar interaction. The time scales of these motions (the correlation times) can be established by measuring nuclear relaxation times.

However, the measurement of these quantities for anisotropic systems such as membranes does not lead directly to correlation times. Both the amplitudes and the rates of motions affect relaxation times. The literature contains many examples. The ^{2}H-spin–lattice relaxation rates T_{1z}^{-1} of [$^2H_{62}$]-DPPC (both *sn*-1 and *sn*-2 chains perdeuterated), plotted as a function of the labeled chain position (Davis, 1979), exhibit a profile (especially the plateau of T_{1z}^{-1} up to carbons 9 and 10) almost identical to that determined previously for the segmental order parameter (Seelig and Seelig, 1974). Recently, Dufourc *et al.* (1984a) observed that the high segmental order parameter produced by the presence of a cyclopropane group in the *sn*-2 chain of 1-palmitoyl-2-dihydrosterculoyl phosphatidylcholine (PDSPC), which leads to a large discontinuity in the plot of order parameters versus chain position (Dufourc *et al.*, 1983), is accompanied by a very short T_{1z} at the level of the cyclopropane group.

One of the main problems when analyzing relaxation behavior is in separating ordering from rates of motion. Several models have been proposed to do this on flexible molecules such as phospholipid chains (Brown, 1982) and on rigid molecules such as cholesterol in a fluid membrane (Brainard and Szabo, 1981; Dufourc and Smith, 1986). Working on rigid molecules simplifies the problem and leads in favorable cases (*vide infra*) to the separation mentioned above.

As will be shown, one can describe very precisely in the frame of a simple and realistic model (Paddy *et al.*, 1981) the nature, energy, rates, and amplitudes of the motions of cholesterol in DMPC (Dufourc and Smith, 1986). Analysis of the deuterium longitudinal relaxation times, T_{1z} of appropriately labeled cholesterol will be presented as an example. Unfortunately, a similar level of description cannot be reached for flexible molecules without resort to very sophisticated and computer-time-consuming lineshape analyses (Meier *et al.*, 1983).

A. Theoretical Aspects

Experiments are performed in model membranes, which can be described as lyotropic liquid crystals, with the bilayer normal *n* as the major optical axis of the mesophase. In such a medium, the molecular fragments that bear the deuterium atoms may experience several motions. If the correlation time τ_i of the motions is smaller than the inverse of the static quadrupolar interaction (i.e., $\tau_i < (2/3)(A_Q^{-1}) \simeq 4.10^{-6}$ s), this interaction will be scaled down to give a residual quadrupolar splitting (see Section II.B).

The idea proposed by Paddy *et al.* (1981) is the following: One can describe the dynamics of such a system by a hierarchy in time of N motions (fulfilling the time-scale conditions previously mentioned that correlation time $\tau_i < 4.10^{-6}$ s), each motion being characterized by its correlation time, nature, activation energy, and order parameter. To simplify the analysis, it is assumed that motions are independent, have separated time scales, and possess axial symmetry. Under such conditions one can consider that the *i*th motion reduces the ordering resulting from the action of motions $i-1$, $i-2$, and so on by the amount S_i [see Eq. (7)].

Quadrupolar interactions dominate the spin-lattice relaxation mechanism; hence the longitudinal relaxation time T_{1z} is given by the well-known expression (Abragam, 1961)

$$T_{1z}^{-1} = A[J(\omega_0) + 4J(2\omega_0)] \tag{9}$$

where $A = (3/80)(A_Q)^2$; $J(p\omega_0)$, with $p = 1, 2$, represents the reduced spectral densities (assuming exponential correlation functions and intramolecular motions); and ω_0 is the Larmor resonance frequency. In the case of two motions, the rate of spin-lattice relaxation T_{1z}^{-1} can be written as (Dufourc and Smith, 1986)

$$T_{1z}^{-1} = A\left[(1 - S_1^2)\left(\frac{2\tau_1}{1 + \omega_0^2\tau_1^2} + \frac{8\tau_1}{1 + 4\omega_0^2\tau_1^2}\right) + (S_1^2 - S_{\text{C-}^2\text{H}}^2)\left(\frac{2\tau_2}{1 + \omega_0^2\tau_2^2} + \frac{8\tau_2}{1 + 4\omega_0^2\tau_2^2}\right)\right] \tag{10}$$

where $S_{\text{C-}^2\text{H}}^2 = S_1^2S_2^2$. It is seen from Eq. (10) that the relaxation time depends on both correlation times and order parameters. It goes without saying that the more motions present, the more observables are needed to solve equations of this type.

B. Experimental

To obtain a maximum of observables, T_{1z} measurements have been performed as a function of temperature, Larmor frequency, and position of deuterium labeling for [2,2,3,4,4,6-$^2H_6$]cholesterol in DMPC (3:7 molar ratio, respectively). The stacked plot of Fig. 5 illustrates the inversion recovery technique used for these measurements (i.e., 180° inverting pulse, τ delay, and echo sequence). For each stacked plot, spectra were de-Paked to yield only the doublet for $\beta = 90°$ (Bloom *et al.*, 1981), and the resulting oriented-sample-like spectra were fitted to the equation $M(\tau) = M_0[1 - A\exp(-\tau/T_{1z})]$ as described (Dufourc *et al.*, 1984a; MacDonald, 1980). M_0 represents the equilibrium magnetization, $M(\tau)$ the magnetization at time τ, and A an adjustable parameter to account for imperfections of the inverting pulse. In all T_{1z} measurements, this equation was sufficient to analyze data, within the experimental error. Some results for deuterated cholesterol are reported in Fig. 6, which shows T_{1z} as a function of temperature and position of labeling, at $\omega_0 = 46.1$ MHz.

There is a minimum in T_{1z} at ~35°C for all labeled positions. However, the absolute values of T_{1z} at the minima depend upon the position of labeling. Equation (10) predicts that T_{1z}^{-1} is linearly dependent on the square of the orientational order parameter $S_{\text{C-}^2\text{H}}^2$. To assess this, the quantity $(AT_{1z})^{-1}$ is plotted against $S_{\text{C-}^2\text{H}}^2$ at various temperatures. In Fig. 7 one must plot $(AT_{1z})^{-1}$ instead of T_{1z}^{-1} to account for the A_Q difference between C-^{2}H bonds linked to carbon by single or double bonds, such as C6-^{2}H. The plots show that there is indeed a linear relationship between $(AT_{1z})^{-1}$ and $S_{\text{C-}^2\text{H}}$ in the temperature range of the study. The principal results obtained at $\omega_0 = 46.1$ MHz [i.e., the absolute value of the T_{1z} minimum is dependent

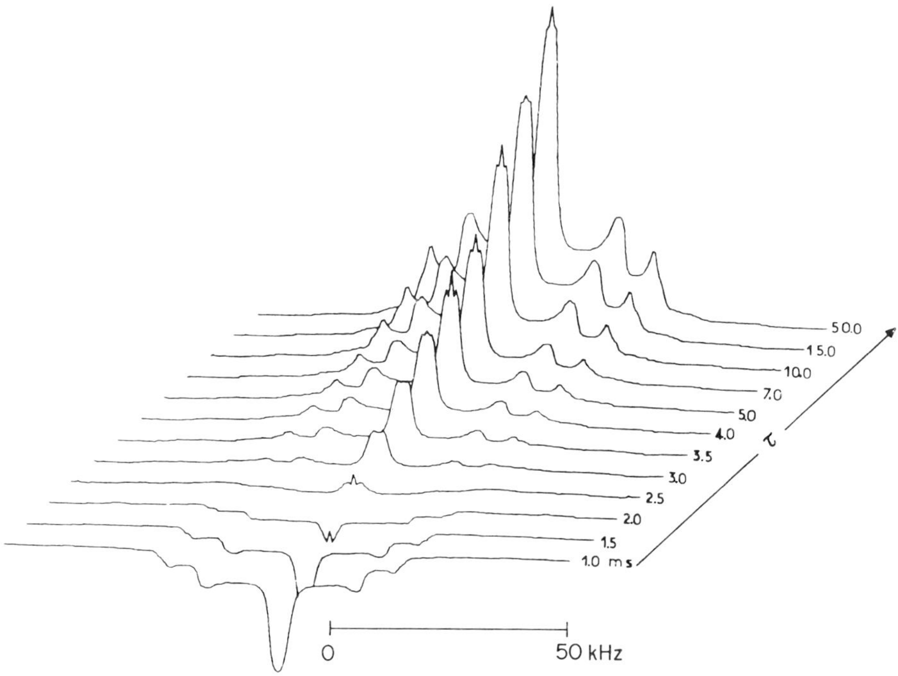

Figure 5 Example of stacked plot of powder spectra resulting from a T_{1z} experiment ($\pi - \tau -$ quadrupolar echo sequence). The data are for [2,2,3,4,4,6-$^2H_6$] cholesterol in DMPC (3:7 molar ratio, respectively) at 46.1 MHz and 35°C. Typical experimental parameters: $\pi/2$ pulse length, 4 μs; pulse spacing in the echo sequence, 60 μs; recycle time, 50–100 ms; spectral window, 500 kHz; 18,000 accumulations for each spectrum. From Dufourc and Smith (1986).

on the position of labeling, and $S^2_{C\text{-}^2H}$ is linearly dependent on $(AT_{1z})^{-1}$] are also observed at $\omega_0 = 30.7$ MHz except that the temperature of the minimum in T_{1z} is shifted down to 25°C. This is illustrated in Fig. 8, where the temperature behavior of T_{1z} for the labeled position [4-^{2}H]$_{equat}$ is monitored at $\omega_0 = 46.1$ MHz and 30.7 MHz.

C. Analysis

The presence of T_{1z} minima in spectra measured at 46.1 and 30.7 MHz indicates that at the corresponding temperatures, the longitudinal relaxation time is dominated by only one motion of correlation time (Abragam, 1961; Davis, 1983), $\tau_i = 0.62\ \omega_0^{-1}$. This leads to $\tau_i = 3.2 \cdot 10^{-9}$ s at 25°C and $\tau_i = 2.1 \cdot 10^{-9}$ s at 35°C. Assuming that this motion follows an Arrhenius-type law of the form $\tau_i = \tau_{0,i} \exp[E_a/RT)$, one can calculate, analytically, the activation energy, $E_a = 32 \pm 5$ kJ·mol^{-1}, and the preexponential factor $\tau_{0,i} = 8.0 \pm 0.5 \cdot 10^{-15}$ s. On comparing this E_a value with those obtained for pure lipid bilayers, under the above assumptions, by Brown *et al.* (1979)

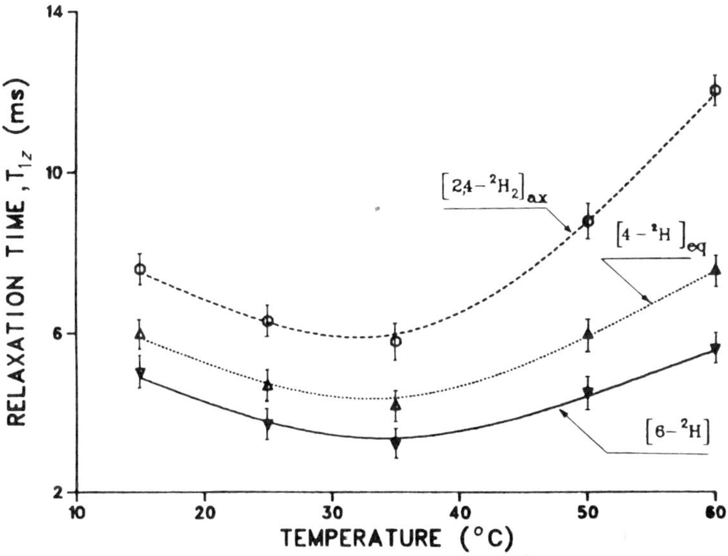

Figure 6 Temperature dependence of the relaxation time (T_{1z}) for the indicated labeled positions of cholesterol, at 46.1 MHz. The bars give an estimate of the experimental error. From Dufourc and Smith (1986).

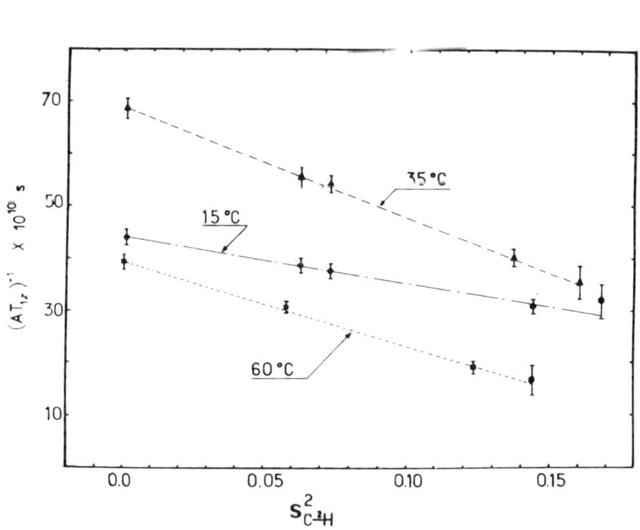

Figure 7 Variation of the normalized relaxation rate $(AT_{1z})^{-1}$ (see text) as a function of the square of the orientational order parameter $S_{C-{}^2H}$ at the indicated temperatures. The data are from relaxation measurements at 46.1 MHz. The bars give an estimate of the experimental error. From Dufourc and Smith (1986).

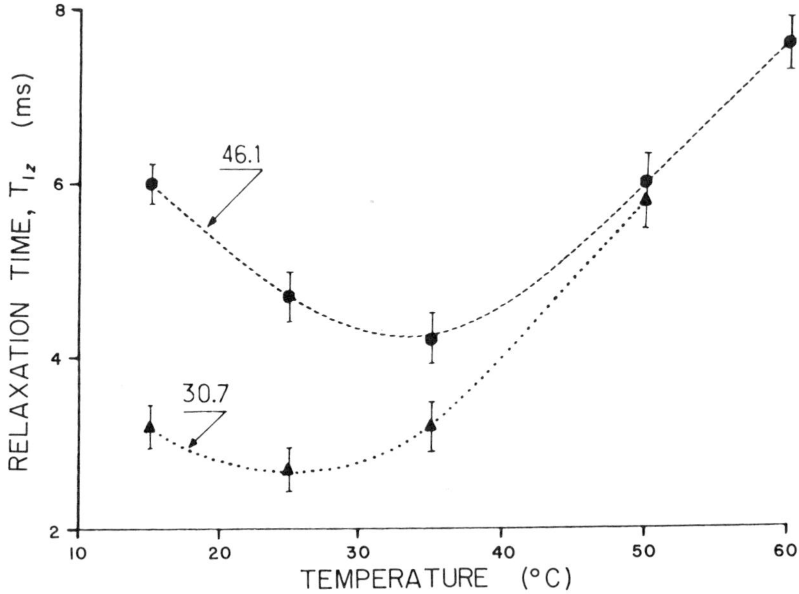

Figure 8 Temperature variation of the relaxation time (T_{1z}) of $[4\text{-}^2H]_{equat}$ cholesterol in DMPC. Figures on curves represent Larmor resonance frequencies in MHz. The bars give an estimate of the experimental error. From Dufourc and Smith (1986).

for DPPC ($E_a = 14.6 \pm 1.3$ kJ·mol^{-1}) and by Dufourc *et al.* (1984a) for PDSPC (lipid containing a cyclopropane group on one of the acyl chains; $E_a = 12.3 \pm 1.0$ kJ·mol^{-1}), one finds a threefold greater activation energy for the motion of cholesterol in DMPC. This high activation energy is an indication that the motion of cholesterol, giving rise to a T_{1z} minimum in DMPC, is much more restricted than are the motions of lipid acyl chains.

Although this motion has been characterized by its temperature-dependent correlation time and by its activation energy, its nature, its rank in the hierarchy of motions, and its order parameter are still unknown. The following will attempt to elucidate the motional mechanism giving rise to the observed nuclear relaxation.

Since one motion dominates T_{1z} in the temperature range of the study, one obtains at the minimum ($\omega_0\tau_i = 0.62$),

$$T_{1z}^{-1}(\text{min}) = 2.85 \frac{A}{\omega_0} \mathbf{f}_S \tag{11}$$

where $\mathbf{f}_S$ is a function of the order parameters S_i. For example, for a hierarchy (in time) of motions, and considering that the first motion is responsible for the observed minima, $\mathbf{f}_S = 1 - S_1^2$. Alternatively, if the second motion leads to the minimum, then $\mathbf{f}_S = S_1^2 - S_2^2$ and so on.

The value of $\mathbf{f}_S$ is an indication of the state of anisotropy of cholesterol in DMPC: $\mathbf{f}_S = 1$ for isotropic motions and $\mathbf{f}_S < 1$ for nonisotropic motions (Dufourc and Smith, 1986). Values of $\mathbf{f}_S$ have been calculated according to Eq. (11) for data at 30.7 MHz and are reported in Table 1.

All $\mathbf{f}_S$ values in the table are <1, indicating that the motion of cholesterol in DMPC is anisotropic. This is not surprising since this model membrane system is a liquid crystal, intrinsically anisotropic by definition.

To determine the rank (in hierarchy of motions) of the motion responsible for the observed minima, one has to envisage several cases, One may assume first that it is the fastest motion and obtain, according to Eq. (10),

$$\mathbf{f}_S = 1 - S_I^2 = 1 - S_{C\text{-}^2H}^2$$

S_I values for all labeled positions can then be calculated from relaxation data and compared with the $S_{C\text{-}^2H}$ values obtained from measurement of quadrupolar splittings on spectra. Table 1 indicates a total disagreement between these two sets of data. The fastest motion is therefore not responsible for the minima. Alternatively, one may associate the observed minima with the second-fastest motion and have

$$\mathbf{f}_S = S_I^2 - S_I^2 S_2^2 = S_I^2 - S_{C\text{-}^2H}^2$$

S_I and S_2 values are then calculated from $\mathbf{f}_S$ and $S_{C\text{-}^2H}$ (Table 1). One obtains $S_I = 0.79 \pm 0.04$ at 25°C and values of S_2 that vary with the position of labeling.

Now one must look for a motion resulting in such a peculiar variation of S_2. Since all C-^{2}H bonds have a fixed orientation with respect to each other, it is reasonable to think that the rotation of cholsterol around its molecular long axis may play this role. The location of this axis in the cholesterol molecule has already been calculated by combining the quadrupolar splitting of each individual C-^{2}H bond with X-ray data

Table 1 T_{1z} Minima values, derived order parameters, and $\mathbf{f}_S$ values for cholesterol in DMPC as a function of the position of labeling

Labeled Position	T_{1z}	$\mathbf{f}_S$	S_I^a	S_I^b	S_2^b	$S_{C\text{-}^2H}$
[3-^{2}H]	3.8	0.42	0.76	0.77	±0.54	0.41
[2,4-$^2H_2$]$_{axial}$	3.8	0.42	0.76	0.75	±0.51	0.38
[4-^{2}H]$^c_{equat}$	2.7	0.59	0.64	0.81	±0.31	0.25
[2-^{2}H]$^c_{equat}$	2.7	0.59	0.64	0.81	±0.33	0.27
[6-^{2}H]	2.3	0.65	0.59	0.81	±0.03	0.027

Note: Values determined at 30.7 MHz and 25°C. T_{1z} is in milliseconds. Accuracy of values is 10%, except for that of position [3-^{2}H], which is 20%.

Source: Data are taken from Dufourc and Smith (1986).

[a] Assuming that the fastest motion is the axial rotation of cholesterol (see text).

[b] Assuming that the second-fastest motion is the axial rotation of cholesterol (see text).

[c] Assignment could be reversed (Dufourc *et al.*, 1984b).

(Dufourc *et al.*, 1984b; Taylor *et al.*, 1981). The salient feature of this determination is that the angle made by the C6-^{2}H bond with respect to the axis of motional averaging of cholesterol is close to the magic angle ($\beta_2 = 54.7°$). Such a value leads to an S_2 value close to zero ($S_2 = (3\cos^2\beta_2 - 1)/2$). Table 1 indicates that this is indeed the case. Angles β_2 for other labeled positions have been calculated from S_2 values and agree, within the experimental error, with those obtained by Taylor *et al.* (1981) and Dufourc *et al.* (1984b).

It can therefore be concluded that the axial rotation of cholesterol is responsible for the observed minima and is the second-fastest motion of correlation time τ_2. The fastest motion of correlation time τ_1, which cannot be determined accurately with the present data, could possible be librational, involving the wobbling of cholesterol, which is too fast to contribute significantly to T_{1z}(i.e., $\omega_0^2\tau_1^2 \ll 1$), but reducing the ordering to a value $S_1 = 0.79 \pm 0.04$. The order parameter associated with this fast motion has already been determined by Dufourc *et al.* (1984b) on the same system and at the same temperatures, but using a different approach. These authors found a value of 0.80 ± 0.03 at 25°C for this order parameter, which agrees very well with the S_1 values found in Table 1. It is worthwhile mentioning that S_1 and S_2 correspond to S_α and S_γ described in Section III.

The results obtained from ^{2}H-NMR relaxation data can be compared with those of Brainard and Szabo (1981) and Brainard and Cordes (1981), who calculated correlation times and order parameters for cholesterol in egg phosphatidylcholine vesicles from ^{13}C-T_{1z} measurements. They also describe the anisotropic motions of cholesterol in the bilayer membrane as a rotation about the long molecular axis and a wobbling of the molecule. At corresponding temperatures and concentration of cholesterol in the membrane, they found a value of $0.14 \cdot 10^{-9}$ s for the correlation time associated with the axial rotation and an order parameter for the wobbling of 0.71. The order parameter compares well with the value of $S_1 = 0.79 \pm 0.04$ just discussed. However, the correlation time does not agree with the value of $3.2 \cdot 10^{-9}$ s found from ^{2}H-NMR data. This discrepancy deserves a comment. The ^{13}C-NMR measurements were analyzed under the hypothesis that cholesterol motions were in the so-called fast correlation regime (i.e., correlation time τ_i such that $\omega_0^2\tau_i^2 \ll 1$). The ^{2}H-NMR measurements indicate that this assumption is not fulfilled for the axial rotation of cholesterol. Moreoever, it must be emphasized that correlation times that are obtained from ^{2}H-NMR relaxation data are determined straightforwardly, without need for a model. Modeling of data by a hierarchy in time of motions is needed only to obtain the nature, rank, and order parameter associated with these motions.

V. CONCLUSION

Solid-state NMR can lead to a very detailed analysis of the motional behavior of cholesterol in biomembranes. The dynamics of cholesterol in model membranes have been characterized by two motions: (1) axial rotation with a high energy of activation and a nanosecond correlation time at physiological temperatures and (2) a faster motion (possibly the wobbling of cholesterol) that reduces the static quadrupolar interaction by 20%. One can also remark that small structural modifications in the sterol molecule can lead to considerable changes in its own ordering properties as well as in those of the medium. Both the rigid structure and its orientation perpendicular to the bilayer surface appear to be the requirements for cholesterol to play a regulatory role in the membrane for motions of flexible molecules, thus providing an increase in membrane stability with regard to external perturbations.

ACKNOWLEDGMENT

EJD is grateful to the CNRS-NRCC exchange program for financial support during his stay in Canada.

REFERENCES

Abragam, A. (1961). "Principles of Nuclear Magnetism." Oxford Univ. Press, London and New York.

Bloom, M., Davis, J. H., and Mackay, A. (1981). *Chem. Phys. Lett.* **19**. 198–202.

Blume, A., Rice, D. M., Wittebort, R. J., and Griffin, R. G. (1982). *Biochemistry* **21**, 6220–6230.

Brainard, J. R., and Cordes, E. H. (1981). *Biochemistry* **20**, 4607–4617.

Brainard, J. R., and Szabo, A. (1981). *Biochemistry* **20**, 4618–4628.

Brown, M. F. (1982). *J. Chem. Phys.* **77**, 1576–1599.

Brown, M. F., Seelig, J., and Häberlin, U. (1979). *J. Chem. Phys.* **70**, 5045–5053.

Chana, S. R., Cushley, R. J., Wassall, S. R., Smith, I. C. P., and Dufourc, E. J. (1985). *Chem. Phys. Lipids* **37**, 345–356.

Davis, J. H. (1979). *Biophys. J.* **27**, 339–358.

Davis, J. H. (1983). *Biochim. Biophys. Acta* **737**, 117–171.

Dufourc, E. J., and Smith, I. C. P. (1986). *Chem. Phys. Lipids* **41**, 123–135.

Dufourc, E. J., Smith, I. C. P., and Jarrell, H. C. (1983). *Chem. Phys. Lipids* **33**, 153–177.

Dufourc, E. J., Smith, I. C. P., and Jarrell, H. C. (1984a). *Biochemistry* **23**, 2300–2309.

Dufourc, E. J., Parish, E. J., Chitrakorn, S., and Smith, I. C. P. (1984b). *Biochemistry* **23**, 6062–6071.

Emsley, J. W., ed. (1985). "Nuclear Magnetic Resonance of Liquid Crystals," NATO ASI C141. Reidel Publ., Dordrecht, The Netherlands.

Gorrissen, H., Mackay, A. L., Wassall, S. R., Valic, M. I., Tulloch, A. P., and Cushley, R. J. (1981). *Biochim. Biophys. Acta* **644**, 266.

Kelusky, E. C., Dufourc, E. J., and Smith, I. C. P. (1983). *Biochim. Biophys. Acta* **735**, 302–304.

MacDonald, J. C. (1980). *J. Magn. Reson.* **38**, 381.

Mantsch, H. H., Saitô, H., and Smith, I. C. P. (1977). *Prog. Nucl. Magn. Reson. Spectrosc.* **11**, 211–272.

Mehring, M. (1983). "Principles of High Resolution NMR in Solids." Springer-Verlag, Berlin and New York.

Meier, P., Ohmes, E., Kothe, G., Blume, A., Weidner, J., and Eibl, H. J. (1983). *J. Phys. Chem.* **87**, 4934–4912.

Murari, R., Murari, M. P., and Baumann, W. J. (1986). *Biochemistry* **25**, 1062–1067.

Oldfield, E., Meadows, M., Rice, D. and Jacobs, R. (1978). *Biochemistry* **17**, 2727–2740.

Paddy, M. R., Dahlquist, F., Davis, J. H., and Bloom, M. (1981). *Biochemistry* **20**, 3152–3162.
Rance, M., and Byrd, R. A. (1983). *J. Magn. Reson.* **52**, 221–240.
Seelig, A., and Seelig, J. (1974). *Biochemistry* **13**, 4839–4845.
Seelig, J. (1977). *Q. Rev. Biophys.* **10**, 353–418.
Singer, S. J., and Nicolson, G. L. (1972). *Science* **175**, 720.
Taylor, M. G., Akiyama, T., and Smith, I. C. P. (1981). *Chem. Phys. Lipids* **29**, 327–339.

16

Use of the Fluorescent Sterols Cholestatrienol and Dehydroergosterol to Monitor Cholesterol Behavior in Membranes and Serum Lipoproteins

Philip L. Yeagle
Department of Biochemistry
State University of New York (SUNY) at Buffalo
Buffalo, New York

Analysis of Sterols and Other Biologically Significant Steroids

I. INTRODUCTION

The study of cholesterol in cell membranes and serum lipoproteins has long been a subject of intense interest because cholesterol is known to be essential for the growth, differentiation, and proper function of mammalian and other cells. In opposition to these essential roles, cholesterol can also be lethal to humans in its participation in plaques that cause coronary artery disease.

A serious impedance to understanding the roles of cholesterol in biology has been the lack of adequate techniques for monitoring cholesterol in cells. Cholesterol possesses no physical or structural attributes that can be readily exploited to observe its behavior directly. For example, it has no particularly useful absorbance or fluorescence properties.

The situation is further complicated by the fact that small changes in the sterol structure significantly change the behavior of the sterol. For example, changes in the sterol tail alter the ability of the sterol to inhibit passive permeability of lipid bilayers. Inhibition of passive permeability is a characteristic of cholesterol. Furthermore, changing the 3-β-hydroxyl to a 3-α-hydroxyl also significantly alters the behavior of the sterol (Demel *et al.*, 1972). Even changes in the methylation of the steroid ring system change the packing of the sterol in the membrane (Yeagle *et al.*, 1977; Yeagle, 1985; Dahl, 1981).

One method of making cholesterol amenable to study involves structural derivatization. The most obvious sites of derivatization of cholesterol, for the purposes of introducing optical chromophores, for example, are the hydroxyl and the tail. As noted, structural changes in these regions can be expected to produce a molecule with a behavior different from that of cholesterol. Therefore, most sterol probes that have been used to date must be viewed with considerable caution. In many cases, their similarity to cholesterol has been proposed purely on the basis of structure and not on standard characterization of cholesterol-like behavior.

The one nonperturbing approach to studying cholesterol behavior that has been successful is nuclear magnetic resonance (NMR). Both ^{2}H-labeled cholesterol and ^{13}C-labeled cholesterol have been used. (Yeagle, 1981; deKruijff, 1978; Gally *et al.*, 1976; Oldfield *et al.*, 1978; Kelusky *et al.*, 1983). Although these are powerful probing methods and have provided considerable information on cholesterol behavior in lipid bilayers, they are in general, too insensitive for extensive use in biological systems, particularly in cell membranes.

Therefore, there has been a serious need for essentially nonperturbing, highly sensitive methods for the study of cholesterol in biological systems. This need has been met by two fluorescent sterol probes: ergosta-5,7,9(11),22-tetraene-3β-ol (dehydroergosterol) and cholesta-5,7,9(11)-trien-3β-ol (cholestatrienol). The former is a derivative of ergosterol, the latter of cholesterol. These fluorescent sterols contain a conjugated triene in the fused-ring structure. As can be seen in Fig. 1, their structures are similar to those of the parent compounds. It would be expected that they would be similar in behavior to their respective naturally occurring sterol parents; as is described later in detail, this expectation is realized by recent experimental data.

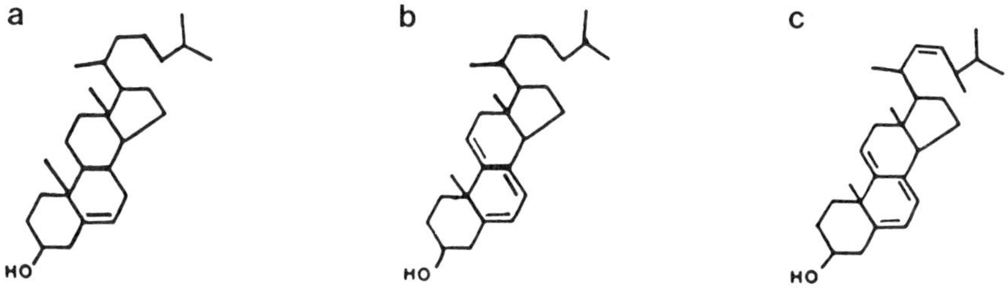

Figure 1 Structure of (a) 5-cholestene-3β-ol (cholesterol), (b) cholesta-5,7,9(11)-triene-3β-ol (cholestatrienol), and (c) ergosta-5,7,9(11)-22-tetraene-3β-ol (dehydroergosterol).

Fluorescence measurements are several orders of magnitude more sensitive than the NMR measurements referred to previously. Therefore, these minimally perturbing fluorescent sterols enable us to pursue questions of cholesterol behavior into biological systems that are not amenable to the NMR approach. As will be seen, detailed molecular dynamics can be studied using the fluorescence measurements, including correlation times for molecular motion and order parameters characterizing cholesterol motion.

This chapter reviews all the available information necessary for using these powerful new probes of cholesterol and discusses some of the applications to which they have been applied. This is a new field, and it is expected that the use of these fluorescent sterols will grow dramatically.

II. DEHYDROERGOSTEROL AND CHOLESTATRIENOL: SYNTHESIS, PURIFICATION, CHARACTERIZATION, AND STRUCTURE

A. Synthesis and Purification

The synthesis of dehydroergosterol and cholestatrienol derives from reports of 30 to 50 years ago (Windhaus and Linsert, 1928; Morton *et al.*, 1930; Ruyle *et al.*, 1953; Antonucci *et al.*, 1951; Zuercher *et al.*, 1954). Dehydroergosterol is synthesized directly from ergosterol by dehydration with mercuric acetate (Smutzer *et al.*, 1986). Two grams of ergosterol were reacted with 3 g of mercuric acetate in 20 ml of chloroform and 17 ml of glacial acetic acid at 37°–40°C in the dark under a nitrogen atmosphere. After 24 h, the material was twice filtered to remove mercurous acetate and concentrated to less than 5 ml in a rotary evaporator. The product was then recrystallized in warm/cold ethanol, filtered, washed with ice-cold ethanol, and then dissolved in ether. The dehydroergosterol solution was refiltered through Whatman No. 1 filter paper, and the filtrate was placed under a stream of nitrogen in the dark to remove the ether. The product was then recrystallized in warm/cold ethanol for several hours, dried overnight under vacuum, and then directly used or passed through a Beckman high-pressure liquid chromatography (HPLC) system equipped with a reverse-phase C-18 preparatory HPLC column (Ultrasphere-ODS, 10 mm × 25 cm). The column separated any unreacted ergosterol from dehydroergosterol and was equilibrated with methanol/acetonitrile (1:19 v/v). Flow rates were 3 ml/min, and dehydroergosterol eluted from the column 24 min after injection as a single peak. Dehydroergosterol can be stored successfully in the dark under nitrogen at −70°C.

Cholestatrienol is synthesized from 7-dehydrocholesterol in a similar manner (Fischer *et al.*, 1984). Reactions were performed in the dark under a nitrogen atmosphere. Two grams of 7-dehydrocholesterol were dissolved in 50 ml of acetic anhydride warmed to 90°C for 3 h. 100 ml of methanol were added and the reaction cooled to 4°C. The acetate was collected as a precipitate and washed with cold methanol. This was then dissolved in 50 ml of chloroform, added to 100 ml glacial acetic acid containing 6.2 g mercuric acetate. The mixture was stirred for 18 h at room temperature. The material was then filtered, and the filtrate was evaporated to dryness. This was then dissolved in 30 ml of chilled diethyl ether and let stand on ice for 15 min to further precipitate mercurous acetates. The material was again filtered and dryed. The cholestatrienol-acetate product was dissolved in 30 ml of chloroform, saponified for 4 h at 35°C by addition of 1 N KOH in methanol/water (9:1). The alcohol product was collected and purified by passage through a C-18 reverse-phase (RP) HPLC column. Rechromatography of the isolated fraction produced a single peak, with only a hint of a second peak at less than the 1% level. The cholestatrienol should always be rechromatographed before storage. Then it can be stored at −70°C successfully.

The HPLC purification is essential for two reasons: (1) Fluorescence is a sensitive technique, and impurities can distort the results; and (2) cholestatrienol is not stable unless it is pure and will degrade rapidly, even at −70°C, if impurities are not removed.

B. Characterization and Structure

The dehydroergosterol product has a melting point 145°–149°C (Windhaus and Linsert, 1928; Morton *et al.*, 1930; Zuercher *et al.*, 1954; Fischer *et al.*, 1985a). It has characteristic absorption and fluorescence emission spectra, which appear in Figure 2. In addition to the purity indicated by HPLC, Schroeder has suggested that the ratio of absorbance 282 nm/324 nm is an indicator of purity, with a value of 0.35 indicating 99% purity with respect to the starting compound, ergosterol, the main contaminant in this reaction (Fischer *et al.*, 1985a). Mass spectral analysis and ^{1}H-NMR and ^{13}C-NMR spectra show that the position of the new carbon-carbon double bond is in the 9–11 position in the steroid ring system (Fischer, *et al.*, 1985a).

Cholestatrienol has similar chemical properties to dehydroergosterol. The primary criteria for purity is HPLC. Again, Schroeder has suggested the absorbance ratio 282 nm/324 nm to be a useful indicator of purity (Fischer, *et al.*, 1984). The mass spectrum and ^{1}H-NMR and ^{13}C-NMR verify the location of the additional double bond in the 9–11 position in the steroid ring system (Fischer, *et al.*, 1984). The absorption and emission spectra are virtually indistinguishable from those of

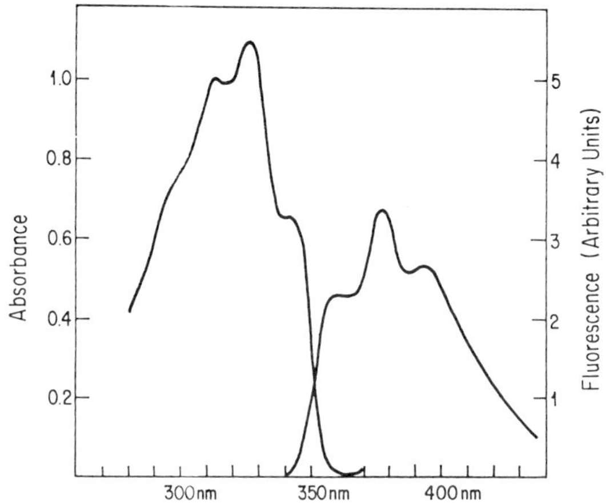

Figure 2 Absorption and emission (uncorrected) spectra from dehydroergosterol in sonicated egg phosphatidylcholine vesicles. Used with permission from Yeagle *et al.* (1982b).

dehydroergosterol since both molecules have the same chromophore and the structural differences are confined to the tails of the sterols.

III. SPECTRAL PROPERTIES OF DEHYDROERGOSTEROL AND CHOLESTATRIENOL

The spectral properties of dehydroergosterol have been carefully characterized to date, so they will be emphasized, with available information added for cholestatrienol. First, the chromophore has been shown to be stable to UV irradiation in a spectrophotometer, though for storage purposes it is recommended that the compound be kept in the dark. One experiment incorporated cholestatrienol at 2 mol % in 1-palmitoyl,2-oleoyl phosphatidylcholine liposomes and continuously exposed the sample to UV light in the spectrometer. After 2 h, at least 96% of the original fluorescence remained (Fischer, *et al.*, 1984). Another experiment measured the fluorescence lifetime as a function of irradiation time, and no effect was observed over a period of 600 min (Smutzer *et al.*, 1986).

Table 1 presents the spectral properties of dehydroergosterol in a variety of solvents. The data indicate an absence of a Stokes shift as a function of solvent polarity. A considerable shift in the emission maximum in aqueous media is noted, however.

Table 2 presents the extinction coefficient of dehydroergosterol in a variety of solvents. Little sensitivity to solvent is noted.

Table 3 presents the relative quantum yield of dehydroergosterol as a function of solvent. Considerable variation in quantum yield is noted, though it does not bear a simple relationship to solvent polarity. Also presented in Table 3 are the fluorescence

Table 1 Spectral properties of dehydroergosterol solutions

Solvent	Absorption, max (nm)	Emission, max (nm)	Stokes Shift (cm^{-1})	Δf^a
Cyclohexane	325.6	372.5	3867	0.001
Benzene	327.6	375.0	3869	0.004
Chloroform	327.8	378.0	4051	0.016
Eether	324.3	373.0	4026	0.167
Ethyl acetate	325.2	373.0	3941	0.201
Pyridine	329.6	—	—	—
DMSO	328.6	378.0	3977	0.262
1-Butanol	325.2	373.0	3941	0.265
2-Propanol	324.8	372.5	3943	0.274
Methanol	324.4	372.5	3981	0.310
DMF	327.3	—	—	—

[a] Δf, orientational polarizability.

lifetimes of dehydroergosterol as determined by time-resolved fluorescence. The lifetimes are very short. In solvents such as methanol, cyclohexane, ethanol, 2-propanol, and benzene, only a single lifetime can be detected. This indicates a relatively simple photophysics for this fluorophore. In other solvents, a second, very minor (1% or less) lifetime component appears to exist, whose origin is at present unknown.

The lifetime has been shown to be independent of excitation wavelength and independent of emission wavelength (Smutzer *et al.*, 1986). These data suggest a lack of excited-state isomerizations, again suggesting a simple excitation and emission behavior for this sterol.

Table 2 Extinction coefficients of dehydroergosterol solutions

Solvent	Extinction Coefficient ($M^{-1}cm^{-1}$)
Cyclohexane	10,100
Benzene	11,500
Chloroform	11,200
Ether	11,700
Ethyl Acetate	10,200
DMSO	10,400
1-Butanol	10,600
2-Propanol	10,600
Methanol	10,500
DMF	11,000

Table 3 Quantum yield and fluorescence lifetime of dehydroergosterol and fluorescence lifetime of cholestatrienol in organic solvents

Solvent	Quantum Yield	τ_1 (ns)	Relative Amplitude[a]	τ_2 (ns)	Relative Amplitude	Chi-Square
A. Dehydroergosterol						
Acetone	<0.001	0.33	98.8	4.68	1.2	2.54
Chloroform	0.003	0.33	98.9	5.00	1.1	2.58
Methanol	0.024	0.18	100.0	—	1.2	1.21
Cyclohexane	0.032[b]	0.20	100.0	—	—	1.21
Ethanol	0.040	0.18	100.0	—	—	2.24
Ether	0.051	0.20	99.7	4.37	0.3	1.12
2-Propanol	0.051	0.27	100.0	—	—	1.24
		0.25[c]				1.91
Benzene	0.058	0.32	100.0	—	—	1.00
DMF	0.058	0.39	99.5	6.12	—	1.31
B. Cholestatrienol[d]						
Ethanol	—	0.24	100.0	—	—	1.56
2-Propanol	—	0.28	100.0	—	—	1.30
Acetone	—	0.28	97.6	2.22	2.4	1.48

[a] Normalized to 100%

[b] From Smutzer and Yeagle (1985).

[c] Data from picosecond laser; dehydroergosterol concentration = 10 μM.

[b] Cholestatrienol concentration = 25 μM.

Viscosity of the solvent does apparently have an effect on the fluorescent properties of dehydroergosterol. Table 4 presents the lifetime of dehydroergosterol in mineral oil as a function of temperature. Also presented are the rotational correlation times calculated from the time-resolved anisotropy decays. These data indicate that the motional properties of the sterols are reflected in the dynamic measurements obtainable from time-resolved fluorescence studies.

Table 4 Fluorescence lifetimes and fluorescence anisotropy decays of dehydroergosterol in mineral Oil

Temperature	Lifetime[a] (ns)	Chi-Square[b]	Rotational Correlation Time (ns)
6.0	1.04	2.16	Not measured
10.2	0.85	1.56	8.20
19.8	0.65	1.01	5.54
24.0	0.58	1.35	3.89
30.1	0.46	1.31	2.31

[a] Measured at 54.7°C.

[b] Derived from lifetime analysis.

IV. TIME-RESOLVED FLUORESCENCE MEASUREMENTS

A. Data Analysis

In the previous section, fluorescent lifetimes were reviewed for a variety of isotropic solvents. Both the fluorescence lifetimes and the decay of the anisotropy are simple in isotropic media but become more complex in biological systems, in which motion is not isotropic. In this section, the analysis of such data for anisotropic biological systems is considered.

Although the details of the accumulation of data describing the decay of the total fluorescence and the decay of the anisotropy are beyond the scope of this review, the data may be obtained from time-resolved decays of fluorescence emission from laser-based or flash-lamp–based systems, or from phase-modulation data. Obtained from such data are parameters such as fluorescence lifetime, residual anisotropy r, and correlation times for the motions leading to fluorescence depolarization. In the case of the time-resolved decay of the total fluorescence, the data can be analyzed according to a decay law of the following form.

$$F(t) = \sum_i F_i e^{-t/\tau_i}$$

where $F(t)$ is equivalent to the observed decay without the instrument function (i.e., the contributions from the light source). This fitting produces lifetimes and preexponential factors that provide a measure of the relative contribution to the overall decay of individual components with individual correlation times.

For time-resolved fluorescence anisotropy measurements, the decay of the polarized components $I_{vv}(t)$ and $I_{hv}(t)$ are collected. These data are fit by

$$r(t) = \frac{I_{vv}(t) - QI_{hv}(t)}{I_{vv}(t) + 2QI_{hv}(t)}$$

where I is the intensity, v the excitation or emission polarizer in the vertical position, respectively, and h the excitation or emission polarizer in the horizontal position, respectively. From this fit, the correlation time characterizing the motion leading to the decay of the anisotropy is calculated.

At times long compared with the lifetime, the anisotropy may not approximate zero but may in fact remain a finite value, r_∞. This indicates that there is restriction on the motion of the fluorophore; that is, the fluorophore is not experiencing isotropic motion on the time scale (or faster) of the fluorescence lifetime. This implies that the fluorophore is experiencing some motional order. An order parameter can be calculated to describe the behavior of the fluorophore.

$$S = \left(\frac{r_\infty}{r_0}\right)^{1/2}$$

where r_0 is the limiting anisotropy in the absence of motion. For dehydroergosterol, r_0 has been measured to be 0.385 (Fischer, *et al.*, 1985a).

B. Motions Important to Fluorescence Anisotropy Decay

To derive meaningful information from the fluorescence anisotropy decay of dehydroergosterol and cholestatrienol in anisotropic biological systems, an appreciation of the most likely contributions to that decay is required. Consider the case of one of the fluorescent sterols in phospholipid bilayers. Motions that are to be important to the anisotropy decay must be characterized by correlation times near or shorter than the lifetime of the excited state of the fluorophore. Motions with much longer correlation times do not contribute because the excited state will have already decayed. This means that, since the fluorescence lifetime of dehydroergosterol and cholestatrienol is in the nanosecond range in phospholipid bilayers (see below), only relatively rapid motions need be considered.

For a lipid in a bilayer, three types of motion are most likely to contribute to rapid reorientation of the molecule or portions of the molecule (Brainard and Szato, 1981; Meier *et al.*, 1986). These motions are rotational diffusion about an axis perpendicular to the membrane surface, time-dependent reorientation of the director for axial diffusion (wobble), and segmental motion within a molecule due to trans-gauche isomerizations about molecular bonds.

For dehydroergosterol and cholestatrienol, this model can be simplified. The fluorophore is in the B- and C-rings of the fused-ring system of the sterol. This fused-ring system is essentially incapable of the rapid trans-gauche isomerizations that characterize carbon-carbon single bonds along the hydrocarbon chains of phospholipids. Therefore, segmental motions can be ruled out as significant contributors to molecular motion for dehydroergosterol and cholestatrienol

Recently, the orientation of the transition dipole for these fluorescent sterols was discussed in the context of the work of Hudson *et al.* (1982). It was concluded that the transition dipole was oriented nearly parallel to the long axis of the sterol (Smutzer *et al.*, 1986). Therefore, axial diffusion of the molecule is incapable of significantly contributing to the decay of the fluorescence anisotropy.

This analysis suggests that only one motion of dehydroergosterol and cholestatrienol is capable of significantly contributing to the decay of the fluorescence anisotropy in lipid bilayers. Time-dependent reorientation of the director, or wobble (as it will be referred to in the remainder of this chapter) should be the major contributor to fluorescence anisotropy decay in membrane studies. In most of the experiments reviewed here, energy transfer is not expected to be a major contributor to the anisotropy decay because the fluorescent sterols are generally used at low effective concentrations (about 1 mol % with respect to the lipids).

V. BIOLOGICAL PROPERTIES OF DEHYDROERGOSTEROL AND CHOLESTATRIENOL

If dehydroergosterol and cholestatrienol are to be used as probes for cholesterol behavior in biological systems, then it is important to assess the ability of these sterols to mimic the behavior of cholesterol in well-defined systems. The chemical structures would suggest similar behavior, but fortunately, considerable effort has been expended to test this hypothesis.

Dehydroergosterol has been shown to be similar to (though not identical to) cholesterol in water permeability studies (Roger *et al.*, 1979), in glucose permeability studies (Yeagle *et al.*, 1982a), in its ability to order membrane lipids (Yeagle *et al.*, 1982a), and in its ability to eliminate the highly cooperative phase transition of dipalmitoylphosphatidylcholine (Hale and Schroeder, 1982). The critical micelle concentration (CMC) for dehydroergosterol is 25 nM (Fischer *et al.*, 1985b), which is similar to the CMC for cholesterol (25–40 nM) (Haberland and Reynolds, 1973). The maximum solubility in aqueous media is 1.3 μM for dehydroergosterol (Fischer *et al.*, 1985b), compared with 4.7 μM for cholesterol. Dehydroergosterol has been shown to be nontoxic to *Tetrahymena pyroformis* (Rogers *et al.*, 1979), to *mycoplasma* (Archer, 1975), and to the growth of LM fibroblasts (Hale and Schroeder, 1982; Schroeder, 1981). Three organisms synthesize dehydroergosterol as a natural product, the yeast *Candida tropicalis* (Sica *et al.*, 1982), the mycelial fungus *Gibberella fujikuroi* (Nes and Heupel, 1986), and the Red Sea sponge *Biemna fortis* (Delseth *et al.*, 1979. However, dehydroergosterol is a poor substrate for cholesterol oxidase (Hale and Schroeder, 1982), and is likely to mimic ergosterol behavior better than cholesterol behavior.

Cholestatrienol contains the cholesterol side chain and may mimic cholesterol behavior under certain physiological conditions. This suggestion is supported by the observation that cholestatrienol is capable of inhibiting HMGCoA reductase in cultured fetal lung cells (Shakespeare and Wilton, 1980). Furthermore, cholestatrienol can be incorporated at up to 80% of total sterol in LM fibroblast plasma membranes without affecting cell growth or the activity of Na^+K^+ATPase (Farias *et al.*, 1975; Whetton and Houslay, 1983; Schroeder *et al.*, 1985). Cholestatrienol is more efficiently incorporated into sonicated unilamellar vesicles of dipalmitoylphosphatidylcholine than is dehydroergosterol (Schroeder *et al.*, 1985). Cholestatrienol has been reported to provide a similar result for the transbilayer distribution of cholesterol in sonicated unilamellar vesicles (Schroeder *et al.*, 1985), as was obtained through exchange experiments using ^{3}H-labeled cholesterol (Pozansky and Lange, 1976).

This discussion suggests that cholestatrienol will better reflect the behavior of cholesterol in membranes than will dehydroergosterol, which presently dominates the literature because it was the easier compound to prepare in stable form. However, cholestatrienol can now be easily prepared and after purification, is stable; therefore, it is highly recommended that future work use cholestratrienol whenever the behavior of cholesterol is being monitored and reserve dehydroergosterol for studies in which the behavior of ergosterol is under examination.

VI. USE OF DEHYDROERGOSTEROL AND CHOLESTATRIENOL TO MONITOR CHOLESTEROL BEHAVIOR IN MODEL MEMBRANES

In this section, the current literature on the use of dehydroergosterol and cholestatrienol to monitor cholesterol behavior in model membranes will be briefly reviewed. The use of these fluorescent sterols to examine the transmembrane distribution of cholesterol will not be considered because that has been the subject of a recent review (Schroeder, 1985). A more general review of fluorescent sterols is also available (Schroeder, 1984).

A. Steady-state Anisotropy Studies

The most extensive steady-state anisotropy studies that have been published concern the dimyristoylphosphatidylcholine/cholesterol system (Smutzer and Yeagle, 1985). Dehydroergosterol was used at about 1 mol % in this study. The partitioning of dehydroergosterol between the membrane and the aqueous phase was found to highly favor the membrane, as expected. The liposomes were prepared by dissolving the phospholipid, cholesterol, and dehydroergosterol in chloroform, followed by drying to a thin film and hydrating with buffer, with vortexing.

Steady-state anisotropy measurements were obtained as a function of temperature. The fluorescence anisotropy was calculated according to the following equation:

$$r = \frac{I_{\parallel} - GI_{\perp}}{I_{\parallel} + 2GI_{\perp}}$$

where $I_{\parallel}$ and $I_{\perp}$ are the fluorescence intensities with the emission polarizer parallel and perpendicular, respectively, to the excitation polarizer, and G represents the ratio of the sensitivities of the detection system for vertically and horizontally polarized light (Lakowicz, 1983). Background fluorescence, determined from an identical sample but without dehydroergosterol, was substracted from both the parallel and perpendicular components of the emission.

Figure 3 shows a typical run. It is interesting that there is an increase, small but highly reproducible, in the steady-state anisotropy as the temperature is increased from temperatures below the gel-to-liquid crystalline phase transition of dimyristoylphophatidylcholine to temperatures above the phase transition. The change is sharp, occurring over less than one degree in many cases. The magnitude of this increase, but not the degree of sharpness of the transition, is sensitive to the cholesterol content of the membrane. The largest net change in anisotropy is observed in the absence of cholesterol. As cholesterol is increased, the net change in fluorescence anisotropy of the dehydroergosterol is decreased in magnitude (Figure 4). In the same system, the steady-state anisotropy of parinaric acid undergoes a decrease from the gel state to the liquid crystal state. This change persists until about 20 mol % cholesterol is reached. These data suggest there is a phase separation of cholesterol-rich phases at very low cholesterol in these membranes.

It is worthwhile returning to the observation of an increase in the steady-state anisotropy of the dehydroergosterol through the phase transition. By analogy to other fluorescent probes, including paranaric acid, one would expect an increase in freedom of motion of fluorescent probes from the gel state of a lipid to the liquid crystal state of that lipid, and one would expect that this would be accompanied by a decrease in the steady-state anisotropy. Thus, the data from dehydroergosterol provide something of an anomaly. Furthermore, the sharpness of the transition

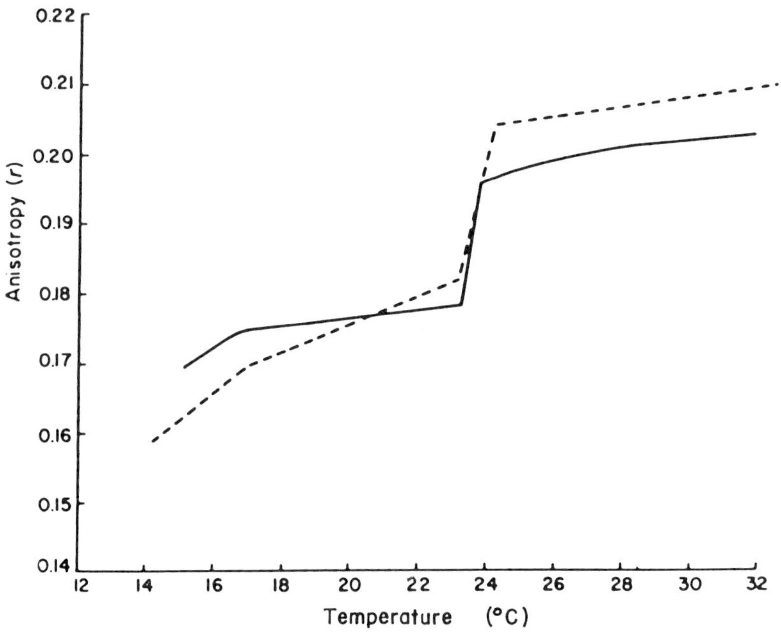

Figure 3 Fluorescence anisotropy of dehydroergosterol as a function of temperature, 0.88 mol % in dimyristoylphoshatidylcholine. Solid line, heating curve; broken line, cooling curve. Used with permission from Smutzer *et al.* (1986).

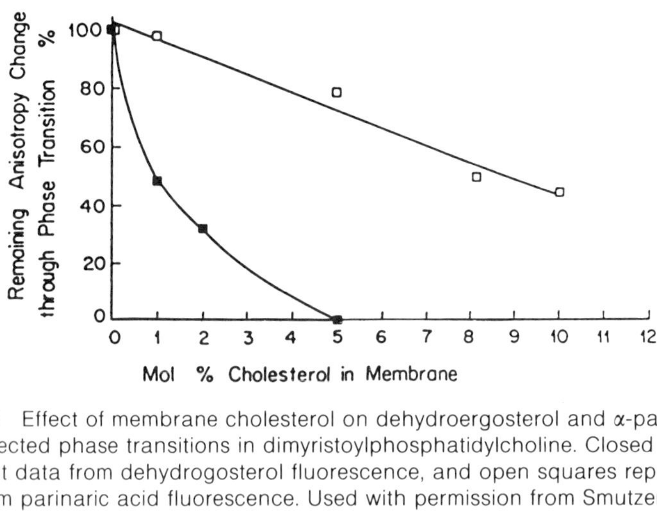

Figure 4 Effect of membrane cholesterol on dehydroergosterol and α-parinaric acid-detected phase transitions in dimyristoylphosphatidylcholine. Closed squares represent data from dehydrogosterol fluorescence, and open squares represent data from parinaric acid fluorescence. Used with permission from Smutzer *et al.* (1986).

detected by the fluorescent sterol is also an apparent anomaly because cholesterol has been shown to broaden the gel-to-liquid crystalline phase transition of phospholipids.

One possible explanation of these results is that the dehydroergosterol is partitioning between sterol-rich and sterol-poor phases. In the sterol-rich phase, the fluorescence is self-quenched because of aggregation of the sterols and does not significantly contribute to the observed fluorescence. Therefore, what is observed is simply the residual dehydroergosterol in the sterol-poor phase, which is still undergoing a cooperative phase transition. At 5 mol % cholesterol, the dehydroergosterol is essentially totally confined to the sterol-rich phase and no longer detects the phase transition.

The increase in anisotropy through the phase transition can be partially understood in the following terms. In the gel state, the dehydroergosterol is more highly phase-separated into a phase with greater freedom of motion than in the liquid crystalline state, in which it is more dispersed among the phospholipids and is thus more motionally ordered. This might lead to more motional freedom below the phase transition of the lipid and less above the phase transition.

One other possibility is that a change in lifetime through the phase transition might affect the steady-state anisotropy. This has been measured (see below) and is not likely a factor. Finally, preliminary results indicate that, under the same conditions, cholestatrienol behaves in the same fashion. At this time, a satisfactory explanation of the increase of the dehydroergosterol fluorescence anisotropy from the gel state to the liquid crystal state is lacking.

B. Time-resolved Fluorescence Studies

Fluorescence lifetimes, r_∞ values, order parameters, and correlation times from anisotropy decays have been determined for dehydroergosterol in several model systems. Table 5 presents a summary of available data, from which several interesting observations can be made. One is that the fluorescence lifetime of dehydroergosterol is nearly an order of magnitude longer in the membranes than in isotropic organic

Table 5 Dynamic fluorescence of dehydroergosterol solutions

System	Lifetime (ns)	r_∞	S	ϕ(ns)
PBS buffer	2.3	—	—	—
DHE in micelles	0.57, 5.26	—	—	—
SUV DMPC 10°C	2.3	0.268	0.83	0.89
SUV DMPC 37°C	1.2	0.162	0.65	0.71
SUV DSPC 37°C	2.8	0.098	0.50	1.21
SUV DSPC 65°C	3.3	0.031	0.28	1.54
Egg PC MLV 20°C	1.4	0.12	0.55	1.0
LM plasma membrane	2.0	0.97	0.48	1.17
Bound to SCP	12.4			

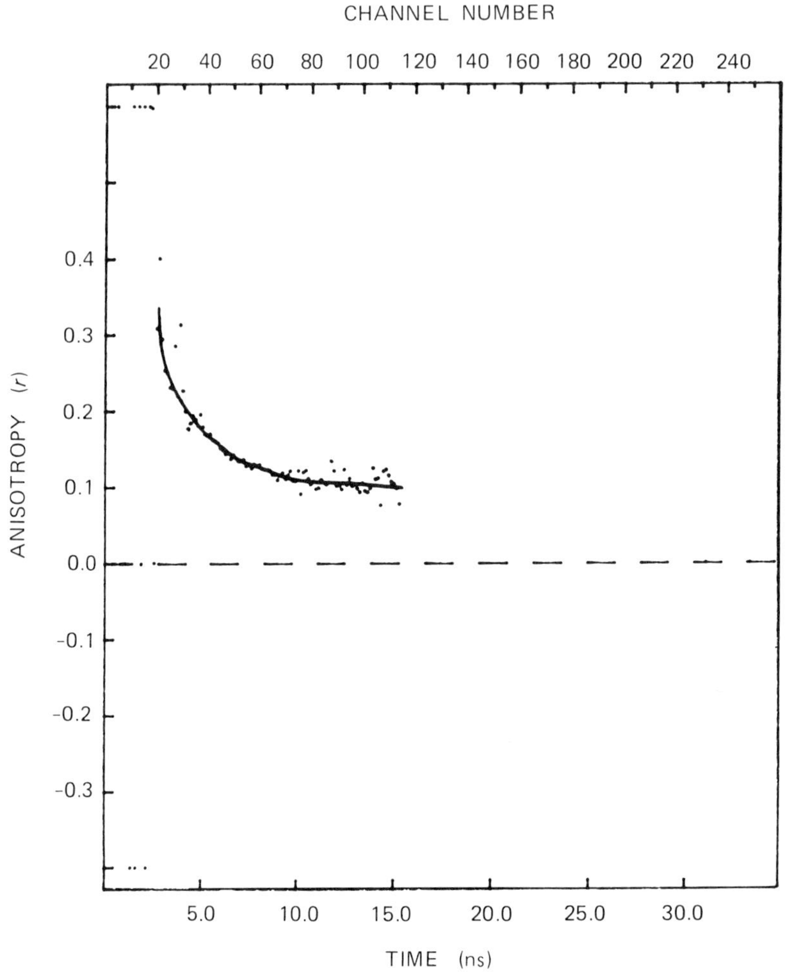

Figure 5 Decay of fluorescence anisotropy of dehydroergosterol in egg phosphatidylcholine multilamellar liposomes.

solvents (compare Table 3 with Table 5). This is likely due to the ordering effect of the membranes. In isotropic solvent, the anisotropy decays to zero during the lifetime of the excited state; in membranes, the anisotropy decays to a finite value (Fig. 5 shows an example). From this residual anisotropy r_{∞}, an order parameter can be calculated; this is also displayed in Table 5.

The correlation times obtained from the anisotropy decay are all very similar for these model membrane systems. As noted earlier, this correlation time reflects the wobble of the sterol about the normal to the membrane surface.

The lifetime for dehydroergosterol has been measured as a function of temperature in dimyrstoylphosphatidylcholine through the gel-to-liquid crystalline phase transition. The major lifetime component decreases about 15% at the phase transition temperature.

VII. DEHYDROERGOSTEROL AND CHOLESTATRIENOL AS PROBES TO MONITOR CHOLESTEROL BEHAVIOR IN BIOLOGICAL MEMBRANES

A. Steady-state Anisotropy Measurements

Only a few studies have been made of the steady-state anisotropy of either dehydroergosterol or cholestatrienol in biological membranes; an example of the steady-state anisotropy of dehydroergosterol in rabbit muscle sarcoplasmic reticulum as a function of temperature appears in Fig. 6. The fluorescent sterol was incorporated into the biological membrane by incubation of the sarcoplasmic reticulum with sonicated vesicles containing the dehydroergosterol.

The details of the procedure are as follows. Egg phosphatidylcholine was mixed with dehydroergosterol in a 1:1 mole ratio in chloroform and dried thoroughly to a thin film. This film was hydrated with 10 mM histidine, 150 mM NaCl, and 1 mM EDTA at pH 7 and vortexed vigorously. The resulting liposomes were then sonicated to clarity and centrifuged at 49,000 rpm for 30 min. The phospholipid small unilamellar vesicles in the supernatent were then adjusted to a concentration of 2 mg/ml in phospholipid. Equal volumes of the vesicles and a dispersion of sarcoplasmic reticulum vesicles (1.5 mg/ml) were incubated in the dark for 2 h at 23°C, under nitrogen, with gentle agitation. The sarcoplasmic reticulum was separated from the vesicles by centrifugation at 40,000 rpm for 15 min. Either a nonexchangeable marker or an analysis of the phospholipid/protein ratio in the biological membranes should be used to ensure that none of the donor vesicles were incorporated by the biological membranes.

The absolute value of the anisotropy of dehydroergosterol in sarcoplasmic reticulum is similar to the values observed for dehydroergosterol in model membranes in the liquid crystal state with low cholesterol. This is reasonable because the sarcoplasmic reticulum is also in the liquid crystal state and is low in cholesterol. The temperature dependence shows no deviations from linearity within the temperature

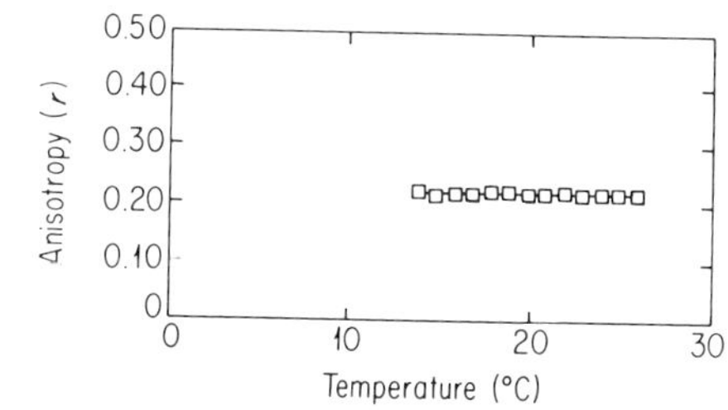

Figure 6 Steady-state fluorescence anisotropy of dehydroergosterol in rabbit muscle sarcoplasmic reticulum membrane.

range measured, which is again expected because there is no known phase transition in the sarcoplasmic reticulum in this temperature range.

It is interesting to compare this result with that obtained from the human erythrocyte membrane. The value of the steady-state anisotropy was about 0.28, substantially higher than for the sarcoplasmic reticulum (unpublished observations). Although this may be due to the much higher cholesterol content of the erythrocyte membrane, further experimentation is necessary to fully understand these results. Likewise, the steady-state anisotropy for cholestatrienol in the rod outer segment disk is also distinctly different from (in this case substantially lower than) that of the sarcoplasmic reticulum membrane (A. Albert, personal communication).

What is clear from these data is that these fluorescent sterols are exquisitely sensitive to differences in environment. The challenge in this field is to understand the information these probes are providing.

B. Time-resolved Fluorescence Studies of Dehydroergosterol in Biological Membranes

The results of the only study in which the lifetime of dehydroergosterol has been measured in a biological membrane is presented in Table 5. These are data for dehydroergosterol in LM cell plasma membranes. The data show a similarity to the data obtained from model systems, but too little information is yet available to adequately describe cholesterol behavior in biological membranes.

C. Experiments on Energy Transfer between Protein Tryptophans and Dehydroergosterol in Biological Membranes

Because of the overlap between the emission of protein tryptophans and the absorption of dehydroergosterol, fluorescence energy transfer is feasible, providing the interchromophore distance is suitable. Such energy transfer has been observed with dehydroergosterol incorporated into the human erythrocyte membrane and in basal lateral membranes from bovine kidney cortex (unpublished observations). However, interchromophore distance calculations are not meaningful in such cases because of the uncertainty of location of donors and acceptors.

VIII. USE OF DEHYDROERGOSTEROL AND CHOLESTATRIENOL IN THE STUDY OF CHOLESTEROL INTERACTIONS WITH STEROL CARRIER PROTEINS

Two studies have been published that explore the interaction of the fluorescent sterols with sterol carrier protein as a model for cholesterol interactions with sterol carrier protein (Fischer *et al.*, 1985b; Schroeder *et al.*, 1985). Since the two studies are very similar, only the study with dehydroergosterol will be described. In this study, the interesting observation was made that the lifetime of dehydroergosterol changed significantly upon interacting with the sterol carrier protein. Instead of a lifetime of 1–2 ns as seen in most other biological systems, a lifetime of about 12 ns was reported. No explanation was provided for this large change. However, it does suggest that interactions of these sterol probes with proteins may be detectable through the introduction of long-lifetime components.

In this study, energy transfer was reported between protein tyrosines and the fluorescent sterol. One sterol per protein was bound. The efficiency of energy transfer was converted into a distance measurement. However, the lack of knowledge of the spatial distribution of the donors makes this determination difficult to interpret.

IX. USE OF DEHYDROERGOSTEROL AND CHOLESTATRIENOL IN STUDIES OF SERUM LIPOPROTEINS

Fluorescence data have been obtained from cholestatrienol in very low density lipoprotein (VLDL) secreted from perfused rat liver. The fluorescence intensity did not show any sensitivity to the phase transition of the core of VLDL. Fluorescence quenching studies suggested with trinitrophenylglycine suggested that the probe was near the surface of the lipoprotein (Schroeder *et al.*, 1979).

In LDL, the oleate ester of cholestatrienol detected the phase transition of the core, in contrast to the results with the cholestatrienol in VLDL (Sklar *et al.*, 1982). This would suggest that free sterol might preferentially partition towards the surfaces of the lipoproteins and might be in low abundance in the core of cholesterol esters and triglycerides. This is in good agreement with a recent ^{13}C-NMR study on cholesterol in LDL (Lund-Katz and Phillips, 1986).

X. CIRCULAR DICHROISM OF DEHYDROERGOSTEROL

In asymmetric environments, the chromophore of dehydroergosterol exhibits optical activity and gives rise to a circular dichroism (CD) spectrum. This has been observed in model membranes (Yeagle *et al.*, 1982b) and in LDL. (Yeagle *et al.*, 1982a). In small unilamellar sonicated vesicles, the intensity of each of the CD bands increases with cholesterol content. This can be rationalized on the basis of motional ordering of the sterol. The greater the cholesterol content of the membrane, the greater the ordering of the sterol. The greater ordering of the sterol then leads to less motional averaging of the local electronic environment of the chromophore, thus increasing the time-average asymmetry of the dehydroergosterol chromophore environment. This in turn leads to an increase in the intensity of the CD bands.

XI. SUMMARY

The history of the use of dehydroergosterol and cholestatrienol is young, yet already it is clear that a wealth of information regarding sterol behavior in biological systems can be tapped through fluorescence studies of these sterols. At the same time, it is clear that further model work is required to interpret the results from biological systems.

ACKNOWLEDGMENTS

The work of the author reported herein was supported in part by a grant from the National Institutes of Health (HL23853) and through a Research Career Development Award from NIH (HL00937).

I thank Dr. F. Schroeder for providing reprints of his work.

REFERENCES

Antonucci, R., Bernstein, S., Giancola, D., and Sax, K. J. (1951). $\Delta^{5,7}$-Steroids. VII. The conversion of $\Delta^{5,7}$- to $\Delta^{5,7,9}$-steroidal hormones. *Org. Chem.* (*N.Y.*) **16**, 1159–1164.

Archer, D. B. (1975). The use of a fluorescent sterol to investigate the mode of action of amphotericin methyl ester, a polyene antibiotic. *Biochem. Biophys. Res. Commun.* **66**, 195–201.

Brainard, J. R., and Szabo, A. (1981). Theory for nuclear magnetic relaxation of probes in anisotropic systems: Application to cholesterol in phospholipid vesicles. *Biochemistry* **20**, 4618–4628.

Dahl, C. E. (1981). Effect of sterol structure on acyl chain ordering in phosphatidylcholine vesicles: A deuterium nuclear magnetic resonance and electron spin resonance study. *Biochemistry* **20**, 7158–7161.

de Kruijff, B. (1978). ^{13}C NMR studies on [4-^{13}C] cholesterol incorporated in sonicated phosphatidylcholine vesicles. *Biochim. Biophys. Acta* **506**, 173–182.

Delseth, C., Kashman, Y., and Djerassi, C. (1979). *Helv. Chim. Acta* **62**, 2037–2045.

Demel, R. A., Bruckdorfer, K. R., and van Deenen, L. L. M. (1972). The effect of sterol structure on the permeability of liposomes to glucose, glycerol, and Rb^+. *Biochim. Biophys. Acta* **255**, 321–337.

Farias, R. N., Blog, B., Morero, R. D., Sinerez, F., and Trucco, R. E. (1975). Regulation of allosteric membrane-bound enzymes through changes in membrane lipid composition. *Biochim. Biophys. Acta* **415**, 231–251.

Fischer, R. T., Stephenson, F. A., Shafiee, A., and Schroeder, R. (1984). $\Delta^{5,7,9(11)}$- cholestatrien-3β-ol: A fluorescent cholesterol analogue. *Chem. Phys. Lipids* **36**, 1–14.

Fischer, R. T., Stephenson, F. A., Shafiee, A., and Schroeder, F. (1985a). Structure and dynamic properties of dehydroergosterol, $\Delta^{5,7,9,(11),22}$-ergosta traen-3β-ol. *J. Biol. Phys.* **13**, 13.

Fischer, R. T., Cowlen, M. S., Dempsey, M. E., and Schroeder, F. (1985b). Fluorescence of $\Delta^{7,9(11),22}$-ergostatetraen-3β-ol in micelles, sterol carrier protein complexes, and plasma membranes. *Biochemistry* **24**, 3322–3331.

Gally, H. U., Seelig, A., and Seelig, J. (1976). Cholesterol-induced rod-like motion of fatty acyl chains in lipid bilayers. A deuterium magnetic resonance study. *Hoppe-Seyler's Z. Physiol. Chem.* **357**, 1447–1450.

Haberland, M. E., and Reynolds, J. A. (1973). Self-association of cholesterol in aqueous solution. *Proc. Natl. Acad. Sci. U.S.A.* **70**, 2313–2316.

Hale, J. E., and Schroeder, F. (1982). Asymmetric transbilayer distribution of sterol across plasma membranes determined by fluorescence quenching of dehydroergosterol. *Eur. J. Biochem.* **122**, 649–661.

Hudson, B., Kohler, B. E., and Schutter, K. (1982). Linear polyene electronic structure and potential surfaces. *Excited States* **6**.

Kelusky, E. C., Dufourc, E. J., and Smith, I. C. P. (1983). Direct observation of molecular ordering of cholesterol in human erythrocyte membranes. *Biochim. Biophys. Acta* **735**, 302–304.

Lakowicz, J. R. (1983). "Principles of Fluorescence Spectroscopy." Plenum, New York.

Lund-Katz, S., and Phillips, M. C. (1986). Packing of cholesterol molecules in low-density lipoprotein. *Biochemistry* **25**, 1562–1568.

Meier, P., Ohmes, E., and Kothe, G. (1986). Multi-pulse dynamic nuclear magnetic resonance of phospholipid membranes. *J. Chem. Phys.* **85**, 3598–3614.

Morton, R. A., Heilbron, I. M., and Spring, F. S. (1930). XIX. Absorption spectra in relation to vitamin A. *Biochem. J.* **24**, 136–140.

Nes, W. D., and Heupel, R. C. (1986). Physiological requirement for biosynthesis of multiple 24,3-methylsterols in *Gibberolla Fujikuroi. ARCh. Biochem. Biophys.* **244**, 211–217.

Oldfield, E., Meadows, M., Rice, D., and Jacobs, R. (1978). Spectroscopic studies of specifically deuterium labelled membrane systems. Nuclear magnetic resonance investigation of the effects of cholesterol in model systems. *Biochemistry* **17**, 2727–2740.

Poznansky, M., and Lange, Y. (1976). Transbilayer movement of cholesterol in dipalmitoyllecithin-cholesterol vesicles. *Nature (London)* **259**, 420–421.

Rogers, J., Lee, A. G., and Wilton, C. (1979). The organization of cholesterol and ergosterol in lipid bilayers based on studies using non-perturbing fluorescent probes. *Biochim. Biophys. Acta* **552**, 23–37.

Ruyle, W. V., Jacob, T. A., Chemerda, J. M., Chamberlin, E. M., Rosenberg, D. W., Sita, G. E., Erickson, R. R., Alimonosa, L. M., and Tishler, M. (1953). The preparation of $\Delta^{7,9(11)}$-allosteroids by the action of mercuric acetate on Δ^{7}-allosteroids. *J. Am. Chem. Soc.* **76**, 2604–2609.

Schroeder, F. (1981). Use of a fluorescent sterol to probe the transbilayer distribution of sterols in biological membranes. *FEBS Lett.* **135**, 127–130.

Schroeder, F. (1984). Fluorescent sterols: Probe, molecules of membrane structure and function. *Prog. Lipid Res.* **23**, 97–113.

Schroeder, F. (1985). Fluorescence probes unravel asymmetric structure of membranes. *In* "Subcellular Biochemistry" (D. Roodyn, ed.), p. 51. Plenum, New York.

Schroeder, F., Goh, E. H., and Heimberg, M. (1979). Regulation of the surface physical properties of the very low density lipoprotein. *J. Biol. Chem.* **254**, 2456–2463.

Schroeder, F., Dempsey, M. E., and Fisher, R. T. (1985). Sterol and squalene carrier protein interactions with fluorescent $\Delta^{5,7,9(121)}$-cholestatrien 3β-ol. *J. Biol. Chem.* **260**, 2904–2011.

Shakespeare, V., and Wilton, D. C. (1980). The inhibition of cholesterol biosynthesis in MRC-5 fibroblasts in culture by cholesta-5,7,9-trien-3β-ol. *Biochem. Biophys. Res. Commun.* **94**, 1242–1251.

Sica, D., Boniforti, L., and DiGiacomo, G. (1982). *Phytochemistry* **21**, 235–236.

Sklar, L. A., Mantulin, W. W., and Pownall, H. J. (1982). Fluorescent cholesteryl esters in the core of low density lipoprotein. *Biochem. Biophys. Res. Commun.* **105**, 674–680.

Smutzer, G., and Yeagle, P. L. (1985). A fluorescence anisotropy study on the phase behavior of dimyristoylphosphatidylcholine/cholesterol mixtures. *Biochim. Biophys. Acta* **814**, 274–280.

Smutzer, G., Crawford, B., and Yeagle, P. L. (1986). Physical Properties of the fluorescent probe dehydroergosterol. *Biochim. Biophys. Acta* **862**, 361–371.

Whetton, A. D., and Houslay, M. D. (1983). 5′-nucleotidase is activated upon cholesterol-depletion of liver plasma membranes. *FEBS Lett.* **157**, 70–74.

Windhaus, A., and Linsert, O. (1928). Uber die ultraviolett-bestrahlung des dehydroergosterins. *Justus Liebigs Ann. Chem.* **465**, 148–166.

Yeagle, P. L. (1981). Cholesterol rotation in phospholipid vesicles as observed by C-13 NMR. *Biochim. Biophys. Acta* **640**, 263–273.

Yeagle, P. L. (1985). Lanosterol and cholesterol have different effects on phospholipid acyl chain orientation. *Biochim. Biophys. Acta* **815**, 33–36.

Yeagle, P. L., Martin, R. B., Lala, A. K., Lin, H., and Bloch, K. (1977). Differential effects of cholesterol and lanosterol on artificial membranes. *Proc. Natl. Acad. Sci. U.S.A.* **74**, 4924–4926.

Yeagle, P. L., Bensen, J., Greco, M., and Arena, C. (1982a). Cholesterol behavior in human serum lipoproteins. *Biochemistry* **21**, 1249–1254.

Yeagle, P. L., Bensen, J., Boni, L., and Hui, S. W. (1982b). Molecular packing of cholesterol in phospholipid vesicles as probed by dehydroergosterol. *Biochim. Biophys. Acta* **692**, 139–146.

Zuercher, A., Heusser, H., Jeger, O., and Geistlich, P. (1954). Uber Umwandlungen in den Ringen B, C und D des Ergosterins. *Helv. Chim. Acta* **37**, 1564–1581.

Index